HUMAN BRAIN $\&$ HUMAN LEARNING

3rd Edition

Leslie A. Hart

Books For Educators, Inc.
We do the research for you!
Covington, Washington

HUMAN BRAIN AND HUMAN LEARNING
THIRD EDITION

© 2002 Books For Educators, Inc.
Third Edition 2002
Printed in the United States of America

ISBN 1-929869-00-2

By Leslie A. Hart
Contributing editor, Karen D. Olsen
Graphics by Kristina Roe

Published by Books for Educators, Inc.
17051 SE 272nd Street, Suite 18
Covington, Washington 98042
888/777-9827; Fax: 253/630-7215
E-mail: books4@oz.net
www.books4educ.com

Published originally in 1983 by Longman, Inc.
White Plains, NY

Published 1983, 1992, 1995, 1998, 2002

To those many educators, at all levels,
who out of deep concern for children,
students, communities, and nation,
have dared to work and fight for change.

CONTENTS

FOREWORD

The future of teaching and learning lies in the study of the brain.

Only in this strange world of nerve cell and synapse will we someday untangle the mysteries of how people learn.

Human Brain and Human Learning makes a major contribution to our grasp of how the brain works. It may well become the basis for important educational reform and for reexamining all we do in schools, including the organization of curricula and the management of learning. We must understand brain functions and operations before schools can be significantly improved.

Leslie Hart's major thesis is that today's educational practice is based on assumptions that relate little to desired student outcomes. He correctly claims that there has been no coherent theory of **human** learning — most of our practices have been based on research conducted with small animals.

In his earlier book, *How the Brain Works*, Hart presented what is known as Proster Theory, dramatically different from conventional theory in that it centers on the brain and explains the learning process in terms of the brain's nature, history, and modes of operation. In the present book, Hart carries his refreshingly new theory forward, relating it specifically to education and particularly to schools. He has also presented Proster Theory in style and language that invites the reader with even minimal technical or scientific background to read with enjoyment and full comprehension. (Those who prefer a moderately technical but still highly lucid substantiation will find it, additionally, in the earlier work.)

Most important to me is that *Human Brain and Human Learning* begins to build a bridge between theory and practice, and offers a broad guide for translating brain research into design and decisions in our schools. On that count, it should arouse intense interest among educators, parents, school board members, and educational researchers. With new knowledge of how the brain functions, of what it demands, and of how learning takes place, we can at last create school environments that will far more successfully help all learners to achieve. Teaching can become congruent to learning.

There emerges from this book a whole new way to look at learning and so a base for a new system of teaching, with the teacher becoming a more dramatic and important "creator" of learning than one who merely instructs. The learning stems from the student's own brain and activities rather than resulting from "being taught." In "brain-compatible" learning—a strikingly new concept—there is a shift "from reliance on raw authority to a far more sophisticated approach of recognizing differences and responding to them in a way that sharply reduces conflict while achieving better outcomes."

While experienced educators will find in the book welcome support for intuitions they have long held (that in fact go far back in the history of education), the reader must be prepared for what can be at first a distressing departure from old and conventional ideas. One must remember that coming at schooling or training from a brain viewpoint is truly new. But Hart draws from a huge amount of present scientific knowledge in a range of relevant disciplines. He builds on the findings and insights of leading brain investigators. In addition, he uses an intimate familiarity with the realities of schools to relate this large body of new knowledge to one's common experiences and observations. The theory he offers and the suggestions he puts forward rest on a solid foundation.

Read and studied carefully, *Human Brain and Human Learning* can have a tremendous impact on education. It should be read by everyone interested in improving our schools, not in small increments, but in a quantum leap. Hart may have developed what all of us have been looking for: The key to greatly improved learning, the basis and methods of reestablishing public confidence in the schools, and designing human environments for human learners.

What is vital now is that Hart's concepts be tried and explored. This is not a "how to" book but the brain-compatible approaches he suggests seem thoroughly practical guides to action. Reality testing of the possibilities he presents is urgently needed. If, as appears likely, learning can be dramatically improved when educational practice centers on understanding how the brain works, the sooner that is done the more students will be effectively educated in the schools and other institutions of our nation.

One thing is certain now: This is an enormously stimulating, penetrating, significant book, demanding attention. It may well prove a landmark in educational thought. And while deeply critical, it also offers more hope for major solutions of our problems than most we have seen for a long time.

Dr. M. Donald Thomas
Superintendent of Schools
Salt Lake City, Utah

PREFACE

The core problem faced by educators today is how to bring about learning. This book is addressed to that question; it is intended for teachers and instructors, administrators, planners, legislators, curriculum developers, and all concerned with effective and humane education and training, including parents. Since failure to learn brings additional problems in discipline, crime, mental health, and social alienation, readers active in these areas may find this discussion of some value.

Because our schools present the most acute needs, and our ideas about schooling color all educational effort, schools are given much attention here. But the brain-based principles of learning put forward, contrasting sharply with conventional views, can be applied at any level and in any learning situation.

We have many brilliant neuroscientists and neuropsychologists at work, and their contributions in recent years have been magnificent. We have, too, many thoughtful, creative educators with intimate knowledge of schools and training—but almost no modern knowledge of the brain. My hope is that this book will help bridge the lamentable gap that exists between these two fields, and bring to educators some sense of the fresh, exciting new vistas that open up when one takes a brain approach to the problem of human learning.

I must stress, however, that this is not an effort to contribute in anyway to the neurosciences, except perhaps as it may increase the awareness and interest of some brain researchers with respect to the practical learning problems typical of schools. Also, this book takes a deliberately simplified, holistic approach to the brain, seeking to add to educators' understanding of what the brain is for, and of its overall architecture and broad modes of operation. To do so, it attempts to synthesize from many disciplines in addition to the neurosciences. There is no effort made to deal with learning on a molecular, cellular, or synaptic level. This is an area of brain knowledge in which mystery still prevails; and it seems to me most unlikely in any case that breakthroughs on this micro level would importantly affect dealing with the brain on a macro level, as must those who labor to bring about student learning.

Our schools, I believe, are not ineffective because they do not know what happens at synapses or the chemistry of neurotransmitters, but rather because they have yet to address the brain's role in learning and to fit instruction and environment to the "shape" of the brain as it is now increasingly well understood. We know that as the consequence of long evolution, the brain has modes of operation that are natural, effortless, effective in utilizing the tremendous power of this amazing instrument. Coerced to operate in other ways, it functions as a rule reluctantly, slowly, and with abundant error.

As we realize this, we can focus on the problem of matching settings and instruction to the nature of the brain, rather than trying to force it to comply with arrangements established with virtually no concern for what this organ is or how it works best. The term *brain-compatible* seems appropriate for education designed to fit the brain. It seems reasonable to assume that moving from brain-antagonistic settings to brain-compatible schooling and training could produce strikingly better outcomes.

We know amply enough about the human brain as the organ for learning, I submit, to begin making this transition, now. Working out the best detailed methods and related needs will of course require the contributions of a great many creative and knowledgeable people over years to come.

Leslie A. Hart
New Rochelle, NY

FROM THE EDITOR

I first suggested to Leslie Hart that he consider updating this book in 1993. After all, given the explosion in brain research studies using breakthrough technologies during the decade since the book was first published, surely there was much rewriting to be done. He assured me that little needed to change except updating the footnotes and other source materials data.

At the time, I found his remark quite surprising and, quite honestly, shrugged it off as a bit of author's pride. Surely, I thought, by the time he finished, he would have made sweeping changes.

By 1995, Leslie had completed most of the textual changes. And I was surprised again. Given Leslie's level of synthesis and the fact that he had based so much of his research on firsthand sources rather than second and third hand reporting that take some time to trickle down to the public, *Human Brain and Human Learning* did in fact need but minor rewriting except for one area: the triune brain theory.

A year later, the urban smog of the Northeast was continuing to raise havoc with Leslie's eyesight so he asked me to take over the task of updating footnotes and source materials. With his notes and my reading, the second edition was completed in 1998. Editing on the first update was minimal, only to soften the edges of his frustration or, occasionally, to clarify points that may be new to readers; headers were added to speed search for information. Updating for this third edition reflects brain research made possible due to the more sophisticated technologies now available to study the brain in action. However, Leslie's keen insights still hold. This is his book. My contributions appear in a different type font—that of this sentence.

As an educator who has spent 30 years looking for a point of attack and a long enough lever sufficient to move our public education system, it is my belief that both the target and the leverage can be found in brain research. In these pages lie hope and challenge in equal measure.

Human Brain and Human Learning is the most comprehensive and understandable version of brain research for educators and parents that I have ever seen. I feel privileged to have played a part in its updating and re-release.

Karen D. Olsen
Oroville, Washington

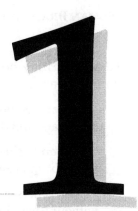

FRUSTRATIONS: THE NEED FOR A NEW FOUNDATION

> The symptom that a particular branch of science or art is ripe for a change is a feeling of frustration and malaise, not necessarily caused by any acute crisis in that specific branch . . . but by a feeling that the whole tradition is somehow out of step, cut off from the mainstream, that the traditional criteria have become meaningless, divorced from living reality, isolated from the integral whole.
>
> — Arthur Koestler[1]

"I taught them, but they didn't learn."

That is the classic remark, usually sadly uttered, of the teacher who tried hard to produce the intended student learning but didn't succeed.

Rare is the classroom teacher who hasn't often felt frustration of this kind, even after presenting an especially well-prepared lesson or unit with skill and enthusiasm.

"At times," remarks a teacher, "it seems as if an invisible glass wall drops down between me and the students, and nothing gets through."

Teachers may well take such failures personally, wondering what they may be doing wrong. Or, since repeated failure can be hard to bear, they may look for others to blame:

"The parents didn't prepare these children for school. They don't encourage and discipline them."

"You can't really expect youngsters from a neighborhood like this to be interested in learning."

"The teachers in the lower grades passed these students along, without basic skills. What can I do with them now?"

"We don't get the facilities and supplies and support we need."

"Schools reflect society. What can you expect? We have to change society first."

Or teachers may join others in deploring television, electronic games, the breakdown of the family, the weakened influence of religion, too little respect for authority, lower moral standards, government interference and red tape, stingy taxpayers, racial and social tensions . . . and much more.

EXCUSES ARE DISTRACTIONS

But we must recognize, when we take a hard look at education, that these "explanations" or excuses serve merely as distractions from the heart of the matter. The schools' first job lies within the schools. Under our system, students are compelled to attend. *The schools must receive them as they are, not as one might wish them to be. And, the school must bring about learning by every student,* not merely giving lip service to "every student can learn," but accomplishing that result.

No one sensibly minimizes the problems: they are varied, difficult, and often profound. But they are problems only the schools can solve and solve them they must. Increasingly, schools are judged on how they cope with these problems. How much public money schools should be allotted, and even whether they should continue in their present form, rest on this judgment. (Charter schools and voucher programs are but two popularly supported options created because the public schools have failed to embrace, and solve, the serious problems that confront them.)

To say "I taught them, but they didn't learn" is of course an absurdity, about equivalent to "we had a wonderful dinner but nobody got anything to eat" or "I took a great vacation trip but I didn't go anywhere." Similarly, in education we know exactly what frustrates teachers—for an entire school year they carry out certain practices and activities in the classroom that are called "teaching" but which in fact work very poorly, even when implemented with commitment and energy, in a manner generally viewed as conventional and appropriate and, in many respects, demanded by authorities. Yet, inescapably, the "teaching" worked poorly if measured against the goal of producing learning for all students. "I taught them but they did not learn."

The Problem . . . Complying

If we point a finger of blame at such teachers, it has to be for complying! But teachers may feel that they have no other option if they want to keep their jobs or be free of continual supervision.

The full import of what has just been stated might evoke profound shock and possibly disbelief. Can one seriously propose that what the great majority of teachers regularly do in the great majority of conventional classrooms brings about massive failure to produce desired student learning? Yes, one can, and in fact must, in the light of recent findings and events. It is a conclusion avoidable only through massive denial of the facts. Within a failure of such appalling scope there is unlimited room for criticism, which often fails to shed light on what is most wrong and which may, in fact, help perpetuate outdated concepts. Persistent attention to factors of minor importance can prevent the needed consideration of major, foundational factors.

An Old Concept:
Learning Automatically Follows Teaching

Teachers, being visible and vulnerable, tend to be the first targets of criticism, however unfair and superficial that may be and however coerced and constrained the teachers were in trying to carry out their assignments. Here we go back to one of the oldest concepts of our whole education system: *if students are put in a room and "taught," learning will follow.* This is a handy idea, appealing in its apparent common sense, but it deflects attention from most of the complexities of the teaching-learning interface and from all the objectives and conditions that affect this interaction. At any level in the world of education, it is shocking to discover how little desire there is, beyond lip service, to probe into such fundamental questions as what we mean by "knowledge," "knowing," "learning, "understanding," or the glib term "achievement." Obviously, here lie the foundations of all successful instruction, yet they are largely ignored.

LEARNING VERSUS TEACHING

Go into an educational library and check the evidence on the shelves. For every volume focused on the topics mentioned above or on "learning" in general, one can find yards of books on *teaching* and *assessment*. Examine the contents of the more broadly circulated publications for school practitioners and the same relationship appears. Look through college course offerings and, again, books on learning are rare.

Even more recent forays into the multiple intelligences and "brain-based" education quickly degenerate into "how to teach it" before their implications for learning are plumbed to any depth. A rare exception is the work of Susan Kovalik & Associates and the care they give to insisting that teachers understand the *why* behind their teaching.

Even more striking (and in a wry sense, amusing) are the urgings and often pompous injunctions of the pundits and politicians *outside* of education who, with the greatest willingness, advise on what is wrong and how to fix it. While the broad assessments of shortcomings are often substantially correct, the more specific suggestions deal with a host of matters from class size and homework to what degrees teachers get and what grades football players must garner to be allowed to play. Every trivial, possibly relevant factor wins examination, but not the obvious crux: How to bring about learning.

Testing, of course, by so-called "standardized" techniques, gets heavy emphasis, on the curious grounds that "we must know exactly where we are" to detect any worthwhile improvement— this after decades of major reports have detailed how desperately bad student attainment is. An analogy here is the ninety-pounds-overweight person who hops on the scales every hour to see whether dieting has achieved another half ounce off.

THE PUBLIC'S CRITICISM OF PUBLIC EDUCATION

The public, and many educators, have been slow to fully realize how desperately poor student learning actually is, as measured by our best evaluative means, in schools with conventional classrooms across the country—not just in inner-city or rural or impoverished schools but in schools everywhere.

Critical Reports by the Hundreds

Since the early 1980s there has been a continuous stream of reports critical of the state of education in the United States. Their findings are disquieting and disturbingly congruent. *A Nation at Risk*,[2] issued in 1983, fell on the American conscience like a bombshell. Only a few dozen pages in all, it included the passage:

"If an unfriendly foreign power had attempted to impose on America the mediocre educational performance that exists today, we might have viewed it as an act of war. As it stands, we have allowed this to happen to ourselves."

The startling document further noted that

". . . individuals in our society who do not possess the levels of skill, literacy, and training essential to this new era will be effectively disenfranchised, not simply from the material rewards that accompany competent performance, but also from the chance to participate fully in our national life."

Members of the panel intended the extreme "act of war" language to win headline attention and jolt the country, especially all concerned with the schools, to realize how seriously they saw the situation. *A Nation at Risk* did seemingly have one lasting effect: it fairly well put an end to a long school tradition of never admitting publicly to significant deficiencies. The topic of much conferencing, writing, and legislation became "Change," soon politely referred to as "restructuring." The report, though the most dramatic in language, was by no means alone; within six years more than a hundred major reports from important sources flooded the scene, almost uniformly supporting and confirming the cry of "disaster!"

Virtually nothing of much weight has appeared on the contrary side—it would be an exaggeration to say that a counter argument has even existed (although a few have attempted to minimize the extent of the gap). A decade and a half later, the nation is still at risk. The great majority of schools continue to operate just about the way they did. Even if their rhetoric has a new sound, little real progress has been made. Despite the intervening 15 years since this book first appeared and subsequent widespread discussion in the popular press, brain research findings rarely get translated into action in schools in comprehensive, coherent ways.

A 1990 summary published by the National Assessment of Educational Progress and widely considered the best such source, bears the prettied-up title "America's Challenge: Accelerating Academic Achievement." Actually the document presents in softened language but firm numbers an overview of the state of learning in the key subject areas. The picture painted by these excerpts is horrifying (emphasis added):[3]

> "Most of the data in this report show that our present education performance is low and not improving. The achievement of 17-year-olds in reading, mathematics, science, history and civics represents only modest performance . . . 81-96% have rudimentary interpretive skills. . . . **Only 5-8% of our 17-year-olds, however, demonstrate those skills we usually associate with the ability to function in more demanding jobs in the workplace or the capability to do college work.**" (p. 3)

> "Despite concentrated studies in mathematics in elementary schools, one-quarter of our country's 9-year-olds failed to reach the beginning level defined by NAEP—a level characterized by the ability to add and subtract two-digit numbers. **Only one-fifth showed a grasp of all four basic numerical operations—addition, subtraction, multiplication, and division.**" (p. 18)

> "That a very small proportion of middle-school students (9%) and only about 41% of high school students can be considered even moderately versed in this subject area [science] is cause for grave concern, **as is the very small percentage (8%) of high-school students with any degree of specialized knowledge in science.**" (p. 21)

> "Across the NAEP findings, cumulative evidence shows that, for any curriculum area, only about half of our high-school seniors may be graduating with the ability to 'use their minds' to think through subject-related information in any depth. **Fewer than 10%** appear to have both an understanding of the specialized

material and ideas comprising that curriculum area and the ability to work with these to interpret, integrate, infer, draw generalizations, and articulate conclusions." (p. 29)

Outcomes on this order, across the board, may well make us gasp. They have changed very little across the last 20 years.

Furthermore:

". . . little seems to have changed in how students are taught. Despite much research suggesting better alternatives, classrooms still appear to be dominated by textbooks, teacher lectures, and short-answer activity sheets." (p. l0)

In 1972 The Rand Corporation issued a still illuminating report on a major study done for the President's Commission on School Finance. Known as the "Averch Report"[4] for its chief investigator, it found, in summary:

"We are saying that research has found nothing that consistently and unambiguously makes a difference in student outcomes."

Further, it observed:

"There is a suggestion that substantial improvement in educational outcomes can be obtained only through *a vastly different form of education.*

The study recognized the difficulties it met, including the major question of how to measure learning achieved. Though it was expertly executed by a respected source (and seems even more impressive in retrospect after 25 years), its message was one that few in education wanted to hear and its impact was small. One factor surely was that at the time no "vastly different form of education" appeared to be available as a candidate. (Though the Montessori approach might have qualified in part, it was perceived as "old" and mainly for very young children.)

Why No Improvement?

One reason for the lack of movement has already been advanced—the widespread reluctance to stop looking at familiar schooling and teaching and start studying what learning is and how it can be brought about. People in any field do not usually yearn to abandon what they view as expertise and useful experience, especially if that requires getting into new and perhaps threatening areas. It is easy enough to vocalize for change, but one must have something to change *to* that is reasonably well understood and ready and waiting for use.

Only the adoption of methods and approaches that do, in fact, sharply increase the acquisition of learning will help. The word "sharply" deserves emphasis — a ten percent gain, or even double that, will make scarcely a dent in the need. (The programs, sometimes much publicized, that produce what are called "significant" gains must be looked at with a cold eye. The significance is often only in the statistical sense: that a difference probably not due to chance was detected. The actual improvement turns out to be trivial.)

LOOKING FOR SOLUTIONS: FOCUS ON BRAIN RESEARCH

Today, I submit, *for the first time in human history* the means to make real change in education is at hand. It is a broad, largely new approach that rests on a newly built, scientifically firm knowledge base: *brain-compatible* education. This is an approach that breaks away sharply from the many current efforts to build upon the stunning failures of the past and modify (instead of root out) the gross defects and upside-down beliefs of an entrenched, obdurate bureaucracy. Because it focuses on the human brain — a fresh field for most educators — it largely avoids being entangled with past judgments and politics as older reform approaches may be.

In short, the door is open. We at last have the truly alternative concepts and practices needed to permit meaningful change. And early application experiences provide strong encouragement. For instance, Susan Kovalik and her associates have been using brain research for the past 15 years as the basis for their view of learning and brain-compatible curriculum and instruction. The rubrics[5] they have developed to assess implementation of brain-compatible strategies and curriculum describe levels of expectation for students that most would say is "pie in the sky" except that students fulfill those expectations. Kovalik's work proves it is doable, that it is happening. And similar results are consistently produced by thousands of ITI teachers in hundreds of schools across the country.

But why only in isolated pockets here and there?

Brain Research Versus Historical Practices

We should note here the paralyzing influence of the very history of schools and schooling. Through many centuries, student learning presented less of a riddle because objectives were simpler. Instruction tended to center around a very few books, which represented accepted and lasting authority. Before printing came into common use, books had to be copied by hand, one by one, and were rare and costly. In most cases, the teacher was the only one who had the book, or had access to a copy or who, as was often the case, had memorized it word for word along with much commentary and interpretation. The teacher's function stood crystal clear: to pass along to students this knowledge of the book. If the student could recite the text, or repeat the official, approved commentary appropriately, learning was judged to have occurred.

The teacher's job was unmistakably to *teach*, in the "hard" sense of being in charge, of dominating, of directing students in all respects, of judging achievement and compliance, and of having the power (usually much used) to punish.

As printing made books widely available, things changed considerably; where there had been a few, "great" books, thousands of high value appeared. At the same time the duration of authority began to shrink. Knowledge became more and more transient and enormously more complex. Our problem today isn't how to obtain information but rather how to cope with the flood that pours out from presses and other kinds of media as well. We know this change has occurred — it is almost a cliche´ to state it — but we have lagged badly in shaping new concepts of what learning is in modern terms. (The yearning for now vanished certainties shows up in part in the demand for testing and "national standards" and other attempts to legislate sameness in the face of human variability).

If we so much as glance at conventional schools almost anywhere, we find obsession with *bits of information*. The so-called "standardized" tests that work so much mischief focus heavily on these snippets, as though ability to recall some of them meant being educated. The idea of education as aimed at better *understanding* of how the world works — how parts relate and interact — seems far distant.

The great bulk of this knowledge explosion, and the accompanying decay of "official" authority, has come about in our own century, and indeed most of it in the last half-century. Our class-and-grade school system, however, goes back to Horace Mann's efforts in the 1850s, a time that in our eyes seems remote, bucolic, stable, and simple. *Obviously, the system we attempt to keep using was never designed to deal with present needs.* It is a relic of the distant past.

As I have suggested earlier,[6] teachers entering their jobs are regularly pushed into a role that makes no sense when analyzed. It consists of far too many tasks, covering a wide range of difficulty and levels. Seldom has the teacher been adequately prepared for the actual conditions that must be met.

TEACHER PRESERVICE PREPARATION . . . INSUFFICIENT TO THE TASK

Particularly jolting is John I. Goodlad's landmark book, *Teachers for Our Nation's Schools*, which sums up the findings of a major survey of college-level interest and effort in preparing teachers. Overall, Goodlad found:

> "These observations support the argument that teacher education today, like medical education at the beginning of the century, is at a critical juncture. Virtually every element common to a profession and necessary to the profession's impact on the common welfare is out of kilter."

Most staggering, however, is Goodlad's broad conclusion that education departments in the larger institutions tend to be far more interested in studying teachers than in preparing them for their work. For faculty members to show interest in the practical working of schools has been a kiss of death, greatly reducing the chances of obtaining tenure or promotion. Teacher education too often seems aimed at preparing the candidates for carrying on classroom instruction in the old, grossly unsuccessful way.

> "In many universities, teaching is no longer the primary mission. Future teachers in college are thus at least as likely as they were in high school to observe teaching methods that should not be replicated."

To discover that the colleges do not do what is needed to ensure teachers are fully prepared and instead teach, if anything, only the practices that have failed so abjectly may seem incredible.

But not so incredible when one considers how wide the discrepancy is between the amount of information about brain research findings appearing in college catalogs versus the popular press. The popular press[7] disseminates far more information—cover stories in *Newsweek, Time* and other mass market magazines; feature stories in daily newspapers, often run as a multi-part series; and numerous books written for the lay public. In contrast, a survey of college catalogs reveals few courses on this vital subject. If some educators cherished any hope that the colleges would lead the escape from the crushing conventional system, it must be abandoned here. Some colleges, of course, are trying but for the most part there is a stunning lack of institutional response to changing times and brain research findings. Instead, such efforts for change are largely being lead by individuals pursuing their personal visions.

LACK OF USEFUL RESEARCH

One more fundamental aspect of schooling as it exists must be looked at—research. Properly engaged, research could tell us why the tentacles of the traditional system are so hard to throw off. Most large enterprises of any nature today take as a given the importance of research, which essentially means learning more about what they are doing, what other people are doing, and what they might be doing to improve their performance. Good research is usually costly but regarded as essential to maintain competitive position and healthful progress. Despite the billions of dollars that pour out for schools each year while taxpayers anguish and states struggle to adopt budgets, research which might bring relief to schools gets the merest trickle, with most of that applied to gathering (unreliable) statistics or conducting (often harmful and misleading) testing. The crying problem is not addressed: How to bring about student learning.

There are several potent reasons why so little research goes to studying what brings about student learning. First, we should note that a huge amount of so-called research is done not for the purpose of finding out anything of value or to answer burning policy questions. Rather, it is largely the result of routine efforts to meet requirements that graduate students and aspiring faculty must perform. The great bulk of the resulting "research" proves of no greater value than one might expect and contributes mainly to clutter.

Another considerable amount of research is "done to order" by more professional and accomplished researchers for whom such assignments directly or indirectly provide living income. Here we move up a level to those who give or inspire the assignment, who may desire a nice, respectable piece of research that will offend no one, upset no applecart, and end with the observation that "more research is needed" before much can be concluded. Foundations, although independent of the educational system, have customarily spent millions on such riskless efforts. Not until recently, pressured by school failures, has research begun to appear that focuses on why effort to improve our schools so consistently fail.

Within the Department of Education, where a tiny fraction of the federal budget supports a research department, some good quality research is supported or at least collected. But any potent findings are handled cautiously with an eye to which way the political winds are blowing.

In most fields outside education, independent and usually obscure research sources sometimes bring forth the bombshells that set investigation and development on new paths, but such sources are few and rare in education. (It might be claimed that the brain-compatible movement is an example.) Most disappointing of all is that valuable research often fails to reach teachers, thus failing to influence the system.

When we come to research that is avowedly addressed to improving outcomes in schools, we find maddening circularity, a circularity that springs from assuming that the structures are givens when in fact they are part of the problem. Chief among these is the universal assumption that *classrooms* are the primary structure of schools. Even some sophisticated researchers seem unable to see the classroom (one teacher and an arbitrary number of students thrust into a closed room for long periods) as the artificial device it plainly is.[8]

As I have suggested many times, to learn about tigers we shouldn't study their behavior in zoo cages and then conclude they are animals that spend their day pacing back and forth, with no interest in hunting or sex. Similarly, students and their teachers when put into classrooms behave, not surprisingly, in classroom ways. Yet endless research efforts focus on behaviors and outcomes in classrooms. Many studies try to isolate one factor ("time on task" is an example) as though it is practical to separate it from the multitude of other, often individual, factors constantly in operation and rapidly changing. The problem becomes even more complicated when attempt is made to set up a "control" classroom for comparison, in an effort to apply the traditional research paradigm leading to statistical treatments.

Stepping back a bit, we can quickly see that studies of how to run a classroom better will—even if successful—never be applicable save in another classroom. The classroom has always been and remains a stubborn obstacle to producing learning, especially individual learning.[9] To study how best to produce learning within a setting antagonistic to learning seems a strange pursuit. Moreover, it pushes everybody involved in precisely the wrong direction: toward the failing, existing system rather than away from it.

Another questionable given is reliance on textbooks whose single, antiseptic, watered-down point of view clashes violently with the basic tenets of our Information Age and use of the internet. Among other problems, the use of textbooks also nurtures mistaken notions of cookie cutter entrance and exit performances of students, e.g., achievement levels students are expected to have when entering and exiting each grade level.

Even our traditional curriculum content ought not to be above suspicion. Whether transmitted via textbooks or delivered through teacher-made curriculum, it powerfully shapes teacher instructional processes toward lecture, the expedient means of covering a lot of material that appears to be unrelated to students' perception of the world they live in, particularly at middle and high school levels.

Failure to Use Research About the Brain and Learning

Even while we remark on the general futility and wrong-headedness of much of the research that is done, we should realistically recognize that research findings are not likely to penetrate the classroom door anyway. First, there is often failure to put the research essence into forms that will engage the teacher and be readily understandable. Second, the teacher may never be exposed to its existence and availability. Teachers have long since learned to depend on themselves, and what scattered, fragmentary input they may get by happenstance, to "learn" to manage a classroom. Their experience with research from outside, and via superiors, has not encouraged them to look in this direction for enlightenment and practical help. They are apt to be skeptical about what little research may be presented in the course of a few hours, or even minutes, of what is purported to be "inservice education." The basic structure of the typical classroom school effectively seals them off from what valid and applicable research findings might be available.

Old Assumptions

In short, "the classroom" embraces so many assumptions and long-frozen relationships—frequently largely unexamined—that it fends off the forces, usually puny, that might exert some pressure for breaking away from the system, a system that holds teachers and students captive in so many ways.

Teacher Vulnerability

The beginning teacher is hardly in a position to introduce major breaks with tradition, and the experienced teacher may well become reluctant to depart from well-established, accepted ways of handling classes. Some who have tried to break away may have become discouraged by outright opposition or worn down by lack of support from principal, parents, board of education, and others. More than one teacher has told me, in substance, "After a lifetime of teaching and trying to change the system, where does it get you? Banging your head against a stone wall, trying to change the system? Why bother? I shut my door and do what I can in my own room."

Blurred Pictures of Change

Even when there is no opposition, the image of *what to change to* may be too blurred, or the means of making the transition too intricate or intimidating, for one or a few teachers to succeed in escaping.

When teachers seek their individual survival, the school crumbles into a collection of little-related units. Adults build their private fortresses; the need for the children to progress continuously gets short shrift. Under the classroom system, teachers come to be almost exclusively concerned with their own rooms and programs and may see their job as one of "covering" the syllabus during the school year. If some learning occurs, well and good. If failures and shortcomings abound, the teacher may simply say, "I did what I was supposed to do." The teacher who moves too far from the syllabus, or who commits the crime of not covering the year's work, may be vulnerable to the point of losing employment. But if learning is poor, as it normally is, that is glossed over, or the students are blamed—or both.

Trouble from Colleagues

And what of the teacher who lets some able learners run ahead? The wrath of the teacher in the next grade can be expected: "Why did you teach them what is in *my* syllabus?" To fit into the system and protect themselves from flack, teachers in traditional settings must spend a good deal of time holding students back or diverting them from coherent, continued learning for which they seem individually ready. ("Gifted and Talented" programs may be at least partly designed to hide what is happening.)

Lack of Feedback

In the present enclosed classroom, lack of feedback presents its own problems. In most human activities, a variety of "scores" tell us how well we have done. The business person can analyze profits and sales, share of market, and the like. The salesperson can look at commissions. The personnel officer can review jobs filled, at what cost, and with what success. On a more personal level, we can enjoy sports in part because we can see the score at the end. After golf or bowling, baseball or tennis, even fishing or birding, we can gauge how well we did by the score or the count.

In teaching, however, the score in terms of genuine learning is harder to find. At present, a great flurry of effort is aimed at finding better, more practical forms of evaluating student progress. An enormous national push to judge our schools is stumbling forward. And the cost is high.

The Antique Classroom Formula

In the meantime, the harried classroom teacher is trying to teach 25 or so very different individuals the same material at the same time in pretty much the same way, as the antique classroom formula demands. With the increased emphasis on highly imperfect, limited-response tests, the teacher gets scarcely any information about how individual students performed on the test, other than a few subset numbers — which may arrive very late, if at all. Oddly enough, those who advocate or defend or tolerate such testing (testing that I consider close to fraudulent) do not seem to care that it minimizes the feedback to the teacher on how individual students are doing and what their specific learning problems may be. With reason, teachers tremble at the prospect of falling scores, not knowing what new pressures that may bring; while a rise in scores brings puzzlement as to cause. Absurdly, news media and local people commonly make much of tiny shifts in scores that mean nothing under sensible examination.

Here again the teacher is put in an unfair and frustrating position; on one hand being held accountable for learning achievement as measured by the tests but, on the other hand, lacking the means to determine what actually happened — why the scores turned out the way they did or what students really know and don't know.

SEARCHING FOR REALITY

Even within their own classrooms, it can be difficult for teachers to ascertain what actually produces learning and what doesn't. Teachers, being as human as anybody, tend to convince themselves that they are doing an effective job; otherwise the level of frustration would drive them from school, however much they might want to work with youngsters. In the study *Looking in Classrooms,*[10] the authors point out that teachers are not trained to monitor their own behavior, rarely receive systematic or useful feedback from supervisors, and in general are so busy that they have little chance to even observe what is transpiring. Commonly, they confuse good intentions with actualities.[11]

Let's not blame the teacher. It is absurd to expect people to concentrate on doing a job and at the same time also to accurately observe themselves doing it. Professional football players spend days after a game reviewing the movies taken during it to see what actually happened. Yet teachers in classrooms, making literally thousands of decisions a day, have neither the equipment nor the time to review their actions. In football, the play occurs and the results can be measured to the inch and replayed. Mostly, the teacher must guess what happened—learning, other than by rote, can be hard to see.

Not only that, but in the graded classroom, the teachers' task of bringing about learning may well be considered hopeless to begin with. There is more than a little evidence that, overall, conventional teaching produces *negative* results: It inhibits, prevents, distorts, and holds back learning and convinces students they are stupid or that school is not a place where they are welcome or can succeed.

No one has wanted to face this grim possibility because there did not seem to be any available alternatives.[12] Only recently has it become marginally permissible to observe aloud that our conventional schools (which of course hold most of our students) may be doing more harm than good on balance. For those working in schools, it still seems risky to admit this possibility. However, *until we have the courage to be honest about the failings of our current system, we will never be able to summon the political will necessary to go forward.*

A NEW ALTERNATIVE

Fifteen years ago we might have despaired at being trapped in a system that patently did not work. Today, however, we have the kind of information about how the human brain learns to justify optimism; at last, a long hoped-for alternative is available to us.

It must be stressed, however, that we are talking about a major *alternative.* If my brief, dispiriting discussion of the conventional classroom system has at all served its purpose, it must be apparent that this outmoded system must go; it is not something to build on. The first step toward effective change or "restructuring" must be to turn our back on the hopeless, destructive old system and face in a new and fresh direction—to look at the human *brain.*

By so doing, we will find ourself in a totally new, fresh, exciting environment that invites teachers and others in schools to become true professionals, on a much higher level.

This does not mean that one or more isolated teachers cannot begin to utilize the striking benefits of the brain approach in their classroom until "conversion" of the school to brain-compatibility can be effected; however, implementation of brain-compatible education by a few teachers rather than the entire staff is not a desirable objective. Half a loaf may be better than none but education is no place for half loaves. *Striving for small changes may require more energy, and bring less progress, than larger aims.*

Nor can we be tolerant of "change" that leaves everybody doing very much what they were doing before. Changing to brain-compatible approaches involves some shocks, some down to the soles of our feet, so to speak. While experienced and intuitive educators will find in the exploration that follows much to nod their heads to, other aspects will call for more soul-searching and getting used to. Some suggested actions may at first blush seem outrageous . . . but there is strong support for brain-compatible learning, scientifically and in educational experience.

I suggest that we can have:

- Schools that are joyful, relaxed, with virtually no discipline problems

- Schools where nearly every student's level of learning will be superior to that of the top five percent of students in most schools today

- Schools where most activities do not go by the clock

- Schools where instruction commonly integrates what are now separate "subjects"

- Schools where teachers do not try to simplify ideas and concepts or present them in "logical" sequence

- Schools in which students are seen as infinitely varied, in brain terms, and are not grouped on the basis of traditional, imagined alikeness

- Schools where teachers work as professionals, applying sound, scientific theory of human learning, on a day-in, day-out basis

Permit me to say here—I hope unnecessarily—that the brain-compatible approach is hardnosed and down-to-earth, has been shown to be thoroughly practicable, and should be fully replicable. There should be no room here for cult, folklore, or warm-fuzzy hopes that lack a brain research foundation. Departing from the bankrupt class-and-grade system does not imply any trip into the wild blue yonder.

NEW OBJECTIVES

Perhaps it will be helpful to the reader if I set down some broad objectives that are consistent with current brain research findings and, I believe, largely acceptable to a great majority of citizens and parents who have done some thinking about education. This explores how these objectives can be attained.

1. Schools are necessary, in some organized form; their success in producing useful learning and helping young people find their responsible and productive place in society is critically important to our democracy and well-being as a nation. We have no reason, however, to hold the prevailing form of schooling as sacred, unchangeable, or not potentially subject to great improvement.

2. Schools cannot effectively operate as an enclave separate and remote from society. They must be integrated with society and especially their communities. They must recognize that learning does not stem only from schooling, nor does in-school learning come only from the official, stated curriculum. The whole school environment has profound effects on students, the more so since the school represents state power, authority, and adult wisdom.

3. The standards that prevail in office, retail store, factory, laboratory or other workplaces and public sites should also apply to the school. We expect certain levels of order, courtesy, respect for all individuals, modern management and communications, integrity, and accountability. These should quite naturally apply in schools as subsets of society. There should be no chaos, disorder, rudeness, disrespect, or regimentation.

4. The day when a case could be made for preparing students for factory employment by training in punctuality, nominal politeness to superiors, and general docility are long gone. We are more aware and accepting of individual differences and capability. The number of occupations in present society has been estimated as high as 90,000; new ones are added daily. In a world changing at dizzying speed, it is futile to speak of "preparing" students in the old sense; preparation must be in broad terms with emphasis on flexibility and continuous learning. (Some definitions of learning will be offered later.)

5. A basic core of learning can be established. However, it needs to be realistically related to present-day needs and not simply tradition. In my view, it should certainly include the ability to read and write, for practical purposes, with ease; a grasp of mathematics and modest skill in computation; at least some familiarity with the meaning and methods of science; some introduction to the arts, literature, history, and the geography of the world; practical skill in communications; some sense of how families work, child rearing and marriage; the law, the fundamentals of business, employment, and taxes; and the responsibilities and procedures of citizenship.

But the old concept of a "canon" or specific body of knowledge, beliefs, or rules has clearly been drowned out by the fluidity of the modern world. Efforts to find or specify a canon for schools quickly prove futile and at times even comical. At a time when we should be helping our young see into the future, we are instead burdening them with disjointed and not entirely accurate snapshots of the past.

We can have superb schools, if we will go down new paths to get them. We can stay on solid ground throughout our quest. We have enough knowledge of the brain and experience in applying it to start *now* and quickly obtain gratifying results.

NOTES

1 Arthur Koestler, *The Sleepwalkers.* (New York: Macmillan, 1959), p. 520.

2 "A Nation at Risk" stirred America's conscience in the early 80s; its unsugar-coated findings are as true today as 15 years ago.

3 The 1990 report by NAEP of national outcomes is as relevant as a measure of our public education system now as it was when first reported. Reports of outcomes in our popular press such as *Newsweek, USA Today, Time Magazine,* consistently reaffirm the findings reported here.

4 Harvey A. Averch and others, *How Effective Is Schooling?* (Santa Monica, California: The Rand Corporation, 1972), pp. x, xiii. A similar finding appears in Christopher Jencks and others, *Inequality* (New York: Basic Books, 1972): "We can see no evidence that either school administrators or educational experts know how to raise test scores, even when they have vast resources at their disposal." (p.95)

5 Editor's Note: A common reaction of those reading about brain research for the first time is "But what would it look like in the classroom?" The rubrics, and other books and videos, created by Susan Kovalik and Associates help answer those questions in concrete and practical ways. See Appendices A and B for a glimpse of brain research in action.

6 Leslie A. Hart, *The Classroom Disaster* (New York: Teachers College Press, Columbia University, 1969), particularly Chapter 5. The book remains one of the few detailed analyzes of the classroom and its effects as a form of organization.

7 Editor's Note: Coverage of recent brain research findings in the popular press are surprising in their frequency and depth. The following represent just a sampling from recent years: the multi-issue, Pulitzer Prize-winning series in *The Chicago Tribune* which served as the basis for the book entitled *Inside the Brain: Revolutionary Discoveries of How the Mind Works* by Ronald Kotulak, 1996; "Your Child's Brain" by Sharon Begley, *Newsweek,* February 19, 1996; "Controlling Computers with Neural Signals" by Hugh S. Lustad and R. Benjamin Knapp, *Scientific American,* October, 1996; "Dyslexia" by Sally E. Shaywitz, *Scientific American,* November, 1996; A Head for Numbers" by Robert Kunzig,

Discover, July, 1997; and *Newsweek, Special Edition, Your Child: From Birth to Three,* Spring/Summer, 1997.

8 Hart, Leslie A. *The Classroom Disaster.* New York: Teachers College Press, 1969.

9 Editor's Note: The classroom as culprit in reproducing the system's dismal educational results is a firmly held conviction of Hart's, born of his thorough research for *The Classroom Disaster.* As he visited schools over the years, Hart grew even more adamant. He and I had several heated discussions about it in the late 1980s. At the time, I, like most educators, could not see past my pictures and paradigms about classrooms. After all, classrooms are so fundamental to schools, what possible alternative could there be? Now able to understand what he saw, I, too, have come to share his conviction. He truly has been a man of few illusions and ahead of his time.

10 Thomas L. Good and Jere E. Brophy, *Looking in Classrooms* (New York: Harper and Row, 1973). See particularly Chapter 2, "Teacher Awareness."

11 When John Goodlad and his associates visited classrooms to see how much could be observed in practice, they found almost none. See *Looking Behind the Classroom Door* by John I. Goodlad, M. Frances Klein, and associates (Belmont, California: Wadsworth Publishing, 1974). See p. 82. This brief book, based on visits to over 200 classrooms, provides a calm but chilling documentation of the real conditions obtaining in classroom as contrasted with pious talk.

12 Recent changes seem aimed more in the other direction, influenced by the budget squeezes and the "back to basics" cry. School boards and legislatures seem to be growing more conservative. But schools seldom change substantially, however much there may be talk of change, in whatever direction of whatever kind, so long as they can continue to operate in the old ways.

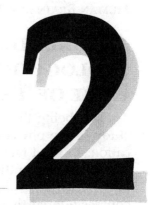

WRONG PATHS: MANN'S FACTORY TO BEHAVIORISM

Over the years we have been presented with all kinds of learning principles and theories which were considered basic for understanding human social behavior. In fact, since almost every school teacher has been required in his training to take a course in learning, he was exposed to ideas based almost exclusively on the learning of individual rats. Nobody has ever demonstrated in anything resembling a compelling manner that these principles and theories were or are relevant to learning in the social matrix of a classroom.

–Seymour B. Sarason[1]

The human body contains many organs, each of which has one or more functions. One of those functions is the production of so-called "informational substances" that, together with the processing of the brain, carry out what we call learning, a product of the bodybrain. (For more information about this learning as a bodybrain activity, see Chapter 5.)

A CONUNDRUM: WHY ISN'T THE BIOLOGY OF HUMAN LEARNING THE CORE OF TEACHER EDUCATION?

This being the case, and hardly news, we must wonder why study of the physiology of learning isn't the core of teacher education. In hard fact, teachers and administrators usually emerge from their preparation with little or no knowledge of the physiology of learning. As college catalogs show, it is still difficult to find courses offered that provide more than an isolated course or two referring to the brain. The majority of classes offered remain unaffected by recent brain research. Rare are the courses which address how to translate brain research into fundamental, and practical, classroom applications.

The reasons for this anomaly seem worth examination. If we are to advance to far more resultful, brain-based approaches, we must not only adopt new theory and practices but also (and much more difficult) *we must abandon old concepts, beliefs, traditions, assumptions, procedures, and authority that obscure or conflict with brain research*. Most of us have been brought up with these old notions, in private life or in training, or both, and they often prove hard to let go. However, we would be less distressed when discarding them if we have a sound understanding of where they came from, and of the damage they do.

In my experience, the great majority of people engaged in education or training would love to see students learn better. Having somebody learn from one's instructional efforts brings great satisfaction. But we are burdened by our own past. We come to formal education with a store of conceptions on "the way things are" that we began to gather at around age three. For example, as a boy, I knew that our winter heat came from a coal furnace and in the kitchen our food was preserved by blocks of ice in a wooden icebox. It never entered my head that before many years coal would yield to oil or gas and that the burly iceman with his leather back-apron and tongs would vanish as white, electrical Frigidaires took over. I feel sure that if I had thought about these matters, I would have assumed that coal and ice had always been the accepted sources of heat and cold. But I had no reason to think about it. Why question what was "normal" and in use all about me?

We began learning about age three that schools were "normal" and commenced attending them by age six or sooner. It did not occur to us to question why they were as we found them to be or how else they might be. More urgent questions were how to please the teacher and how to work the drinking fountains. In time various aspects of school displeased us; but we likely attributed any distress to the powerful individuals in charge. We didn't question the existence of classrooms, fixed groups, grades, periods, subjects, courses, evaluations, or junior highs and high schools, any more than we questioned lamp posts, fences, green grass, or the warm sun of summer. These things *were*.

Those opting for teaching or related careers come to college with a dozen years of things-as-they-are experience. Most return to the school milieu at around age 22 — a time when real-world experience may be scant and contact with real children at the lowest point. They come not as revolutionaries but to make a living, fit in, get along, survive. After some 16 or more years of status quo exposure to education's structures and procedures, and the ideas that support them, what is is accepted as normal without much question. This is powerful indoctrination. Unlike accountants, mechanics, biologists, police officers, and others who enter their work milieu only after graduation, educators are "brought up" in their field. Little has changed. Old, familiar ideas are hardest to shake. On the job, pressures begin at once, problems are insistent. Looking back, to ask "Why is this as it is?" may seem an unaffordable effort.

Yet look back we must in order to gain insight into why education seems awash in acute difficulties, frustrations, and conflict. Hindsight shows us that education followed two wrong paths, paths that have taken us deeper and deeper into our present troubles.

TWO WRONG PATHS

To understand our current situation, it is essential that we understand two paths that have led us into powerful systemic problems: the impact of the Prussian-based factory model with its class-grade structure and the rise of psychology, particularly behaviorism.

Wrong Path #1: Horace Mann and the Prussia-Based Factory Model

The first of these paths carries us back 150 years to Horace Mann who had so profound and lasting an effect on our school system. In 1837, when Mann was named to his position in Massachusetts—what we would now call Commissioner of Education—he was an attorney, with no children of his own (until late in life), no previous experience with children or with schools, and no special preparation for the assignment aside from interest. The existing schools revolted him. Based mostly on the old schoolmaster pattern, the teaching required the students, mostly boys, to memorize their lesson and then come forward one by one to recite it to the master. The content was often totally irrelevant to the times, the place, and student needs. The whole business was unbearably dull, pointless, crude and mean, with a large overlay of violence: the teacher beat the students constantly if able to and, if not, was frequently beaten and turned out by the larger students if not able to subdue them. For primary grades, a sort of school might be conducted by a local woman in her kitchen, a roomy and warm place, in return for small fees.

Mann, an earnest, able, tenacious, and devoted advocate, quickly recognized the need for a new system that would be adequate to the needs of a growing population. He traveled to Europe seeking a model he could adopt. Probably he saw the Prussian system through the tinted glasses of hope and need—and from that source, almost exclusively, came our class-and-grade system, still in use with its essentials scarcely changed.

Meanwhile, another type of school had arisen and spread widely: the one-room school, an object of legendary regard today. It was an American form, suitable to communities where students were few in number with a wide range of ages. It survived long into the 20th century—its demise due more to the roads and buses of the automobile age than to anything else. When we look back at the miserably small resources such schools had and at the teachers who often possessed some education but no formal training, we must marvel that they were as successful as records seem to suggest. Lacking training, the teachers did what came naturally, working with their charges as individuals without regard to age, grouping them on the basis of their current attainment levels in each subject area, and encouraging some of the more advanced students to help others. They did not have to fight the structure to do this; they had little alternative. In small, raw settlements, their curriculum was, of course, practical and focused on what we now call "basic skills." In those times, we should remember, "book learning" was low on the scale of priorities. Youngsters attended school when there was nothing more important for them to do, in their parents' eyes.[2]

The Prussian Model:
The Class-Grade Structure Wins Out

In older villages, towns, and cities, however, population growth and increasing density were creating pressure that invited new, larger structures. The Prussian system seemed to present answers to several needs.

Minimal Education for the Poor Versus Universal Education for a Democracy. In the 1830s, a good many people acknowledged the need to pay, through "poor rates," for a minimal education for children whose parents or guardians could not provide for it privately, mainly because the citizens believed that children not able to read religious literature would be easy prey for the devil. Public enthusiasm for paying these rates was hardly keen, we may well assume. Mann sought a great deal more: a system of publicly supported schools available to all, not as charity to the poor or orphaned, but as an expression of public policy that universal education was essential to a flourishing democracy. Mann's aims were bold, broad, and well ahead of his day.

The schools Mann inspected revealed the degree of local commitment to formal schooling that existed. They were tiny, ill-kept, poorly heated, furnished with crude benches, and about the only equipment was the inescapable switch for punishment. Many lacked even an outhouse—the woods nearby served, if there were woods. A common view was that "citizenship came by a process of patriotic osmosis,"[3] the result of exposure to communal activities and means of earning a living. The few hours children might spend in school hardly seemed much of a factor. A lawyer like Mann or a preacher might require considerable formal education, but such educational needs were hardly typical.

With his well-developed sense of practical politics, Mann needed no one to tell him he faced great odds, even with his high reputation and deserved fame as an orator.[4] If a new system were to be introduced, it would have to be one that would meet the least resistance. While Mann talked eloquently and in the most optimistic terms (education could be expected to cure all social problems), and undoubtedly was sincere, he was also introducing a system with some canny and timely operating advantages.

Dividing Into Classrooms: A Labor Convenience. By dividing the school into classrooms, a large and rapid increase in population could be accommodated. A room that at first contained 15 students could later hold 30, then 60, and ultimately as many as could be squeezed in physically, sometimes more than a hundred. Expense scarcely increased at all.

Not only that but grading the classrooms also helped solve labor problems. Male schoolmasters were hard to find. But "respectable" females, especially maiden ladies and widows, had little choice of employment. They could thus be hired at far less cost than men and for only as many weeks as required; needing their employment, they could be directed and managed with ease by male supervisors. Further, they could serve if they had enough knowledge for any one grade level, without need for a more general education, if they followed instructions. Thus began the tradition of the meek, genteel, badly-paid schoolteacher.

The Apparent Simplicity of the Factory Model. Added to these critical advantages in economy was the overall *apparent* simplicity and order of the structure. Here again we must recall the temper of the times. The factory system, which came to America a good half century later than to Europe, was taking hold in England as Mann was struggling with his mighty task of rebuilding education. On the whole, new mills and factories (which might even utilize that amazing invention, the steam engine) were admired — by people in no danger of working in them — for their productivity, which was in fact bringing an unprecedented flood of goods and products at lower prices.

By no accident, this model was applied to education. *The new kind of class-and-grade school was plainly a factory.* The students were the raw material, fed in at one end, batch processed, and turned out at the other. The teachers were the factory hands, the principals and supervisors were the foremen and managers. The board of education (which originally had the responsibility of determining who was destitute enough to need assistance from the poor rates) soon became an imitation of a corporation's board of directors.

The model, understandably, had remarkable appeal to communities which, if forced to expand public education, much preferred the cheap and presumably simplest means.[5] The pressures of growing population could not be ignored—especially since each wave of immigration brought a new variety of poor, "inferior" newcomers, deemed desperately in need of the moral direction the new schools were intended to deliver. (It was supposed, then as now, that the weakness of the home was the primary cause of the lamentable state of morality.)

The class-and-grade system and its factory school spread with remarkable rapidity. Other states soon followed the same path, at least where population was dense enough to warrant larger school units.

Mann wrote to a number of friends extolling his exciting new, broader concepts of education: "Under the soundest and most vigorous system of education which we can now command, what proportion or percentage of all children who are born, can be made useful, exemplary men—honest dealers, conscientious jurors, true witnesses, incorruptible voters and magistrates, good parents, good neighbors, good members of society?" Some replies seemed to confirm his optimism, suggesting a failure rate of below one-half percent, another predicted not a single case of failure.[6] To the best and wisest people, it seemed manifest that the schools would teach and the children would learn. How could there be problems?

Problems with the Factory Model

Very soon after the new kind of schools came into use, however, problems showed up. The first basic flaw was that the children were not inert raw material. They persisted in being individuals, differing enormously. Many did not "process" well. Yet despite the evidence, schools, then and down through the years, followed standard factory procedure whenever possible: *Make* the material fit the factory machinery. If the material is "defective" or does not process properly, throw it out on the scrap heap.

Factory Mentality: Children Can Be Processed at a Uniform Rate. Another error lay in supposing that the children could be processed successfully at a *uniform* rate. Learning was seen as a function of time: in two years a child should learn twice as much as in one year. When it soon became evident that this did not happen, many plans for modifying the rigid system were experimented with. Some actually helped. But overall the class-and-grade instructional plan was fundamentally flawed. Yet, the economic advantages won out and self-deception became a tacitly accepted way of life for school people. *One could preserve the system only by ignoring, distorting, or disclaiming responsibility for the results it produced.* For decades huge numbers of students were tossed out on the scrap heap. While such students came to be called "dropouts," the term "pushouts" was often more accurate, the more so as the years of schooling increased. As long as there were a variety of jobs available for those who did not process well, no crisis arose. The schools served as a sieve that separated "better" and "nicer" people from the contemptuously regarded recent immigrants and Native American, Afro-American, and Hispanic "minorities." The "better" and "nicer" group, which held power, found this an acceptable arrangement.[7] Other views were suppressed or brushed off.

Faith in the Public System Obscures Myths. Only a few years ago anyone writing such a summary of the history of our schools would have been called a nasty radical, a bitter cynic, or a poor patriot. As many have noted, Mann did his propaganda work so well that faith in the schools eventually acquired virtually a religious quality, a good deal of which still supports myths. Finally, however, that unquestioned belief is now painfully crumbling. But if we focus on learning,[8] we see that the class-and-grade system was adopted on naive assumptions.

Few questioned that if students were educated they would become model citizens and admirable individuals. Also, it was widely assumed that teaching would automatically and reliably produce learning. The basic teaching method derived from the centuries-old "learn the book" approach would surely result in a simple transference of knowledge from the teacher's head to the student's. Much learning would be achieved by rote and enforced by beating children as often and as cruelly as seemed required. (Mann was a kindly person, opposed to this torture, but an exception among the many who approved inflicting pain as a means of enforcing compliance.) The great bulk of instructional effort was directed toward training students to give "right answers" to standard questions. The spelling bee was enormously popular, handwriting had to be executed in a precise, official style, arithmetic was done by unvarying algorithms, geography meant storing facts like an atlas or gazetteer.

Although the more modern ideas of Pestalozzi, Froebel, Herbart, and others had won some following in Europe, they had little importance in America until much later. The discipline of psychology was far in the future; any thinking about learning that was done was largely the concern of philosophers who were not addressing practical applications. Though Mann had insights and intuitions far ahead of his day and saw the conflict between individuals in a free society and masses of youngsters grouped in schools,[9] he threw his weight behind the mass approach. The vision was clear: the schools would teach, the students would learn, the social problems would evaporate. Those trashed from the system would find gainful work.

As for the brain, it was then almost completely a mystery. Not until 1850 would instruments be developed to prove that nerves did indeed carry some kind of electrical pulse. (Mann had encountered *phrenology* on his travels, the notion that the shape and bumps of the head signified possession of various capabilities and aptitudes; he was fascinated by this quite wrong but later popular idea.) *Knowledge of the brain had nothing to offer education for over a century to come.*

The class-and-grade system had taken hold. At the time it was a triumph for the concept of free education for democracy but it put us on a wrong path for education, one that we are still struggling to leave behind.

WRONG PATH #2: RIDING THE RISE OF PSYCHOLOGY

A second reason why study of the brain was not a concern to educators lies in the rise of psychology, a science little over a century old if we date it from Wundt's pioneer laboratory at Leipzig.

Wrong from the Start

In America, behaviorist views gradually became dominant. The behaviorists had a sound aim: to get away from introspection, from dubious ideas such as phrenology and worse, and from the inaccessible, baffling brain in general—to try to make the new science more "scientific." A deliberate course was set **to stay outside the brain** and to concentrate on what subjects *did* that could be observed in accordance with the procedures for scientific observation currently in vogue.

Like the class-and-grade system, this sounded sensible at the time but it too, I suggest, has proved a disaster. Psychology became the study of rats, mice, cats, pigeons, and other creatures convenient to deal with in a laboratory. Primates received relatively little attention, and humans even less. The practice of avoiding the brain continued; even today it is given only superficial examination.

Ausubel, a dissenting psychologist influential in the 1960s, pointed out:

> The more scientifically conducted research in learning theory has been undertaken largely by psychologists unconnected with the education enterprise who have investigated problems quite remote from the type of learning that goes on in the classroom. The focus has been on animal learning or on short-term and fragmentary rote or nonverbal forms of human learning, rather than on the learning and retention of organized bodies of meaningful material.

Further, Ausubel noted that educational psychologists concerned themselves with measurement, group dynamics, counseling, and such and that, despite "the self-evident centrality of classroom learning and cognitive development," these areas were both theoretically and empirically ignored.

Little has changed to invalidate these observations. In general, psychologists who were heavily interested in learning in the first half of this century lost interest as the elaborate theories they had developed or explored broke down and interest shifted to new and perhaps more fruitful fields opened by stunning new advances such as DNA. The old behaviorism still survives in many college introductory courses, perhaps due to inertia (as if it must seem a shame to throw out such a huge amount of work). Even today psychologists seldom pay attention to schooling applications. Educational psychology texts freely confess to understanding little about learning and psychologists working in schools have tended to busy themselves in other directions, especially testing.

The Failure of Behaviorialism. The distaste and dissatisfaction teachers commonly express toward the educational psychology they have been forced to study appears to be well grounded. Massive as the effort has been, *it has contributed almost nothing to a useful understanding of learning and how to encourage it.*[10]

On the contrary, it has inhibited and distorted insights by persistently trying to transfer findings from contrived experiments with rats and other small animals to humans — at times with the caution that this should not be overdone, at times without it. Simultaneously, a vocabulary that is a large part of the problem had become conventional among educators: *stimulus, response, motivation, association, mediation, reinforcement, reward,* and more. Such terms embody antique and wrong ideas, as we shall see, yet they are so commonly used that they seldom are subjected to scrutiny.[11] In my view they are primitive, ill-defined, obsolete terms that continually tend to throw us off a productive track. Some people in educational research and decision-making are so dependent on them that they would be almost speechless and without direction if deprived of this jargon!

If this very brief review of a long period of educational history has served its purpose, we can see that we are saddled with out-of-date school structures and largely useless, confusing psychological precepts. *They do not provide foundations on which we can build,* only a thick overlay of historical debris that we must push aside if we are to make progress.

Time to Move On

Some people, I realize, will be outraged by my blunt and sweeping evaluation of conventional behaviorist psychology in relation to education. The past — especially those ideas that we have all been brought up with — is not easily or unemotionally cast off. However, I don't think that we dishonor the memory of the many outstanding people who labored in this field if we now recognize that their contributions have not panned out and that the structures they erected have tumbled down. New discoveries have been made, new ideas have emerged, and weaknesses in the old have become too evident to gloss over.

THE LEGACY OF MISTAKEN BELIEFS

In part, perhaps, we are all to blame. We have assumed that if valuable insight into human learning was to come, it would be from conventional psychology. We have paid scant heed to how few psychologists have been deeply interested in school learning, to how carelessly the results of animal studies have been applied to humans, and to the possibility that much more insight might come from other disciplines—especially from the study of the human brain, an area that behaviorists found inconvenient.

And we continue to use Mann's class-and-grade system, endlessly trying to patch it rather than face up to its inherent, incurable conceptual errors. As a consequence, schooling has become almost totally an elaborate, fiercely expensive ritual, divorced from learning outcomes, even while some two million well-intentioned and usually committed people work hard under dismaying conditions.

Notes

1 *The Creation of Settings and The Future Societies* (San Francisco: Jossey-Bass, 1972), p. 259.

2 In 1839 Mann persuaded the Massachusetts legislature to establish a minimum school year of six months. For many years, though, attendance remained far below present standards of regularity, especially in more rural areas. Reasons included weather, lack of suitable clothing, illnesses, family needs and circumstances, and child labor outside the home.

3 Jonathan Messerli, *Horace Mann* (New York: Alfred A. Knopf, p. 1972), p. 253. This excellent biography of Mann illuminates the period and Mann's remarkable abilities and personality.

4 Although a master of oratory, Mann at times felt discouraged in his prodigious efforts to sell the concept of public education. "I seem to myself as if I were standing, on some wintry day, with the storm beating upon me, ringing the door bell of a house that no one lives in, or perhaps where the dwellers are all sound asleep, or too much absorbed in their own minds to hear the summons of one who comes to tell them that a torrent from the mountains is rushing down upon them." Quoted from Horace Mann, *On the Crisis in Education*, Louis Fuller, ed. (Yellow Springs, Ohio: Antioch Press), 1965, p. 14.

5 At the time, the factory system, then new in America, had few negative connotations. The human suffering it could produce became evident some years later.

6 Jonathan Messerli, *Horace Mann* (New York: Alfred A. Knopf, 1972), p. 444.

7 In general, school boards afforded immigrant and minority groups — including women — little or no representation. The idea that "anyone can go to college" is very recent. It was long assumed that youngsters from poorer homes would seek jobs, at the latest after high school graduation (which most did not achieve). For a challenging view of the role of the schools in serving immigrants, see Colin Greer, *The Great School Legend* (New York: Basic Books, 1972).

8 For a full discussion of this view, see *Class, Bureaucracy, and the Schools: The Illusion of Educational Change in America* by historian Michael Katz. (New York: Praeger Publishers, 1971).

9 Historian Lawrence A. Cremin has pointed out Mann's struggle with the inner conflict between leaning toward kindly, individualized treatment of young learners and his drive for a socially effective "common school." He observes: "Mann by no means solves this problem but, to his great credit, he recognizes it. He is one of the first to try to work out the pedagogical implications of a universal education for freedom." See Horace Mann's Legacy, in *Horace Mann: The Republic and the School* (New York: Teachers College Press, 1957), p. 17.

10 David P. Ausubel, *Educational Psychology, A Cognitive View* (New York: Holt, Rinehart and Winston, 1968), p. 9.

11 In *The Psychology of Learning Applied to Teaching*, 2nd Edition (Indianapolis: Bobbs-Merrill Co., 1971). B.R. Bugelski observes: "The fact that many educational practices lack a scientific foundation is not solely the fault of educators. The very nature of their business, learning or teaching, is not really well understood even by those who have attempted to study it under refined laboratory conditions. The psychology of learning is marked by great gaps and theoretical controversies" (p. 15). Bugelski quotes several sources in agreement. For a more recent evaluation, by a number of distinguished psychologists, see *Psychology and Education: The State of the Union*, edited by Frank H. Farley and Neal J. Gordon (Berkeley: McCutchan Publishing Corp., 1981). Farley suggests that one might conclude from the reports given at research conventions that: "Cognition bears no relation to the nervous system; that personality, emotion, and motivation have no major bodily aspects; and that an organism could be effectively studied in complex situations without consideration of its evolutionary and biological structural and functional character, including those processes that might serve or control psychological matters" (p. 10).

12 William S. Shakian notes: "Psychology of learning has throughout the first half of the twentieth century been dominated by stimulus-response learning to the virtual exclusion of any other orientation." *Instruction to the Psychology of Learning* (Chicago: Rand McNally Co., 1976), p. xvii.

THEORY: SEEING WITH NEW UNDERSTANDING

> If we think that we already know how learning takes place, we are not likely to learn anything new about the process, particularly if the new concepts are contradictory to what we already "know." Therefore, popular beliefs about learning have to be unlearned or set aside if we are to gain any new insights. Unfortunately, most of the teaching and education planning that takes place throughout the world is based on outmoded, ineffective concepts of the teaching/learning process. The fact that students do learn is ordinarily taken as evidence that traditional/conventional theories about learning "really work," but evidence shows that they are highly questionable and that students often learn in spite of teachers' theories, rather than because of them.
>
> –Henry Clay Lindgren[1]

At times I have been introduced to teacher audiences as a theorist. The term causes foreheads to wrinkle: What is a theorist? Who needs theory? What will theory do for me Monday when there is a large, unruly, or bored class to face, in a school where morale is falling apart day by day? What will theory do for the budget threatened with still further cuts. What will theory do to quiet parents who want, or oppose, censorship of books in the library with impolite words in them or the teaching of "creationism," or programs for the gifted, or more art and music, or strictly basics and no frills?

THE USE OF THEORY: FOREIGN TO EDUCATION

So-called working educators, meaning those who have direct contact with and responsibilities for students (also often described, revealingly, as "those on the firing line"), tend to take a dim view of theory , even of the word itself. Theory may be instantly rejected or ridiculed, brushed aside, or possibly distorted to support, very superficially, the practices the educator had decided to use anyway. Or to impress parents, certain buzzwords in fashion may be tossed into the conversation ("applying Piaget" or stressing "thinking skills").

Here and there, to be sure, charismatic trainers of teachers claim to offer theory that teachers can apply in their regular classrooms "on Monday." The ideas may have value for stimulating thinking in the right direction but the theoretical foundation may be far less than rigorously scientific and the scope limited to small areas of interest. The claimed successes that application supposedly produces rarely stand up when investigated and the initial enthusiasm does not survive long. Characteristically, these thrusts do not seek to produce broad basic theory from which applications may *later* develop through the work of many who have learned about it. Sometimes, the theory ties closely to proprietary uses for commercial gain.

Discomfort With Theory: Not Without Reason

In general, working educators and many at "higher" levels feel uncomfortable with theoretical approaches. Even the great bulk of educational research that absorbs large sums of money and produces avalanches of published reports does not attempt to build theory. As Broudy has put it, "researchers do whatever interests them or whatever project can be funded."[2] Many others have made similar observations.

There are a variety of reasons for this. In their training, most educators were exposed to weak, fragmentary theory, often derived from animal studies, and found almost useless in classrooms. Few educators possess much scientific background (including some who teach science). Still fewer have had actual experience in fields where the primacy of theory has long since been accepted (today, virtually all fields except education). And rarest of all are those who have been involved in efforts to work from basic theory to practical applications.

Foshay, a prominent educator, put it bluntly:

Most school practice arises from tradition, ritual, and the context within which schools are conducted. Only during this century has scientific learning theory had an influence and then only in a fairly minor way. The school is a kind of subculture in which are preserved the relics of former times, with a few practices added or subtracted because of contemporary thought.[3]

A Change in Attitude Is Needed

I believe we can no longer afford these attitudes toward theory. Hot spotlights focus on schools today. If they reveal to a now dubious public a subculture rich in "relics," support can be expected to tail off even faster. People assume that within human limits accountants, doctors, plumbers, engineers, tailors, business managers, and others with skills or professions *know what they are doing* because an established body of "how to do it" exists. *To discover that traditional education lacks basic theory and proved expertise, and that few are seeking to build and use such a foundation, is jolting.* Debate and dispute rage in education because everyone has an opinion. The discussion begins and ends on the level of opinion, without ever moving to any sound basis or demonstrated results. Aukerman's well-known compendium of reading methods, for example, reviewed more than 100 approaches currently in use![4] The confusion, the lack of established theory, could hardly be better illustrated. Small wonder that teachers often respond to a flood of opinion-based advice by withdrawing into their classrooms, closing the door, and implementing their own opinions and methods.

Substantial theory (especially theory of learning) welded to practice stands at the top of schools' most urgent needs. With the tolerance of those readers who may be sophisticated in the concept and use of theory, let us consider some aspects of theory that relate most directly to education but are rarely discussed.

THE FUNCTION OF GOOD THEORY

The prime function of good theory is to cut through a morass of opinion and miscellaneous knowledge, or supposed knowledge, by *organizing* what is firmly known, observed, or with solid reason believed, into a unified structure, a structure that is substantially coherent and consistent. Essentially, a theory explains how things work.

Explanations, of course, can be dead wrong and yet hold sway in their day. Epilepsy, for example, was long thought to result from demons invading the victim's body. (We still say "God bless you" to guard against this when someone's mouth is open during a sneeze—earlier viewed as a great opportunity for an alert demon to hop in.) The treatment favored by even the best-educated people was to beat the patient severely, to make the demon so uncomfortable it would leave. Since epileptic seizures usually are of short duration, the treatment at times seemed to work and thus the theory endured for centuries. Similarly, blood-letting was the solution of the day for a wide range of ailments. Many times the treatments did more harm than good.

Wrong theory, we should note, results in counterproductive efforts; worse, it *harms* those it's supposed to help. A contemporary example of wrong theory applied can be found in conventional early reading instruction which is based on analytical, "logical" theory that reflects no more understanding of the brain than beating for epilepsy.

Other theories may be called "dead end" in that they do not advance understanding. In past ages, for instance, people believed earthquakes were caused by the anger of various gods. Offerings, ceremonies, and contribution had limited practical value. In contrast, our present theory, based on the interactions of tectonic plates, seems to be gradually moving toward ability to predict severe quakes and so lessen disasters.

One major evaluation of a theory stems from demanding skeptically, "So what?" A good theory should be intensely useful. *It should strongly suggest what to do* or at least in what directions to investigate. And, just as importantly, it should strongly suggest what not to do and directions to avoid.

What may be called *word-theory* plagues education and human relations fields generally and proves equally impractical. A word-theory is verbal or "armchair" discussion that never touches ground, never becomes tangible or substantial enough to ever be subjected to hard-nosed trial; it remains in the realm of words—speech or writing. To me and certainly many others, Freudian theory provides a mammoth example.[5] While Freud's often fantastic word-explanations proved enormously valuable in opening up new areas of investigation, one may well ask if they produced more confusion than direction. A good theory should not lead us to expend a lot of energy in wrong directions. Yet, efforts to use Freudian word-theory to treat psychosis or severe anxiety, for example, have produced outcomes as much disputed as the theory itself. To accept Freudian ideas, one must have a deep belief, akin to religious faith, that they have validity.

Theory: A Construct to Be Challenged, Not Believed

As scientific method has come to dominate our times, good theory has become more and more a construct to be challenged rather than believed — virtually a target put up for others in the field to try to shoot down. That can be done by showing it is not internally consistent, or does not fit well with observations, or, by cleverly devised tests, is shown to be fragmentary or having some weakness. In education, which deals with highly complex interactions, small-scale trials may show whether outcomes move in the right or wrong directions. Even when a theory stands up well, begins to prove useful, and applications produce impressive outcomes, we scientifically accept a theory only on a tentative basis, as the best working explanation we have for a year or a century but subject to disproof or replacement by a better explanation at any time.

Practice Without Theory . . . No Understanding of Why

Today, almost all technology depends on theory. Before such a base existed, however, craftsmen relied on ritualistic procedures. Splendid Samurai swords, for example, were made by processes handed down through the generations, executed with prayer or ceremony at each step. Early Egyptian glass makers could produce beautiful objects but attempts often failed because control of material, temperatures, and air moisture content was weak. Failures were blamed on "unclean" participants, astrological influences, or divine displeasure.

With no theoretical insight into what they were doing, people had to rely on the slow emergence of detailed methods that often required centuries of effort full of successes and failures. There was still little ability to explain why the process produced good results.

But this kind of "do it without understanding why it works" approach has little usefulness in modern education, where the "raw materials" vary so enormously, the conditions are always in flux, and needs shift so rapidly. Over time, most teachers acquire "a bag of tricks," such as cooperative learning strategies, how to teach short vowels, and so forth, that they believe work in certain circumstances. But, in general, the set procedures, when looked at closely, prove to be mainly rituals and traditions that fail much more often than they work so far as observable or measurable learning outcomes are concerned. Many relate only to pupil control to maintain an orderly classroom.

With over 45 million students and more than two million classrooms, we have a huge opportunity each year for superior methods to emerge but that does not happen. We have a vast store of bits and pieces of knowledge, or supposed knowledge, about teaching and learning and equally vast room to observe; but out of this has come only a mass of conflicting opinion and almost no theory, no coherent "why" explanations. Without guiding theory, education flounders, often going around in circles by discovering "new" methods that some historical research may show were "new" 20 and 40 and 60 years before.

GETTING ONTO A NEW PATH

With the brain as a focus, however, it becomes possible to get onto genuinely new paths. Using information never previously available, we can arrive at a kind of theory that does explain what learning is and how it comes about, theory described sharply enough to be tested in many ways.

A theory, of course, does not have to be perfect to be very useful if it brings together our best knowledge, fits pretty well with what we observe actually happens, and introduces solid knowledge—rather than adding fancy words that sound impressive but merely cover up ignorance. A theory can help us in practical ways though later it may need revisions and improvements. Take for example the theory that folk dances of people in relatively simple societies reflect the way they make their living, such as by hunting, herding, or agriculture. Its ideas help us see the dancing with "new eyes," discerning relationships never considered before.

ANATOMY OF A GOOD THEORY

A good theory of learning will help us look for, and perhaps find, relationships in the processes of education that previously were largely ignored, or not understood, or perhaps not generally noted at all. The theory we will explore in later chapters, for instance, suggests that *input* and *threat* are among highly important factors, until now hardly observed or considered. (These terms will be explained shortly.)

Usefulness . . . Accommodating for Levels of Expertise and Knowledge Structure

In assessing a theory's usefulness, it may be helpful to consider the learner's *levels of expertise* and the degree of specialization developed as a result of the *structure of knowledge*. The automobile makes a convenient illustrative subject, since most of us have to operate or utilize vehicles.

For example, think of the ground floor of our structure of expertise as occupied by those who do not drive but know what a car is, what it is for, that it has an engine that requires gasoline or other fuel, that it has brakes and lights, and so forth. We can call this the *orientation* level.

On the next floor are the many who can operate a car on a *procedural* basis. They know how to start the motor by turning a key, how to move the gear shift, how to press the throttle to control speed, and so on; but they may have little idea of just what happens when the key is turned and the gearshift lever is moved.

On the third floor are those who have a general grasp of the mechanics of an automobile. This is the *comprehension* level. By knowing to a degree "what is going on" they drive more expertly, detect developing problems, and are able to take simple remedial actions to deal with difficulties.

On the next floor of our structure are the mechanics and skilled amateurs, those whose understanding is deep enough to test and repair. This is the *technical* level.

On the fifth floor are the engineers who employ far deeper knowledge to evaluate materials and parts, direct production, and use sophisticated instruments to test and measure results. This is the lower *engineering* level.

On the sixth floor are various *design* engineers with deep knowledge that permits them to design parts, subsystems, and perhaps an entire vehicle. At this level, more and more of the work is done on paper or on computers, making more and more use of theory.

Occupying the highest floor are specialists, scientists, and researchers; a physicist concerned with the behavior of hot gases in a cylinder, a chemist involved with antipollution catalysts, a mathematician analyzing front-end geometries, all working intensively with theory.

If your car stopped running on a lonely road late at night, you might be luckier to have your garage mechanic come along than one of these higher experts. Yet plainly they have vital roles to play in giving us better performing and more reliable cars to begin with. Although the mechanic must have a good grasp of basic theory to be at all expert on a day-to-day practical level, he or she probably isn't equipped to perform at these higher levels. The higher the responsibility, the greater the need for sophisticated theory.

This kind of structuring of knowledge and the specialization that goes with it, we should note, is quite new in the world. Just a century ago in the United States, many families were largely self-sufficient. They raised their own food; processed and stored it; cared for their livestock, butchered and skinned them, built houses and barns; made soap and candles; spun, wove, knitted, and tailored garments; and made or repaired tools and weapons. Almost all of this was done at the ground floor or procedural levels.

Reliance on Theory Rather Than Tried and True Procedures. Today, our society has become so complex and reliant on technology that we must go to "museum villages" for a glimpse of those simpler times. Where for millennia we did things procedurally, "the way they were always done," we now are far more dependent on theory. As a boy, like many other inquisitive youngsters, I once took a clock apart and got some idea of the works and how they functioned. A child today who takes apart one of the new digital clocks will find nothing inside but mysterious circuits—not a single moving part other than switches! But a three-year-old can procedurally operate a color television, an incredibly complex, precision apparatus, because somewhere there are people at the various structural levels who utilize the theories that are the foundation for television, theories needed to design user-friendly TVs requiring no technical knowledge whatsoever.

Lack of Knowledge Structure in Education

As shocking as it may be, we must realize that we have not had a parallel knowledge structure in education. Education's "higher ups" do not *necessarily* have more grasp of theory. A viable theory of learning and theory of teaching just hasn't existed to any extent! The procedures that are widely used in schools do *not* rest on sound, substantial theoretical foundations. In that sense, education has never entered the twentieth century. It is still fundamentally back in prescientific times with more people suffering the consequences.[6]

WHY WE DON'T APPLY SCIENTIFIC AND TECHNICAL APPROACHES TO EDUCATION

The argument that schools deal with people and that therefore we can't apply modern scientific and technical approaches is, I submit, largely an excuse. We make cars and typewriters and frozen foods and synthetic textiles and antibiotics not to lie in warehouses but to be used *by people.* People staff offices, drive trucks, program computers, operate factory machinery, and conduct experiments in laboratories, just as people work in and attend schools. Businesses spend billions each year training their employees to use the best theories available which help explain what makes people tick, be it shopping or shoplifting, giving to charity or breaking the law. Our technologies *to great extent reflect our current people-needs.* The main complaint about schools is that they don't!

Even if the theories that now exist were perfect, most of us in education would be hard pressed to know what to do with them because *we have never before worked from theory to practice.* We have to learn and acquire expertise in this new way (new to education) of dealing with needs and problems; we cannot expect a theory itself to solve our problems, any more than new understanding of a disease will of itself effect cures. The understanding has to be applied.[7] At the same time, the old ways, based on tradition and ritual and often unsupported opinion, have to be terminated and discarded. And letting go can often be harder than taking hold.[8]

NOTES

1 *Educational Psychology in the Classroom*, 6th ed. (New York: Oxford University Press, 1980), p. 262.

2 Harry S. Broudy, *The Real World of the Public Schools* (New York: Harcourt Brace Jovanovich, 1972), p. 104.

3 Arthur W. Foshay in *The Elementary School in the United States*, 72d Yearbook of the National Society for the Study of Education (Chicago: University of Chicago Press, 1973), p. 197.

4 Robert C. Auderman, *Approaches to Beginning Reading* (New York: John Wiley and Sons, 1971).

5 For a very critical view, see Martin L. Gross, *The Psychological Society* (New York: Random House, 1978); see also *Mainstream Psychology* (New York: Holt, Rinehart and Winston, 1974) and various articles by Benjamin M. Braginsky and Dorothea D. Braginsky. No amount of criticism, of course, should dim the enormously important contributions of Freud in calling attention to unconscious aspects of the brain, the influence of early childhood experiences, parent-child relationships, and individualism.

6 This view is noted widely throughout the literature, as for example, George W. Denemark in *Education for 1984 and After*, report of Study Commission on Undergraduate Education and the Education of Teachers (Paul A. Olson, Director, University of Nebraska): "Much of what currently passes for theory is simply outdated specific knowledge–for which there should be little room in the teacher education curriculum" (p. 142). Martin Haberman refers to "a few generalizations that we pass off as theoretic principles. . . ." (p. 223).

7 Perhaps it is not too early in this discussion of learning to caution the reader not to expect neat recipes, offered for use Monday. The work to apply theory requires the efforts of many, over a considerable period. While the author and his associates have studied at least some applications for years, and investigated some in test and practice, this book seeks to deal with aims and principles that, if substantial and scientifically supported, can guide much wider efforts.

8 Peter F. Drucker, in *The Age of Discontinuity* (New York: Harper and Row, 1969), remarks: "The most difficult and most impor-

tant decisions in respect to objectives are not what to do. They are, first, what to abandon as no longer worthwhile and, second, what to give priority to and what to concentrate on. . . . The decisions about what to abandon are by far the most important and the most neglected." Drucker is speaking here of organizations in general, including schools (p. 192).

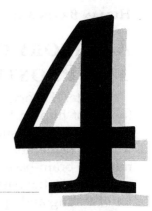

PROSTER THEORY: COMPREHENSIVE NEW SYNTHESIS

> Schooling in the United States can and must be revitalized. This cannot be done, however, by adding an innovation here or there. Systematic conceptualizations of what is required followed by systematic, step-by-step reconstruction are called for. The major educational challenge of our time is to reform our existing schools and school systems.
>
> — John I. Goodlad and M. Frances Klein[1]

In this book I present *Proster Theory* in terms I hope will be readily understandable and useful to all who are concerned in any way with teaching and training.

Introducing the theory will require a number of chapters, as the various findings and concepts that form its foundations are dealt with. The neologism "proster," pronounced "pross-ter," short for program structure, will be explained in Chapter 10.

A THEORY OF LEARNING: THE PROSTER THEORY

Proster Theory, which I have been developing since 1970, is *a* theory of human learning. It appears to be the first comprehensive, brain-based such theory to be published[2] and it has by now won a considerable amount of attention and interest. The fact that now one brain-based theory can be constructed implies that others can be, too — the basic information is available to all.[3] It will take a lot of testing and application experience[4] to move any theory into being, at least temporarily, "the" leading theory. But the practical beauty of a theory, if well and carefully conceived, is that it can be immediately useful in suggesting direction: what to examine and what to test.

Origins of Useful Theory

Typically, a useful theory does not come from the laboratory type of discovery or from long, original research in a limited area. Rather, it is likely to stem from pulling together knowledge and findings from a wide range of sources and arranging information and ideas into a coherent *system* so that we get a *whole* rather than a litter and jumble of fragments. In doing so, however, we must guard against falling victim to the neat appeals of *world theories* which result from stretching research implications beyond their original scope.

An example of a world theory long-dominant in education is the vision of the "trained mind," so strengthened and sharpened by hard study, instruction in logic, and "exercise" through mastery of Latin and mathematics that there would be "transfer" to all other fields. The system, however, had nothing to it but some impressive-sounding words. When tested, it utterly failed. Evidence to the contrary was overwhelming: What was learned transferred only to very similar applications.[6] Although this world theory collapsed half a century ago, it is still not unusual to hear a school board member, for instance, spouting this doctrine that sounds so reasonable but has been proved to be fallacious.

As we shall see, Proster Theory touches earth at many points, in two main ways. First, it easily fits into place and accounts for a great many frequently repeated observations of how people and learners do behave. Second, it fits with much that we now know about the physical nature of the brain and its history and development.

A Workable Theory Must Have a Broad, Deep Base in Brain Research Findings

To the reassurance of the reader, Proster Theory is grounded in multiple sources. Generated by deliberately looking in many disciplines, instead of just one or two, for findings that might apply, the roots of Proster Theory include the fields of:

- Anthropology and archeology, particularly the early pre-history of humans and the rise of civilization

- Evolutionary science and the general principles of the development of species

- Ethology, the study of creatures in their normal, natural environment rather than in laboratories or in confinement

- The neurosciences, which variously emphasize the physiology, electrochemistry, pathology, and other aspects of the brain, including neuropsychology

- Evolution of the human brain, about which a great deal is known

- Computer science, which has contributed enormously to understanding the brain as a kind of computer (to a considerable degree computer science has itself benefited by the comparison and contrasts)

- The newer "information processing" or cognitive psychologies and modern communication theory

- Primate studies, especially those involving the larger apes, the closest relatives of the human species

- Behaviorist psychology, in the sense that findings of experiments in many cases held significance, often distorted or obscured (or ignored) in the effort to build non-brain systems

- Educational experience, particularly in the contrast between widespread inadequate outcomes and a few notable successes

In generating the Proster Theory, the problem I faced was not one of having to scratch for useful evidence but of sorting out the solid materials from a great mass and then synthesizing it. As is common knowledge, scientists and researchers in different disciplines all too rarely cross their borders to make common cause. Adding to this fragmentation are the jargons that tend to make such mutual efforts even more difficult. Translation into something closer to plain English was a large part of the task.

Recent progress in the neurosciences played the crucial role in my work. In the last 35 to 40 years the achievement in these fields has been stupendous, largely reflecting the availability of new means of investigation—new tools that have been brilliantly used. Many of these achievements stemmed from progress in electronics: the computer in various forms which not only served as a model but made possible acquisition of huge amounts of data; the electron microscope and its scanning version that permitted a new range of magnification; probes so tiny they could be inserted even into single neurons of experimental animals; and an array of high-tech scanning devices such as PET, MRI, fast MRI, and the like.[7] At the same time, direct information on the human brain could be obtained as a by-product of medical procedures that utilized these and other new resources. Any criticism we may feel inclined to make of earlier investigators must, in fairness, be modified by realization that they lacked the key tools that are of such great value today—in some cases converting speculations to fact and, in others, producing surprises.

Because of these quite recent discoveries, we can feel far more certain that we are indeed entering into never-before-explored territories rather than recycling yet another time through some earlier educational ideas.

A THEORY OF INSTRUCTION MUST BE BASED ON A THEORY OF LEARNING

It is not too much to say that with this body of new information on the human brain we can now attain an unprecedented understanding of human nature. *A theory of learning overlaps a theory of behavior to a large degree because most human behavior is learned. A theory of instruction obviously must be based on a theory of learning* if there is to be a solid foundation. Yet in the entire, vast literature of education there is not enough on instructional theory (as opposed to descriptions of practices) to fill half a section of library shelf! In the absence of learning theory of sufficient substance, effort to develop general instructional theory has had to be speculation or declarations of personal beliefs or philosophies. Psychologists have contributed even less. Gage once noted that: "In comparison with learning, teaching goes almost unmentioned in the theoretical writings of psychologists."[8]

Even those who have written about learning directly for educators, after surveying the whole field, have offered little in terms of theory for teaching. Even practical advice for instructors has been inexplicably scarce. For example, the well known and properly admired book *Essentials of Learning* by Travers[9] gives virtually nothing in the course of about 500 pages. Nor does *Theories of Learning* by Ernest J. Hilgard and Gordon H. Bower, a somewhat more detailed survey.[10] In *The Psychology of Learning Applied to Teaching,* Bugleski does end with a brief chapter on "Practical Applications" that include but a few paragraphs of theory that he describes as "incomplete" and for which "primitive" might be a fair word.[11] The chapter includes a list of 59 "suggestions" which are provided as a summary and self-test of points made in the text, not as a coherent structure. In my view, the list does not contradict the admirably frank declaration in the introduction that "at the present time there is little to offer by way of practical advice to the harassed teachers."[12]

Essentially, these distinguished authorities are testimony to the paucity of useful knowledge and theory found in the classroom system. Happily, it is now possible to turn to a wealth of new information and theory, offering striking potentials, and to build on scientific foundations the older material so poorly provides.

The new body of material is *not* an addition to the old. It must be viewed as *replacement*—something like moving to vaccines and antibiotics from old drugs that merely soothed symptoms. To abandon concepts that one has spent much time, labor, and money to acquire must be painful—but less so than trying to cling to ideas and procedures that cause agony to both teacher and student, while serving society badly.

The arrival of brain-based learning theory, I suggest, forces all engaged in instruction or administration to make a choice, one which we have never faced before. The choice is between holding to the past—familiar, however inadequate—or breaking sharply away to enter quite new areas which will inevitably suggest and lead to development of new concepts of instruction and settings for learning.

To get to brain-based theory, we must go by way of the brain.

NOTES

1 John I. Goodlad and M. Frances Klein, *Looking Behind the Classroom Door* (Belmont, California: Wadsworth, 1974), p. v.

2 Proster Theory is presented in considerably more detail in Leslie A. Hart, *How The Brain Works* (New York: Basic Books, 1975). Most chapters are not technical; those that are have been kept free of jargon and shouldn't present difficulties to readers with some scientific background or interests.

3 Editor's Note: In the past 20 years, the amount and sophistication of brain research conducted has grown exponentially, with the number of studies now doubling two to three times a year. Reported both in the popular press and in quasi-scientific media as well as in the expected science and medical journals, there is no shortage of materials that explain the findings in very understandable terms. There are numerous bookstores on the internet that specialize in supporting educators wanting to learn about and implement brain research in their schools and classrooms. Books for Educators has one of the most useful listings of resources. See Appendix C

4 Editor's note: While Leslie Hart's Proster Theory has been studied and used by many educators over the years, the most long-term, consistent, and sizeable effort to implement the Proster Theory has been through the work of Susan Kovalik & Associates, Inc. and their ITI (Integrated Thematic Instruction) Model. There are also numerous large-scale, long-term projects based upon the ITI model and training. For information about ITI schools in your area or for information about formal research studies conducted on ITI schools, contact Susan Kovalik & Associates, Inc. See Appendix C.

5 Editor's note: The ITI model, developed by Susan Kovalik and her associates, is a concerted and sustained effort to translate the Proster Theory (and other relevant brain research findings) into a comprehensive, doable model for teachers and administrators. There is nothing "new" about the elements of the model: Good teachers have, through intuition, identified most of the strategies over the years. What is new, though, is that the ITI model puts old strategies into a new framework in order to accomplish a new purpose (the implementation of the Proster Theory). Teachers often remark that it would be easier to imple-

ment the ITI model if everything were new; using old tools in new ways is very difficult, requiring much unlearning and tossing out of old ideas in order to address the new. See Appendix C for a listing of the ITI model book appropriate to the grade level of your interest.

6 See Robert M. W. Travers, *Essentials of Learning, Third Edition.* (New York: Macmillan, 1972), p. 480: "The studies demonstrated that no particular subject-matter field had special powers to train the mind as the nineteenth-century educators had believed."

7 For a technical but generally lucid glimpse of many aspects of current brain laboratory investigation, see *Newsweek, Special Edition, Your Child,* Spring/Summer, 1997, especially, "How to Build a Baby's Brain" by Sharon Begley, pp. 28-32.

8 N. L. Gage, "Theories of Teaching," in *Theories of Learning and Instruction*, 63rd Yearbook of the National Society for the Study of Education (Chicago: University of Chicago Press, 1964), p. 269.

9 See note 3.

10 Hilgard writes: "It has been found enormously difficult to apply laboratory-derived principles of learning to the improvement of efficiency in tasks with clear and relatively simple objectives. We may infer that it will be even more difficult to apply laboratory-derived principles of learning to the improvement of efficient learning in tasks with more complex objectives." (New York: Appleton-Century-Crofts, 3rd Ed. 1966), p. 542. Teachers, of course, must often deal with extremely complex as well as usually vaguely stated objectives.

11 B.R. Bugleski, *The Psychology of Learning Applied to Teaching*, 2nd Ed. (Indianapolis: Bobbs-Merrill, 1971), p. 279.

12 Ibid, p. vii.

WHERE AND HOW LEARNING HAPPENS

> The brain is a tissue. It is a complicated, intricately woven tissue, like nothing else we know of in the universe, but it is composed of cells, as any tissue is. They are, to be sure, highly specialized cells but they function according to the laws that govern any other cells. Their electrical and chemical signals can be detected, recorded, and interpreted and their chemicals can be identified; the connections that constitute the brain's woven feltwork can be mapped. In short, the brain can be studied, just as the kidney can.
>
> —David H. Hubel[1]

Editor's Note: Perhaps the two biggest fears of any educator or lay person reading about how the brain learns are, first, the dread of being overwhelmed by complexity and unfamiliar vocabulary and, second, the aversion to being dragged into yet another educational fad.

Dread of overwhelming complexity and scientific detail is not unfounded, perhaps even completely justified, because the brain is, in fact, the most complex three pound mass in the universe. And study of the brain is just the beginning in understanding how learning occurs. The aversion to fad, that "Been there, done that, and don't want to repeat another futile, if not foolish, loop," is also well grounded in reality. Add to that the dizzying speed and quantity of emerging brain research and there is reason to doubt whether trying to hang one's hat on a moving target is worth the effort.

Avoiding levels of complexity unnecessary for understanding and finding well-grounded ways for applying the implications of brain research is a central goal of this book, one Leslie Hart has achieved and, as editor, I have attempted to uphold.

Falling prey to fad or being left behind by new discoveries about the brain is a legitimate concern; fortunately, however, the expanding story of the brain over the past 25 years is just that, an expanding story rather than a hopscotch leap from one abandoned theory to another. As the story expands, piggy-backing on new technologies that read like science fiction, old explanations have been found to be not wrong but incomplete. For example, this chapter was originally predicated on the belief that "the brain is the organ for learning." While not a false statement, today we know that learning is a bodybrain function or partnership with a two-way flow of communication between the brain and body, one affecting the other.

Thus, in keeping with this notion of "expansion not invalidation," this chapter will begin with the understandings about the brain of the late 1970s and early 1980s and end with an expanded picture of learning thanks to research through the late 80s, 90s, and early 21st century. This chapter is essentially as Hart wrote it unless noted by the use of the font type of this editor's note. Again, the message here is important: The research of the 1990s and early 21st century has expanded the story rather than invalidated previous work. As Paul Harvey notes, "the rest of the story" changes the context of our earlier understandings. As the context changes, so does our interpretation of the details. And so it is with brain research.

WHAT BRAIN RESEARCH CAN TELL US

With our new knowledge of the brain, we are beginning to realize that we *can now understand humans, including ourselves, as never before and that this is the greatest advance of our century, and quite possibly the most significant in all human history.*

In this discussion, we have the additional justification of wanting to see learning and instruction as aspects of brain nature and activity. Fortunately for those whose curiosity does not lead them into scientific matters, we do not need to get into any great technical depth in this subject. It is not detail we are concerned with but the broader picture. We want to know:

- What the brain is for
- How it functions in health and in ordinary use
- How we came to acquire what is often considered to be the most complex apparatus we know of in the universe
- How it learns
- How best to deal with the brains of others and to use our own.

We can call this a practical, useful, holistic approach, macro rather than micro, since we will look at the brain as a system, considering its interrelations, rather than trying to isolate and focus on one tiny area or function at a time. We will be concerned with the brain in health, not with neurological symptoms and illnesses.

LEARNING—AN OVERVIEW OF THE BRAIN'S ROLE

We can begin by looking at the human brain as a physical organ.[2]

An Introduction

If asked, people generally can give a quite detailed description of the human hand or eye. They may have a less sharp concept of stomach or liver. When it comes to the brain, however, many will simply draw a blank or be able to say only that "It has two sides" or "It's very complicated in there." We don't ordinarily have much reason to study the brain. As I have pointed out, even education is only beginning to give serious, in-depth attention to the brain; for the most part, engagement is still at a surface level suggesting implementation ideas which only tweak the old system rather than use of the information to reinvent curriculum and instruction.

It's Surprisingly Small But Complex. The adult human brain weighs a little over three pounds, or around 1,500 grams, and in volume is a little more than a quart, close to a liter. Individual brains vary considerably but, within a normal range, variations in size do not directly signify greater or lesser ability. On a species basis, however, size does tend to be significant. Among mammals, humans have by far the largest brain, except for porpoises, whales, and some other heavy mammals which we do not as yet have reason to believe surpass us in mental capacities. The ratio of brain to total body weight appears to be a key factor. Women's brains overall tend to be somewhat smaller than men's, to about the degree that the female body tends to be smaller.

The Brain As an Integration Center. We should be clear on what is meant by *brain*. The term implies an *integration* center for the nervous system. The vast majority of creatures do not have any brains at all in this sense because their various subsystems are not unified in a "head office." True brains are largely (but not exclusively) associated with mammals. *The size and complexity of an animal's brain tends to be directly related to that species' survival needs: The more behaviors it needs* to find food and avoid danger and the more *sensitivity to its surroundings it must have, the more brain it requires.* A grazing, herd animal such as a cow will have less in brain resources, especially in proportion to total weight, than a deer, which must be far more alert; the deer needs less than the dog, which must be far more adaptable in order to find and catch its food; and the dog gets along with less than the large apes, such as the chimpanzee, which lead a complex social life.

Humans have no "standard" way of living. We are the jack-of-all-trades of mammals, extremely adaptable and dependent on a great number of behaviors—a means of survival and a way of living that demands a stupendously large brain.

In truth, humans may properly be regarded as brain freaks. We can regard a giraffe as a neck freak and the elephant as even more a nose freak since its snout measures yards rather than inches. But the human brain is millions, even billions, of times more complex than the organ possessed by most other creatures with brains.

The Brain Viewed Over Time. Throughout much of human history the brain was not regarded as being of major importance. The liver, much larger, was long thought to be far more significant as well as the seat of the soul; the heart was quite literally considered the seat of courage and wisdom. Our common speech still reflects this. Though we don't talk much any more about "lily-livered" cowards, we do still say "learn by heart," "listen to your heart, not your head," "he hasn't got his heart in his work," and "let's get to the heart of the matter."[3]

Nature, however, has no such illusions, as we can see by the elaborate developments that give the brain better protection than any other portion of the body. The skull provides a chamber of sturdy bone, lined with a special coating, and filled with a fluid that further cushions against shock. The few pounds of pinkish-gray, jelly-like mass in this armored box get royal treatment in other ways. The brain has a rich blood supply that brings nourishment and oxygen and, in severe conditions in which these are in short supply, the brain has first call on what may be available. It routinely consumes a much larger share than its size and weight would warrant; the brain never "turns off," even in deep sleep.

Realization of the all-dominant role of the brain is even bringing about a new conception of what signals death. The old idea that death comes when the heart stops has been yielding, even in law, to instead considering the degree of brain activity. With modern support apparatus, the heart can be kept going in certain types of coma cases after the brain has in effect stopped functioning.

A Key Design Function. Unlike a bowl of jelly, *the brain has a "design" fully as specific as hand or ear or knee joint but vastly more complicated.* To make any sense at all out of its many, exceedingly intricate structures, we have to bear in mind that our human brain is the product of hundreds of millions of years of evolution. It is not a logical apparatus, like one a computer engineer might design at a drafting table, so to speak. (Today teams of specialists use computers to design new computers!)

That the brain is not a logical apparatus is a fact, a hard fact, of absolutely fundamental importance to learning. The brain is an organ—material tissue, not an abstract concept. We have to deal with it as it is, not as it might be, or as we might wish it, or suppose it. Since behavioral psychologists have long declined to look at it, and have shown hardly the smallest interest in its evolution, or indeed human evolution in general, we should not be too surprised to find that a brain-based theory brings us to some very different insights. And we have to *discard* old misconceptions which have kept us on wrong tracks for ages.

Historical Perspectives About Learning

Up until the 1950s, the study of human learning was largely fragmented and carried forward primarily by laboratory animals and brain trauma patients—the physical study of the brain—and by psychologists and psychiatrists interested in understanding and explaining behavior but who were little concerned with the physiology of healthy brains.

In the 1950s, however, Dr. Paul MacLean put forth the triune brain theory, a model that married aspects of the study of the physical brain with behavior.

Editor's Note: Useful for 40 years, the triune brain theory has recently been replaced by study of a more comprehensive view of the biology of learning that is coming to be referred to as the bodymind connection or, more appropriately I think, the *bodybrain partnership*.[4] A description of MacLean's triune brain theory is retained here in order to provide readers an historical perspective and to assist them in placing the triune brain theory within a useful context until it is retired altogether.

The Triune Brain Theory. MacLean gave us a very useful simplification of overall brain structure, based on a great deal of knowledge available at the time about how animal brains have actually developed over the last 250 million years or so.[5] He suggested we think of the present human brain as composed of three brains, of very different ages.

The oldest brain can be identified as **reptilian**. It may be compared to the kind of brain possessed by agile reptiles (Synapsida) that became the ancestors of mammals and may roughly be dated as perhaps 200 million years old.

The second brain, the **old mammalian**, is many tens of millions of years newer and a far more sensitive and sophisticated brain, common to all mammals as they flourished after most reptiles of the dinosaur age perished and became extinct, about 60 million years ago.

The third brain, the **new mammalian,** relatively speaking came into use only recently—it has been around so few millions of years that in evolutionary terms it may be considered, especially as developed in humans, as brand new. It is enormously more subtle

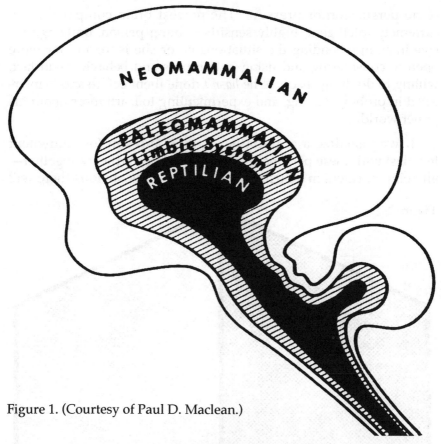

Figure 1. (Courtesy of Paul D. Maclean.)

and resourceful than the old mammalian, and many times as large as the other two brains combined. (See Figures 1, 2, and 3.)

It can be helpful, in considering the roles of these three brains, to be a bit fanciful and view them as so many familiar personalities. The reptilian brain can be related to an elderly person who happens to be very set in his (or her) ways, not too sensitive to what is happening around him (except for life and death situations), and apt to make oversimplified judgments: absolutely yes or absolutely no, very good or awful, content or terribly unhappy. Using the same analogy, the old mammalian section can be seen as more alert, much more discriminating as to the details of what is happening—as some middle-aged person might be. While this brain is not nearly as rigid as the older one, the personality is that of one who has developed accustomed ways of doing things and departs from them only under some persuasion or pressure. The newest brain compares to an extremely intelligent, highly sensitive young person, quite aggressive in comprehending the situations he or she is in, and far more open to considering and using new inputs and behaviors—in fact, willing to do things because he *hasn't* done them before and is interested in probing, testing, and experimenting to learn more about his or her world.

If we visualize a grandfather, father, and son (or equivalent females) with these personalities forced to live and work together—all being partners in a business, let us say—it is obvious there will

Figure 2.

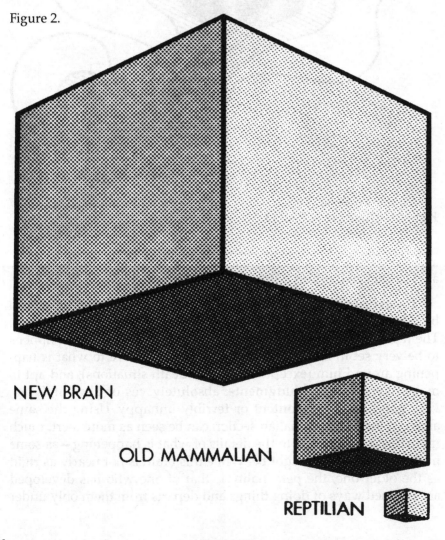

NEW BRAIN

OLD MAMMALIAN

REPTILIAN

be constant conflict and contention. This is one of the key aspects of the mid-century understanding of the human brain that MacLean brought more clearly into view: Emotions significantly affect brain functions and thus learning, memory, and behavior. The brain, not a harmonious whole as a result of evolution, was seen as working through a precarious, constantly changing balance of these three "partners."[6] This concept helped throw new light on human behavior, making it far more understandable and, for the first time, connecting learning and behavior to functions of specific brain structures.

MacLean's work, although now seen as an oversimplification, was paradigm breaking at the time. For a society long-steeped in a belief in logical, sequential, linear thinking processes as the bedrock not only of "hard" science but for a total societal worldview, suggesting that emotion played an important role in the operation of the cerebral cortex was a bit of a surprise. As educators, it's important to understand the roots of the groundbreaking work now being done on the origins and operations of emotions, research into what Dr. Candace Pert calls the "molecules of emotion," the "information substances" of the bodybrain partnership.[7]

The Triune Brain In Operation. The triune brain was seen as resulting from nature's parsimony. In evolution, old structures are rarely cast off. Rather, they are modified, improved, or added to (as seal legs became flippers or the delicate bones of our inner ear were remodeled from ancient gill structures). Thus the reptilian brain was retained even as something better evolved and the newer brain was placed more or less on top of and around the older one. When a still better kind of brain evolved, it again took form over and around the older two.

MacLean used Figure 1 on page 63 to diagram this relationship. We should bear in mind that this whole discussion is a simplification to a great degree; but for our present lay purposes it can help us get oriented rapidly to major and only recently understood aspects of the fabulous apparatus we are considering. In this diagram, the bulge off the brain stem represents the *cerebellum,* or "little brain," a specialized structure, tiny but a most effective computer that has long been known to coordinate physical movement. For example, as we learn a new dance, we are at first clumsy but with some practice the cerebellum gradually smoothes out the muscular activity and then stores the program for future use. If one learned to ride a bicycle as a child and then got on one after a forty-year lapse, the skill would be quickly brought back into use—proof that it has indeed been stored in the brain. More recent research suggests that the cerebellum also plays important roles in a wide range of brain functions including memory, spatial perception, language, attention, emotion, nonverbal cues, and decision-making.[8]

Figure 2 on page 64 suggests, very roughly, the great differences in size and "power" of these three brains. As we see, the old mammalian has many times the resources of the oldest or reptilian brain; and the newest brain—we loosely use the terms *neocortex* and *cerebrum* in referring to it—dwarfs the others.

In Figure 3 on page 67, the cerebrum is shown with a gray tone. Here we are looking up from below at the relatively huge neocortical "cap" of newest brain. It accounts for about five-sixths of the entire brain. In all the animal kingdom, there is nothing like this structure. More than any other, it makes us uniquely human.[9]

Virtually all of the learning we are concerned with in formal education involves this cerebrum.[10] The two older brains have no speech beyond sounds and cries and, in a sense, some expletives. All the language and symbols that we use, written or oral, and our ability to act, plan, and review abstractly—out of the presence of the people or things or events we are dealing with—stem from this newest brain.

We can readily see the basic limitation of trying to learn much about higher human capacities and typically human behaviors by studying cats, rats, hamsters, or other small laboratory animals. If we found engineers studying horse-drawn wagons in the hope of coming to know more about automobile engines, we might well think them mad. Yet generations of behaviorist psychologists who have written about humans have based their experimental work very heavily on animals whose brains are hundreds of times smaller to begin with and that have only the merest trace of this new kind of brain tissue that dominates the human brain. (The danger in this is well illustrated by MacLean who showed that when such animals' neocortex is prevented from developing during gestation, their behavior without it scarcely changes at all; this suggests that animal behavior is driven primarily by the older structures.)

Figure 3.

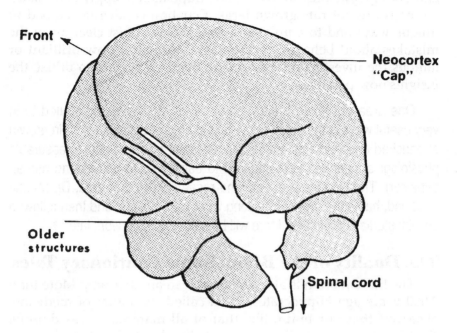

The two older brains by no means are unimportant in human affairs—quite the contrary: we are only beginning to grasp their full influence and roles. But enough is known about the human brain to say bluntly that the kind of learning *teachers* are concerned with involves *the great cerebrum that humans have and small animals lack.*

A Word About Rats. The rat psychology of the behaviorists, still taught in the great majority of colleges that give courses in psychology, is often applied to humans, sometimes with and sometimes without apology. It is hardly surprising that it has provided us with a large supply of misleading answers and distortions, and a vocabulary, that now put roadblocks in the way of coming to understand human learning in terms of human brains. For example, many uses of "stimulus" suggest a passive person who must be influenced by outside events, rather than an active, goal-oriented person who selects inputs to a great extent.[11] "Motivation" suggests the rat in the box must be starved into action the experimenter wants rather than being impelled by inborn and acquired goals that don't have to be externally provided. Such terms, I suggest, mislead and should be avoided by those unwilling to preserve errors of the past.

As we shall see, there are other reasons why study of rats can and does grossly mislead us if it is extrapolated to apply to humans. Humans are not rats grown large. Our brains have developed in unique ways and to a unique degree and we must clear away the mistakes about behavior of the past—no matter how brilliant or famous the investigators who made them—if we are to utilize the insights now possible.

One area of human brain research that rats have contributed to in very useful ways is the study of the actual physical effects on brain growth of enriched environments and of impoverished environments (measurable physiological changes as compared to using rats to understand human behavior). The pioneer and long-time researcher in that area, Dr. Marian Diamond, has done ground-breaking work with rats first and then followed up with studies of humans. More will be said about her work later.[12]

The Duality of the Brain: Some Cautionary Tales

The human brain is also remarkable in another way. More than 2,000 years ago Hippocrates, often called the father of medicine, observed that our brain, like that of all mammals, was double. That is, as we see in Figure 4, it quite clearly has two cerebral hemispheres, left and right, which are roughly (but not exactly) mirror images; and the older structures also tend to divide or duplicate left and right.

Generally, in animals that have backbones, this dual formation reflects symmetrical organization of the body and limbs on either side of the backbone, except that there is a crossover: The left side of the brain, in motor areas, controls the right side of the body, and vice versa. In humans, however, as huge nonmotor areas of the brain have developed, the two sides or hemispheres of the cerebrum have taken on *different* tasks.

In the great majority of people, the left hemisphere is much concerned with language. The right side is concerned with spatial matters, recognition of faces and many visual patterns, and music. But this does not mean the division is complete, neat, or simple. The main connection between the two halves of the cerebrum is a bridge called the *corpus callosum* which consists of 200 million or more nerve fibers. They carry information both ways. Any time we consider the brain, we must bear in mind that it has no truly separate parts—every part is elaborately interconnected with all other parts—and the brain always operates as an intricate system, a whole.[13] Also, how the two sides divide the work *varies widely from person to person.*

Work in the field of hemispherical specialization has given rise to some important findings but also a considerable amount of nonsense and unfounded speculations about "right side" and "left side" aspects of personality.[14] It has been widely suggested that the left side is logical and sequential because it is usually so involved with language. But a moment's thought should show that language is anything but logical, full of often absurd twists and turns, accidents and usages, and words and phrases that have dozens of different meanings in various uses. Nor is listening to speech more sequential than listening to music. *The "two sides the brain" concept has been badly abused, over-applied, and over-simplified.* A healthy human brain is a *whole brain* with considerable inter-communication and duplication.

In education, where modern knowledge of the brain tends to be scant, ill-founded notions of left/right functions have had all too hasty and wide circulation, leading to some bizarre activities and enthusiasms. To be sure, the classroom operates in a highly verbal fashion and so gives rise to the objection that it "educates only half of the brain," as some observers put it. But the brain existed long before classrooms and so can hardly be dependent on what happens in a few hours of school to become "educated."

Editor's Note: Conclusions about how learning takes place which are too simplistic or unanalyzed will only compound errors that have long existed. By unanalyzed, I mean conclusions that jump from a single brain research finding to a presumed way of implementation without being checked for personal or philosophical bias, examined for confirming educational research about its actual effect, or filtered through common sense. In my opinion, dabbling with brain research, rather than committing oneself to acquiring a strong, working understanding, is dangerous—dangerous because the things implemented can be of questionable value for students and because such "fads" distract us from the real issues of the need for fundamental change. Also, implementation of isolated, ineffectual strategies inevitably fails to make a difference. This, in the long run, gives brain research-based efforts a black eye and erodes the public's confidence in them.

Figure 4.

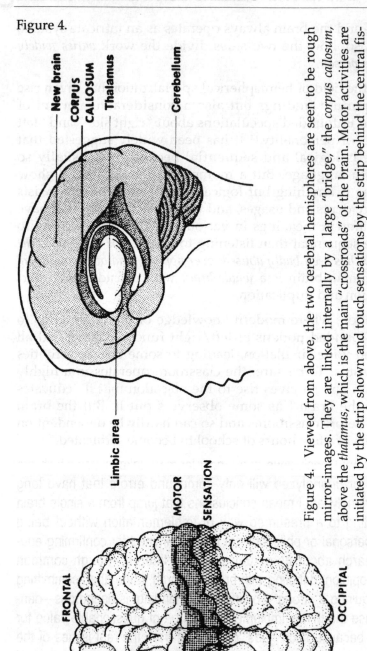

Figure 4. Viewed from above, the two cerebral hemispheres are seen to be rough mirror-images. They are linked internally by a large "bridge," the *corpus callosum,* above the *thalamus,* which is the main "crossroads" of the brain. Motor activities are initiated by the strip shown and touch sensations by the strip behind the central fissure. Vision is processed mainly by the lobes (occipital) on both sides at the very back of the brain. The neocortex or "bark" of the cerebrum is about 1/8 inch thick. The deep folds of the brain allow more surface for its tens of billions of neurons but the area of the entire neocortex is only about that of a large kerchief.

THE BIOLOGY OF LEARNING

Due to fantastic advances in technology, our understanding of how learning takes place, especially in the 1980s and 1990s, has radically expanded. While the story is all fantastically more complex than needed for our purposes here or in the classroom, a simplified accounting of the biology involved provides, I believe, valuable pictures for teachers (and their students). "Just what does go on in there?" is a question of undeniable human curiosity.

The Basic Building Blocks of Learning: Neurons, Dendrites, Axons, and Information Substances

The existence of neurons, dendrites, and axons is old news in science and their roles are understood in considerable detail. Information substances are the new kid on the block. How they function is a story in the unfolding.

Neurons, Dendrites, and Axons. There are, on conservative estimate, 100 billion brain cells (neurons) of various kinds with differing functions, all of which make more than a million billion connections. Because growth of new neurons after birth is limited,[15] it is how they organize themselves and how they connect with others that results in learning and the quality we call intelligence. This organizing and connecting results in real, measurable physiological growth of the brain. For example, Figure 5 on the next page illustrates the increase in complexity of dendrites and axons from birth to age two. As a result, the brain actually becomes denser and heavier (during infancy, the overall size of the skull increases as well).

Such growth and multiple branching of the dendrites and axons is the brain's response to rich sensory input from an enriched environment.[16] In contrast, sterile, boring environments not only result in significantly less growth but in actual shrinking of existing dendrites. A period of drastically reduced enrichment, even as short as four days, can result in measurable shrinkage of dendrites.[17] "Use it or lose it" is powerful advice when it comes to growing a brain. Parents and educators alike, take heed. Your job is to help children (and fellow adults) grow dendrites.[18]

Exactly how learning occurs is still a mystery, hidden at the molecular level. But the story is rapidly unfolding. In simple terms, as depicted on page 73, communication among neurons (brain cells) is an electrical-chemical affair. The sending neuron transmits an electrical signal down its

Figure 5.

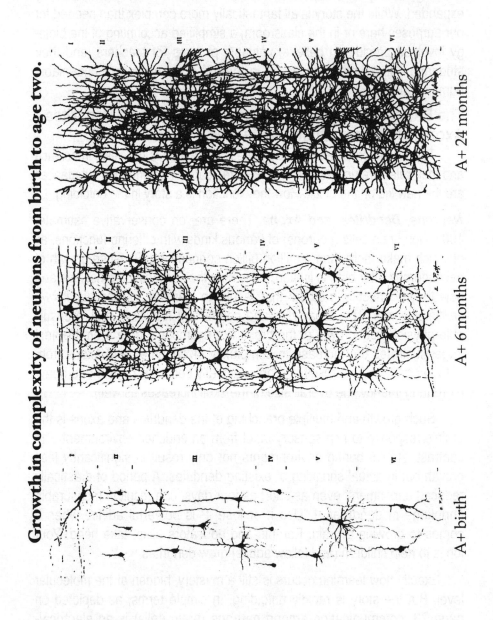

Growth in complexity of neurons from birth to age two.

A+ 24 months

A+ 6 months

A+ birth

Source: *Magic Trees of the Mind* by Marian Diamond, Ph.D.,
and Janet Hopson

Communication of Neurons Across the Synaptic Gap

Figure 6.

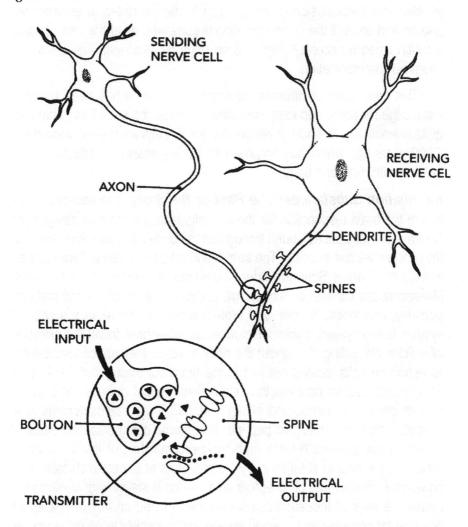

Among neurons, communication is an electrical-chemical affair. Within a neuron and its appendages, it is electrical. Between neurons, it is chemical, taking place across a narrow gap between the sending nerve cell's bulbous axon tip and the receiving cell's thornlike spine on a dendrite.

Source: *Magic Trees of the Mind* by Marian Diamond, Ph.D., and Janet Hopson

axon to its tip which is very close to the bulbous ending on the dendritic spines of the receiving cell. Chemical messengers, neurotransmitters, travel from the axon to the dendrite across the synaptic gap. If the information is compelling enough[19] to the receiving neuron, it in turn will spark an electrical transmission down its axon to the dendrites of another cell and on and on until the communication is complete, all at the rate of up to a billion times a second.[20] Figure 6 on page 81 illustrates this electrical-chemical communication.

This description of neurons, dendrites, and axons has been bedrock knowledge for some decades. Recently, however, the story has expanded quite dramatically. In short, it seems that the Greeks were on to something 2,000 years ago when they emphasized the importance of educating and training both mind and body.

Information Substances: The Rest of the Story. The neurotransmitters in the brain responsible for the synaptic leap are but one category of "information substances" found throughout the body and brain that carry out the process we call learning. The term "information substances" was coined initially by Francis Schmitt, elder statesman of neuroscience from the Massachusetts Institute of Technology, to describe a variety of transmitters, peptides, hormones, factors, and protein ligands that make up a second system. In this system, chemical information substances travel the extracellular fluids circulating throughout the body to reach their specific receptors, receptors on cells located not just in the brain but throughout the body.[21] This second system parallels the conventional model of neuronal circuitry with its dendrites, axons, and synaptic leaps. Some neuroscientists now speculate that less than two percent of neuronal communication actually occurs at the synapse.[22] Less than two percent! Most of the information received by a neuron is taken in by the receptors at the cell's surface. And no wonder. The number of receptors on a neuron is staggering; current estimates are tens of thousands to a million+ per neuron.[23] That's a lot of potential for conversation! It would appear that the ability to perceive understandable patterns and learn from them is so important to survival that it cannot be posited only in one place or with one method of communication—not just one part of the neuron (at the synaptic gap) nor just in the brain. The entire body is involved.[24]

So just what are these "information substances" and what is their role in learning? These molecules, or ligands, are the basic units of a language used by cells throughout the organism to communicate across systems such as the endocrine, neurological, gastrointestinal, and even the immune system. As they travel, they inform, regulate, and synchronize.[25] Peptides are the largest category of information substances; one kind or another is produced in every cell in the body, not just by cells in the brain. Furthermore, every peptide now known to be produced within the body has receptors in the brain, thus qualifying each peptide to be considered a "neuropeptide." This means that the body talks to the brain, giving it information that alters the brain's messages back to the body and vice versa. A true, two-way conversation.

The effect of such "conversations" on the organism is to change physical activity cell by cell and as a total organism, including behavior and even *mood*—the closest word to *emotion* in the lexicon of hard science.[26] Examples of outward manifestation of such inner "conversations" include a "gut feeling" about something; a first impression of someone as untrustworthy; a physical restlessness that something is wrong before you can put your finger on it; a spark in the eye that says, "I get it even though I can't yet explain it"; a passion for one's hobby; deep love for the beauty of nature; the contentment of a quiet hour spent with a special friend. As was foreseen by the now virtually abandoned triune brain theory,[24] core limbic brain structures such as the amygdala, hippocampus, and hypothalamus—which were long believed to be involved in emotional behavior—contain a whopping percent of the various neuropeptide receptors studied to date, perhaps as high as 85 to 95 percent.[28] Now add to that the startling finding that several of the key emotion molecules such as endorphins can be found in single-cell animals as well as on up the evolutionary trail. Peptides, it appears, have been carrying information since before there were brains, leading researchers such as Antonio Damasio to assert that "emotion is the highest part of our mindbody survival kit."[29] One of their key roles is to tell the brain what's worth attending to and the "attitude" with which one attends. Again, as so nicely summarized by Dr. Robert Sylwester, "Emotion drives attention, attention drives learning/memory/problem-solving/just about everything else."[30]

Another important piece of this new view of learning as a bodybrain partnership is the discovery that there are other locations in the body where high concentrations of almost every neuropeptide receptor exist. One example is the dorsal horn (the back side of the spinal cord) which is the first synapse with the nervous system where all somatosensory information is processed. In fact, in virtually all locations where information from five senses—sight, sound, taste, smell, and touch—enter the nervous system, there are high concentrations of neuropeptide receptors. Such regions, called nodal points or hot spots, seem to be designed so that they can be accessed and modulated by almost all neuropeptides as they go about their job of processing information, prioritizing it, and biasing it to cause unique neurophysiological changes. Thus, peptides filter the input of our experiences, significantly altering our perception of reality and the input selected and allowed in during any learning situation. According to Dr. Candace Pert, author of *Molecules of Emotion: Why You Feel the Way You Feel,* "emotions and bodily sensations are thus intricately intertwined, in a bidirectional network in which each can alter the other. Usually this process takes place at an unconscious level but it can also surface into consciousness under certain conditions or be brought into consciousness by intention."[31]

Implications for Teachers

The "How can I help Johnny?" question, from a teacher's point of view, might be re-phrased: "How do I best stimulate the brains of my students to make them grow, to increase the number of connections being made?"

Perhaps the most relevant window on how the brain functions from an educator's point of view comes through the new field of brain enrichment pioneered by Dr. Marian Diamond. The kinds of questions such researchers ask are closely akin to those which educators raise when they ask the time-worn question, "How can I best help Johnny learn X (math or geography or spelling)?" The answers lie in encouraging real physical growth in the brain. Here are several key concepts for educators to hold in mind when developing curriculum and planning instructional strategies.

1. Dendritic spines grow, change shape, or shrink as we experience the world. Therefore, choose the types of input that will produce the greatest physiological change in the brain. Eliminate or drastically reduce low-input materials and processes such as textbooks, worksheets, and working in isolation in absence of large

amounts of sensory input from experiences in the real world. Remember, dittos don't make dendrites!

2. The stimulation of an enriched environment results in significant physiological change in the brain—as much as 20% compared to brains in sterile, boring environments.

3. There is a correlation between brain structure and what we do in life—what we spend time doing and not doing.[32] In other words, how we spend our time—what we ask our brain to do on a daily basis—actually alters its physical structure. Vast amounts of time spent on television and/or video games (4-6 hours daily) wires the brain to do television and video games and does not wire the brain for other things like physical exploration or high facility for initiating and processing language. If students cannot do what you expect of them, take time to build the neural wiring and structures that will enable them to do what your curriculum expects. An analogy is keeping the high jump bar over their heads when they don't have the physical skills for jumping it at waist height. In track sports, this would be instantly recognized as both cruel and a foolish waste of time.

4. Much of the increase in the physical size of the brain (at birth, the brain is one quarter of its eventual adult size) is due to myelination, a process by which fatty tissue forms around the axons of frequently-firing neurons which act like rubber insulation on electrical cords. This allows for speedier and more reliable transmission of electrical impulses thus improving communication among neurons. While much of this process occurs with the unfolding maturation of the brain, much can be deliberately enhanced through ample practice in using the knowledge or skill being learned, particularly in real-world settings which allow for rich sensory input and feedback. See Chapters 9 and 10 for a discussion of a new, brain-based definition of learning which asks that we design curriculum that encourages mastery in real-world applications rather than quick quiz responses that usually stop at ability to *recognize* rather than *use* knowledge and skills.

5. Emotions drive attention, attention drives learning, memory, and problem-solving. Making instruction engaging for the learner is

not a nod in the direction of "competing" with TV and its MTV-like programming. It is a learning imperative. Lack of attention in the face of boring circumstances is not necessarily a sign of attention deficit disorder; it is a normal response of a normal bodybrain partnership. Engage students emotionally, through your passion for teaching and enthusiasm for the topic and through making the content real and useful to the student.

6. In the bodybrain partnership, each sends messages out to the other which alters the messages that are sent back. The brain does not function separately from the body. The quality of relationships in the classroom—teacher-to-student and student-to-student—is critical. Forge a sense of community characterized by absence of threat, inclusion, influence, and affection.[33] See Chapter 11 for more discussion about implementing the implications of the bodymind partnership.

In Summary

If this brief chapter has served its purpose, it will have provided some orientation to the bodybrain partnership—as we know it scientifically today—that can serve to focus teachers and instructors on how to increase learning. It will help readers push aside, I hope, the grossly wrong and misleading mountain of old psychology that has become a major obstacle to improving education.

Suppose I ask you to design a glove, giving you all the resources you may need. You know the shape of the hand, so your glove will emerge, we can feel confident, with provisions for one thumb and four fingers, a palm and wrist, and flexibility to permit finger movement. You will know that the hand's fingers bend forward, but not back, and that the thumb swings in from the side. Because you know the shape of the hand, and its general functions, you can hope to design something that will fit and work on actual human hands.

If next you are asked to design *instruction to fit the bodybrain partnership*, you see immediately that you cannot hope to do that job unless you know the "shape" of the brain, its main functions, and how it collaborates with the body. Without good, hard, realistic knowledge, a design group might labor a thousand years and get nowhere—indeed, in over two thousand years of teaching, a vast amount of effort has produced but fragments of knowledge useful to understanding how humans learn! We see teachers and instructors failing and frustrated wherever we look—now more than ever, because more is being attempted.

But today we have the knowledge to design bodybrain-fitting, *bodybrain-compatible* instructional settings and procedures. The "compatible" concept may startle us, simply because we are not used to it in education. All around us are hand-compatible tools and machines and keyboards, designed to fit the hand. We are not apt to think of them in that light because it does not occur to us that anyone would bring out some device to be used by human hands without being sure that the nature of hands was considered. A keyboard machine or musical instrument that called for eight fingers on each hand would draw instant ridicule. Yet we force millions of children into schools that have never seriously studied the nature and shape of the human brain and its bodybrain partnership, and which not surprisingly prove to be actively bodybrain-antagonistic.

We know less than we might and will; but we already know amply enough, I contend, to bring about instructional environments that, being body and brain compatible, will produce huge gains in learning. In a number of pioneering body brain-compatible schools, this is convincingly demonstrated.

NOTES

1 *Scientific American,* September 1979, p. 45.

2 *The Science Teacher,* April 1978, p. 32.

3 Editor's Note: The number of English language idioms involving the heart is quite fascinating, especially in light of the emerging research on the connection between the heart and brain. According to noted researcher Karl Pribram: ". . . our emotional state . . . affects how our brain matures. . . . Stressful, incoherent emotional states in a primary caregiver impair development and learning in children while positive emotional states enhance coherent maturation and learning." (See "Early Childhood Development and Learning: What New Research on the Heart and Brain Tells Us About Our Youngest Children," an unpublished paper by Karl Pribram (Director, Center for Brain Research, Department of Psychology, Radford, University, Radford, VA and Deborah Rozman (Executive Director, Institute of HeartMath, Boulder Creek, CA). See *The HeartMath Solution* by Doc Childre and Howard Martin (San Francisco: HarperSanFrancisco, 1999).

Also see *The Heart's Code: Tapping the Wisdom and Power of Our Heart Energy* by Paul Pearsall, a fascinating look at new findings about cellular memories and their role in what he calls the mind/body/spirit connection (New York: Broadway Books, 1998).

4 Editor's Note: In coining the term "bodybrain partnership," I am attempting to capture or represent several key concepts from the new brain biology. First, there is no hyphen in bodybrain, just as there is no way to separate the functions of the two as generator and receptor of the dozens of information substances. Second, both are physical entities, not conceptual models such as "mind." Both can be studied concretely, scientifically, to the cellular and molecular levels. Third, both come to school and sit before us; we must learn to deal with them as they are, not as may be convenient for the system. Fourth, *connection* is too passive a term. Survival—for which learning is the first line of offense and defense—requires a proactive, committed collaboration of body and brain—a true "bodybrain partnership."

5 MacLean's triune brain concept has been presented by him in a number of articles, some not readily accessible. See "The

Imitative-Creative Interplay of Our Three Mentalities," in Harold Harris, editor. *Astride The Two Cultures* (New York: Random House, 1975), and "A Mind of Three Minds: Educating the Triune Brain" in *Education and the Brain, 77th Yearbook* of the National Society for the Study of Education (Chicago: University of Chicago Press, 1978). I am here using his concepts freely, based on his writing and conversations with him, and gratefully acknowledge his generous and helpful interest in Proster Theory and my debt to him.

6   Editor's Note: The idea that the cerebral cortex was not wholly in charge of the brain's operation, that there might be a "partner" in the mix, was a significant break with prior thinking (and with the Western world's worldview for some centuries). At the turn of the 21st century, we now know that the partnership is not only among the older and newer parts of the brain but an partnership of the bodybrain and an inseparable one at that.

7   Dr. Candace Pert, then working at the NIMH, did groundbreaking research into the role of chemical messagers produced and received throughout the body and brain, proving learning to be a bodymind partnership. For an extraordinary account of her work in a highly readable autobiography of a neuroscientist, *Molecules of Emotion: Why We Feel the Way We Feel* (New York: Scribner, 1997).

8   At the 1995 Annual Society of Neuroscience Conference, nearly 80 studies were mentioned that suggest such important links of the cerebellum. See Eric Jensen's summary in *Teaching with the Brain in Mind* (Alexandria, Virginia: ASCD, 1998), p. 84. See also *A User's Guide to the Brain: Perception, Attention, and the Four Theaters of the Brain* by John Ratey (New York: Pantheon Books, 2001), especially Chapter 4.

9   As study of the cerebrum continues, the part of the cerebrum that makes us truly human are the frontal lobes, the so-called "executive brain." For a readable and truly fascinating account of this area of the brain, see *The Executive Brain: Frontal Lobes and the Civilized Mind* by Elkhonon Goldberg (New York: Oxford University Press, 2001).

10 Editor's Note: When first published, available brain research supported the statement that, "Virtually all of the learning we are concerned with

informal education **must occur** in this cerebrum." Today's view of the brain supports that "...formal education **involves** this cerebrum." Again, the current view of learning as a bodymind activity expands rather than invalidates our view of how the human brain learns.

11 Editor's Note: Anyone still clinging to the idea that M&Ms, stickers, and other such forms of external rewards and punishments are effective or desirable when working with students for the long haul should read Alfie Kohn: *Punished by Rewards: The Trouble with Gold Stars, Incentive Plans, A's, Praise, and Other Bribes* (New York: Houghton Mifflin, 1993) and *Beyond Discipline: From Compliance to Community* (Alexandria, Virginia: ASCD, 1996).

12 Editor's Note: During the early years of Dr. Diamond's work, critics of her work cautioned that one could not extrapolate findings about the physiological changes in rats brains caused by enriched environments to similar changes in human brains. Sufficient work with human brains has now been done to substantiate her fundamental premises: Enriched environments do produce significant change in the brain: the neuron body increases in size, dendrites grow and further branch, axons further myelinate; such changes increase connections and make communication more reliable, thus resulting in greater intelligence. The converse is also true: a sterile environment results in decreased growth, even shrinking of dendrites. Diamond's maxim, "Use it or lose it," is a scientifically accepted homily for working with the human brain. See Marian Diamond and Janet Hopson, *Magic Trees of the Mind: How to Nurture Your Child's Intelligence, Creativity, and Healthy Emotions from Birth Through Adolescence* (New York: A Dutton Book, 1998). This is a wonderful resource for both teachers and parents—a layman's explanation of the brain by a pioneering brain researcher.

13 For a thorough discussion see Sally P. Springer and George Deutsch, *Left Brain, Right Brain* (San Francisco: W. H. Freeman and Co., 1981). The book can serve as an excellent corrective for many current, oversimplified, speculative, and inaccurate notions. The authors remark: "Our educational system may miss training or developing half of the brain but it probably does so by missing out on the talents of both hemispheres" (p. 192).

14 Dr. Robert D. Nebes of Duke University Medical Center has pointed out: "Many people are now attempting to superimpose upon the anatomical and functional duality of the brain many of the philosophical and spiritual dualisms which have fascinated man over the centuries." See *UCLA Educator* (Graduate School of Education), Spring 1975, p. 16.

15 Editor's Note: For years, it had been assumed that the brain stopped producing neurons at birth or shortly thereafter. However, new discoveries indicate that the hippocampus, where new memories are made, continues to produce new neurons. Also, tantalizing discoveries of the flexibility of building block T-cells suggests that they, under certain conditions, can become neurons. This is currently a hot area of brain research.

16 Editor's Note: For a description of the kinds of input that most stimulate physiological change (learning), see the Kovalik ITI model materials for appropriate to your grade level listed in Appendix C.

17 Editor's Note: Marian Diamond provides an observation about the impact of *boredom* on young and adolescent rats: "A boring environment had a more powerful *thinning* effect on the cortex than an exciting environment had on cortex *thickening.* Young rats are obviously very susceptible to losing mental ground when not challenged, and that shrinkage shows up after just four days. In rodent "teenagers," at least, the shrinkage can begin to be reversed again after four days of enrichment." Given the number of parallels between the affects of enrichment and boredom on the brains of rats and humans that have proven true, this is quite a disturbing observation. Among many things, it should cause us to reexamine the school calendar. It would appear that the traditional agrarian calendar with three months of summer vacation works strongly against those who most depend upon the public schools for learning.

18 Editor's Note: For a powerful, electrifying image of the how dendrites grow in the brain, see ABC News *Prime Time,* "Your Child's Brain" with Diane Sawyer (January 25, 1995).

19 Editor's Note: William Calvin, author of *How Brains Think: Evolving Intelligence, Then and Now,* talks about competing choruses, each

singing its own message or answer and trying to get others neurons to agree. The chorus best able to recruit neighboring neurons into singing its song determines which competing message wins out. An example of this is when we "can't make up our mind." Choice A or B, is it a cheetah or a leopard? (Conversations with William H. Calvin, January, 1997, Covington, Washington.)

20 Diamond and Hopson, p. 26.

21 Pert, p. 139.

22 Ibid, p. 139.

23 Conversations with Dr. Candace Pert, Tukwila, Washington, May, 1998.

24 Editor's Note: An amazing but still mysterious discovery is the presence of cells through the digestive track—from mouth to anus—that are identical to neurons in the brain. Dr. Candace Pert and other scientists wonder aloud if these cells may be the source of our "gut feelings." See *Your Body Is Your Unconscious Mind* by Candace Pert (audiotape) and *The Second Brain: The Scientific Basis for Gut Instinct* by Michael Gershon (New York: HarperCollins, 1998).

25 Pert, pp. 26-27.

26 Pert, p. 38.

27 LeDoux, Joseph. "The Emotional Brain," presentation at Emotional Intelligence, Education, and the Brain: A Symposium, Chicago, IL, December 5, 1997. See also *The Emotional Brain: The Mysterious Underpinnings of Emotional Life* (New York: Simon and Schuster, 1996).
Editor's Note: Given the typical time lag between findings within the brain research community and education, it will likely be some years into the 21st century before reference to the triune brain is abandoned and new ways of talking about, and implementing, the power of emotion in the bodybrain partnership are developed and put into widespread use.

28 Pert, p. 133.

29 Damasio, Antonio. "Thinking about Emotion," presentation at Emotional Intelligence, Education, and the Brain: A Symposium, Chicago, IL, December 5, 1997. See also *Descartes'*

Error: Emotion, Reason, and the Human Brain (New York: G. P. Putnam Sons, 1994).

30 Editor's Note: Robert Sylwester has synthesized a good deal of research into a very useful and memorable phrase: "Emotion drives attention, attention drives learning/memory/problem-solving/just about everything else." Quoted in an unpublished paper entitled "The Role of the Arts in Brain Development and Maintenance." Also see *A Celebration of Neurons: An Educator's Guide to the Human Brain.* (Alexandria, VA: ASCD, 1995), especially Chapter 4.

31 Pert, pp. 141-142. Somasensory refers to any bodily sensations or feelings, whether it is the touch of another's hand on our skin or sensations arising from the movement of our own organs as they carry on our bodily processes.

32 Ibid, p. 33. See also Jane Healy—*Endangered Minds: Why Children Don't Think—and What We Can Do About It* (New York: Touchstone Books, 1990) and *Failure to Connect: How Computers Affect Our Children's Minds—and What We Can Do About It* (New York: Touchstone Books, 1998).

33 Editor's Note: Jeanne Gibbs has synthesized an enormous amount of sociological research into simple ingredients for a sense of community: inclusion, influence (others care about what I say), and affection. See *Tribes: A New Way of Learning Together* (Santa Rosa: California: Center Source Publications, 1994).

6

BAD FIT:
THE BRAIN IN A
TRADITIONAL CLASSROOM

> It is the plasticity of the brain which enables learning and memory to occur and which impresses upon each individual a set of unique and characteristic behaviors, thoughts, and emotions . . . allowing essentially the same brain which once served the cavemen to enable today's men to operate in the vastly more complex environment that they have themselves created.
>
> —Steve Rose[1]

The human bodybrain learning system represents such an incredible achievement of nature that we can best build comprehension of it, I think, by approaching it from many directions, trying to grasp some of its main features, rather than trying to examine it segment by segment under some neat scheme. This chapter examines some main features of the brain important to educators.

PUTTING THE BRAIN IN PERSPECTIVE

Imagine yourself a villager from a remote mountainous region of central Asia. Abruptly, you are transported and set down in the heart of New York City. You have never seen a city or even a paved street, nor automobiles, stores, electric lights, elevators, telephones, electronic devices, railway stations, libraries, business offices, hospitals . . . nothing like this crowded, fevered activity. The 100-story building is hard to comprehend. Automobiles that are moved by motors which burn a liquid like water and can carry you a mile a minute on thousands of miles of paved highways seem nonsensical. Pictures seen on a television screen are actually of events taking place in another country and the voice heard originates not in the box but far away. Such strange and often alarming miracles.

An introduction to the brain as currently understood, after much brilliant scientific investigation, may seem equally fantastic, overwhelming, and difficult to believe. Most of us have almost no notion of how the brain works. When we do find out, the answers may strike us as so unexpected and different from all we ever heard before that it strains our belief.

It may help, though, if we look on the human brain as nature's most fantastic product, one that took at the very least a half-billion years to create. A remarkable amount is known now about its evolution; the patient tracing of its development, I believe, greatly helps understanding (and believing) its present shape and functions.[2] In the same way, understanding something about early humans, how they lived and what they needed to survive, can be extremely helpful as well.[3]

In a modern industrial society, we take for granted living in a highly structured way. If employed, we typically go to a fixed place of work, on scheduled days, for certain prearranged hours. Our home is probably a permanent address for years. Of necessity, ordinary, routine life requires complying with a great many rules and regulations, from staggeringly complex income tax laws to requirements on how and when to put out the garbage for collection. Lawyers, accountants, surveyors, insurance adjusters, and a host of other specialists pore over fine print to decide fine points that may greatly affect our welfare. All of this may be bothersome, and at times exasperate us beyond easy tolerance, but we are used to such demands as a part of living in communities.

Thus, it takes considerable imagination to move back in time, to conditions 15,000, or 30,000, or more years ago. Our forebears lived under sharply different conditions. They existed by gathering and hunting—and in the colder, more difficult climates by gathering and hunting just about anything that might help sustain life. In general, humans developed as nonspecialists (in contrast to most animals), able to find and willing to eat almost anything nourishing and able to survive a great range of climactic conditions in a wide assortment of physical environments.

A Historical Perspective

Study of early humans suggests strongly that in most areas they long lived in bands of around 50 members that had no fixed abode and that moved around as necessary to find food, water, shelter, and materials. (Not until roughly 10,000 years ago did humans settle down and form cities.) We can see why early humans became better able to survive as they developed bigger, more subtle, more flexible brains, capable of an unprecedented amount of learning. We became "brain freaks" because having a certain type of brain, of enormous capacity, meant continuing to live and breed where less brain, or a different shape of brain, could not cope with the struggle.

How long have humans been on earth? New discoveries keep changing the picture but some rough approximations can be advanced. It seems probable now that our evolutionary line branched off from that of apes perhaps six million years ago. Recent findings suggest that creatures that walked fully upright existed about four million years ago (even their well-preserved footprints have been found!)[4] It seems clear that quite a variety of human or hominid species evolved, finding footholds for a while in many parts of the globe. All humans have died out save *Homo sapiens,* which is to say modern humankind, which is to say us.

Our immediate ancestors, often called Cro-Magnon (and best identified as the creators of the magnificent cave paintings in France, Spain, and elsewhere) seem to have arrived relatively suddenly in Europe, probably having come from Africa and the east, although origins are mysterious. These people almost certainly existed a minimum of 50,000 years ago and in all likelihood much longer ago than that.

Neanderthal man, often identified with the brutish cave men of popular legend, apparently coexisted with Cro-Magnons, and we must assume, lost out in a competitive struggle for living space. They were far from being the hunched-over, ape-like creatures they were portrayed to be in the last century—some anthropologists believe that a normally dressed and groomed Neanderthal, alive among us today, would attract no particular notice. Their brain, it is startling to learn, was if anything larger than ours on average—but with a difference. The Neanderthal skull lacked the high, bulging forehead that we typically exhibit. The front of the head was lower and flatter; relatively more of the brain space was further back.[5] This difference may well have been critical as we shall see when we look more closely at the prefrontal lobes of our brain, the portion immediately behind the forehead. It is the part of the brain that handles more intricate and longer-term planning.

The Appearance of the Frontal Lobes. Of vital interest to teachers (and parents) is the fact that this part of the brain does not fully mature until at least the late teen years—for practical purposes, we can say, until adulthood is achieved.

Consider the mental demands of hunting, an activity that appears to have had a powerful influence on our history as a species. There is a huge gap between merely happening upon an animal and killing it for meat and skin versus hunting in the full sense of a planned, organized, directed, and mutual activity involving many individuals and using well-developed weapons, equipment, tactics, communications, and so forth. Only an impressively large and sophisticated brain can conceive and carry out so elaborate an enterprise, or build a fishweir to trap that prey, or go through all the steps of finding suitable stone and fashioning it into exquisitely worked tools.

The ability *to make plans and carry them out is the key aspect of human intelligence*—a truth that becomes strikingly evident when we look at our history as humans. Yet, in conventional schools, instructors complying with usual practice commonly do the planning themselves (or follow that laid down by authorities) while the students, told what to do at every turn, get little chance to use their brains in this basic, human way.

If we look at these ancestors during their long gathering-hunting period, we also observe—with perhaps more than a little shock—

that they had virtually no need or use for what we now commonly term logic, meaning a step-by-step, linear, sequential way of thinking. The concept of logic did not appear for tens of thousands of years. These people slowly but steadily made progress in many areas, developing, for example, clothing, tools, weapons, utensils, housing of various sorts, dance, music, painting, sculpture, ever richer language, religion, social customs, mining, uses of fire and the great invention of cooking, and far more. It can be a shock to realize that in none of these huge areas of achievement—the broad foundations of society, culture, and technology—did they employ or need what today many people commonly tend to esteem as the best, most respectable, most admirable, type of thinking: Greek-type intellectualizing and sequential logic.

Mistaken Notions of the Brain As a Logical Device. We use the term "logical" very loosely in ordinary speech and writing. Logical thinking can mean sensible, or unemotional, or correct, or resultful mental effort, and one can be complimented on a logical presentation, for instance, when more precisely it has been simply thorough or orderly.

Here I am using the term with a specific meaning: The kind of logic in which there is a deliberate progression from fact or observation or statement A to B and then to C, D, E or more, all connected by "therefore" or "it follows that. . . ." This was the broad method we associate—a bit too simply—with the philosophers of the Golden Age of Greece and others who for centuries in Western culture held to related approaches. We find similar chains of reasoning in the more familiar areas of mathematics. And we usually use at least the appearance of such reasoning when reporting findings or studies to others. The businessman who has reached a conclusion after mulling over a complex matter does not tell his board that he woke up one morning feeling convinced that a proposed plant should be delayed. Rather he presents logical arguments to support that position. The scientist who stumbles on a solution to a knotty problem several times before finally realizing that he has something of value typically isn't eager to detail his thinking process, reluctant to admit what now seems his stupidity in not grasping the implications sooner. Consequently, he writes a formal paper, in the standard format, presenting his findings logically.

There seems nothing wrong with this procedure. It serves usually as a convenience to all. But *we are misled if we assume that the decision or discovery was actually **arrived** at logically.*

BREAKING THROUGH TRADITIONAL BELIEFS ABOUT SEQUENTIAL LOGIC

On the other hand, the rise of modern science after 1500 (to use a loose, general date) depended heavily on *breaking away* from this sequential logic. For example, it was long held that God had personally set the planets in their paths; that what God does must be perfect; that the circle is the perfect form; that the planets must then move in circular orbits. For centuries astronomers strongly influenced by this logical word chain failed to make sense of their observations. When finally Kepler saw that undeniably planets move in ellipses, he was dumfounded and horrified, fearful of how authorities might view his discovery. Even Newton, often thought of as the embodiment of logic and mathematical thought, saw the whole universe as a riddle set by the creator. Keynes writes: "By pure thought, by concentration of mind, the riddle . . . would be revealed to the initiate."[6]

In essence, people believed that the way to escape magic and alchemy was through logical, sequential analysis. Today, given current brain research, it is clear that yesterday's solution has become today's problem. Just as early scientists struggled to free themselves of medieval magic and alchemy traditions as they moved toward natural philosophy or science, scientists today struggle to escape the traditional reverence of sequential logic.

Even if "pure thought" of this kind were the highest human achievement (a proposition I, for one, would deplore), plainly it is quite a recent activity — developed within the last 2,500 years. And we need only look around us to see how little a part it plays in literature, arts, politics, economics, science and technology, or our daily life today. It played no part in the lives of our direct ancestors of 10,000, 20,000, 30,000, and more years ago — this kind of logic had not yet been invented.

In mathematics, for example, we need precision and ability to deal with complex problems. They did not exist in gathering-hunting societies, where (we can feel fairly sure from ancient evidence and the study of now-vanishing primitive, essentially Stone Age peoples) they counted only to four or five, then went to a few, many, a lot, a great many, or some similar progression. They owned no land, conducted no business, used no money, had neither lawyers nor engineers, and handled decisions by recourse to traditional ways, permeated by elaborate magic.

How the Old Brain Worked (Still Works)

These ancestors had, to the best of our knowledge, brains virtually identical to those in our heads today. They had taken their shape over millions of years and had reached their present level of development long before "civilization" and the rise of kings and increasingly intricate trade, record keeping, laws, and interfaces.[7] The implications of this must be seen as staggering for anyone engaged in instruction: *The brain we are dealing with — the brain in the heads of students now sitting before teachers — was not "designed" by evolutionary needs for logic, manipulation of symbols, for dealing with tight, sequential structures or word systems, which today constitute the main concern of conventional schooling.* While the flexibility of the brain is so great that it can usually, under duress, and given time, accommodate such matters, they go against the grain — they are *superimposed, not natural.*

In *The Universe Within,* Morton Hunt observes:

> For many centuries, philosophers and others who have studied the human mind have believed that reasoning takes place according to the laws governing logic. Or rather, that it should, but regrettably often fails to do so. . . . Such is the tradition that runs unbroken from Aristotle to Piaget. But the findings of cognitive science run counter to it: logical reasoning is not our usual — or natural — practice, and the technically invalid kinds of reasoning we generally employ work rather well in most of everyday situations in which one might suppose rigorous deductive thinking was essential.[8]

Among those who study the human brain and its workings, this view is hardly likely to cause surprise or disagreement. However, recognition of the artificiality and limitations of logic, so long enthroned, has still not come to general public awareness. The idea can prove upsetting to those who have never had occasion to question or examine a very old and broad tradition.[9] Few people today want to deny the brilliance and energetic "thinking" of Aristotle but we know today that a great many of his conclusions were dead wrong or way off the track. Some of his high-powered, glorified intellectualizing kept whole populations misled and befuddled for a thousand years![10] We still have those (even in education *reform*) who would wrap themselves in the togas of the Great Thinkers and preach the need to teach children "thinking skills," "problem solving," and wise use of "the mind," all the while cherishing a long-erroneous concept of a "logical" brain and ignoring how the real brain in our skull functions.

We may also, in passing, take note of the huge, costly effort over many recent years, involving hundreds of brilliant people dedicated to making digital computers into "Artificial Intelligence" (AI) devices, truly powerful, tireless thinking machines. Alas, overall the effort has floundered badly, as psychologist Howard Gardner has reported well and at length. It is now plain that the real brain and the AI machines differ almost totally—they go off in different directions. (The new, still crude "connectionist" machines, are far more like the real brain.)[11]

WORKING <u>WITH</u> THE BRAIN

Instruction that recognizes and is compatible with the *natural* (precivilization) brain functions will proceed much more quickly and be vastly more successful—much as it is easier to go with the current of a swift river than against it.

For example, the human brain typically does a poor job of routine mathematics. Even the astronomical and navigational tables of premachine days were full of errors. We are delighted to turn such chores over to "stupid" computers that can do them a million times as fast, with very high accuracy. As scientists, engineers, and inventors rid themselves of this symbol-pushing burden, it becomes all the more apparent that major advances in these fields come almost entirely from accidental discoveries, "blunders" that produced unplanned experiments or observations, transfers of ideas and techniques from one field to another, pure serendipity, chance conversations or shared knowledge, fortuitous incidents and above all, intuition. Creative people frequently report waking up in the night with the solution to a problem suddenly "delivered" by the brain or having ideas and solutions "pop into their head" while doing chores or relaxing. "Sleep on it" can be valuable advice: The morning often produces insights or decisions based on nonlogical, nonconscious brain activity.

The brain of our *Homo sapiens* ancestors 50,000 years ago worked well enough to allow humans to survive and become dominant in all habitable parts of the globe. To expect this successful, established brain to change its natural ways of working to conform to schools—a very recent invention—or to readily accept demands that it work logically seems to me obviously absurd. We have all been brainwashed by the undeserved respect given to Greek-type sequential logic. Almost automatically, curriculum builders and teachers try to devise logical methods of instruction, assuming that logical planning, ordering, and presentation of the content matter or skills is the obviously correct and only respectable approach to take. They may have trouble conceiving alternative approaches that do not go step-by-step down a linear progression. Not surprisingly, little research on these alternatives has been encouraged by the establishment, although individual teachers often explore as much as they feel free to do.

A Truism

It can be stated flatly, however, that the human brain is not organized or designed for linear, one-path thought. Most electronic computers do work linearly, one step leading to the next (although most recent, sophisticated types may not remain quite so limited). *But the brain operates by simultaneously going down many paths.* We identify an object, for example, by gathering information—often in less than a second—on size, color, shape, surface texture, weight, smell, movement, any sound it may make, where it is found, what else is with it, any symbolic information with it (such as label or price sign), how other people are responding to it, and so on. All of these investigations by the brain to answer the question "What is this?" go forward along many different and branching paths, among the brain's trillions of connections, *all at the same time.* From the vast knowledge stored, answers or tentative answers get pulled out, then assembled, compared, and interpreted by, if possible, extracting a pattern.[12] The whole miraculous "parallel processing" procedure bears no relationship to linear processing; it helps explain the incredible subtlety and sensitivity of the brain—and why, in recognition, a six-year-old child can with ease outperform the costliest electronic computer devised by a small army of able engineers.

To demand that this brain meekly put aside its mighty resources and go step-by-step down one path is to cripple and inhibit it. We can all too readily see that fundamental error *built into curriculum almost anywhere we look in any classroom where teaching goes on conventionally, uninformed and unguided by knowledge of the brain's real nature.* Experienced teachers agree that the more different approaches they use, the better the learning is apt to be, yet most yield to pressures for single-path, sequential logic.

A Truism Applied

Once we begin to look critically at this notion of teaching in logical sequence, we can see that usually a further giant—and utterly wrong—assumption has been made: that if a subject is fragmented into little bits, and the student is then presented with the bits in some order that seems logical to somebody, the student will be quite able to assemble the parts and emerge with the whole—even though never given an inkling of the whole! Teachers may or may not have some grasp of the whole; certainly there are many who in mathematics or science simply present the parts by following a text or manual. But even if they do possess the large concept, the synthesis they demand of the student may be extremely difficult. We would hardly expect that if we show a young person all the parts of a television, he or she would then be able to assemble the receiver much less grasp how the interrelated, interdependent components work as a system.

One Person's Logic Is Another's Puzzlement. The logic that seemed apparent to the curriculum builder, textbook writer, or teacher may be invisible and incomprehensible to the student. The parameters, the structure, are missing. Consider an ordinary jigsaw puzzle, with a picture of the completed assembly on the box and rectangular edges that provide helpful clues. Most children soon become quite adept at such puzzles. But now substitute a "blind" puzzle, one with no picture and an irregular outer shape. The child has a far harder time—as do most adults. The diagramless type of crossword puzzle provides a similar example. The author knows what the diagram is, but the solver flounders. The brain has a hard time extracting patterns, or making sense, of the effort.

This kind of difficulty, there is much reason to believe, underlies our greatest educational embarrassment, the reading problem. Conventionally students are given a mass of parts, in the form of rules, phonics, and a long list of subskills. Students who have learned to read before school or who have at least grasped what reading is *for* may be able to survive this kind of instruction but the majority become confused and distracted, make little sense of what is going on, and may never in their lifetimes become able to read with ease, confidence, or enjoyment.[13]

The instruction of older, advanced, and sophisticated learners can be "logically" organized with less harm. A group of process chemists, for example, can be taught the functions of a new catalyst this way because they already have an established, broad understanding to which the new material can be related. (Such previous knowledge allows them to "make sense" of the logic within the presentation; however, it would still be hasty to conclude that the logical presentation will necessarily work best to produce the desired learning.)

Most Learning Is Via Random Input. If we look around us at how most learning occurs, we quickly see that it is not by logical sequence or blind assembly. Watch Little Leaguers play baseball, and you can marvel at their skill and grasp of an intricate game, and related knowledge, picked up over years in *random* fashion, mostly by participation as opportunity offered. If the game were to be taught logically, there would be a unit on its origins and history, on terminology, on the playing-field geometry, on hitting, on fielding, on baserunning, and so on down a long list. Obviously, none of the players learned this way. They "picked up" the game by exposure over many years, in an utterly random, unplanned way—perhaps with no formal teaching at all. If they do get coaching, it will likely be on a purely individual basis as needed. For example, after an infielder misses a stop, the coach shows the player how to handle that situation or the coach may work with the catcher to explain how to throw off the mask to catch a high pop foul.

Or, compare how we learn to drive cars, an activity that demands life-and-death expertise. Most of us, from early childhood on, begin learning about steering, braking, obeying traffic signals, parking, and servicing the vehicles, both in the family car and through toys. Even if we take driving instruction, we bring to it a great deal of accumulated knowledge of hazards, types of roads, normal driver behaviors, and much more. We acquire our ability to use and manage cars in a dominantly *random* fashion. Clearly, *the great majority of the major abilities we have acquired came about in just this manner.*

Examples of Misfit

After presenting these ideas to a school's faculty, a teacher asked me whether I would care to be operated on by a surgeon who had had this random kind of training. I pointed out to her that there was no other kind: Surgeons get their real preparation as interns and residents dealing with a variety of cases as they happen to enter the hospital!

This incident suggests how blinded we can be by unexamined conventions. Almost anywhere we look in formal schooling and instruction, we see teachers using plans and curricula that have won approval for being logical and well ordered. Furthermore, they must often submit daily or weekly lesson plans. While many instructors struggle to follow these guides (some resolutely ignoring outcomes that suggest how wrong such guides are), it is scarcely hard to find many others who cheerfully depart from or ignore the plans as soon as the ink is dry. But plans are respectable and mandatory.

Learning Machines and Programmed Learning. The "teaching machine" and programmed learning (and other "teacher-proof" materials that attempt to substitute logical presentation of input for human interaction and real world environments) vividly demonstrate how far off the mark logical presentation can be, even when (or perhaps especially when) the most basic tenets of behavioral psychology are applied. Essentially, the teaching machine is any of many devices that present the material, broken down into small bits, in some logical, sequential manner, providing immediate right-answer/wrong-answer feedback and perhaps some kind of quick "reward." For a period of years, especially during the sixties, millions of dollars were poured into this so-called programmed instruction. (The word programmed should not be confused with similar terms I will shortly be using in another connection.) These teaching machines were hailed as the perfect application of behaviorist psychology and bound to bring striking results.

But the actual outcome was a fiasco. There was little gain in learning effectiveness but much increase in student boredom. Even more devastating was the painful discovery that it seemed to make little difference whether one sequence of presentation was used rather than another, or whether rewards were given, or whether the machines were used in schools (where they might be resented as a threat to teachers' employment) or in commercial applications. The big companies that had hurried to cash in on this bonanza soon hurried to get out and end their large losses; the teaching machine virtually disappeared from sight and thought, leaving behaviorist tenets and notions badly mangled.

Computers. The sharp drop in the cost of small computers over time has encouraged many schools to put in more, although effective use of computers is often elusive. What computers can do, of course, depends on the programs or software available, just as the usefulness of a book depends on its contents. In early years, the software seemed to be an effort to revive the teaching-machine approach in new guise, flying the magic banner "technology!" It is hard to see how small computers fit the natural brain's needs, since they are sequential to an extreme and force the user down a few, fixed paths, one at a time, step by step, and provide but limited sensory input—far from the brain's natural use of parallel processing and "intuitive leaps." One can guess that they are popular with students, at least for a while, because they are interesting machines, under individual control, and thus are an escape from "pay attention to teacher."

While computers clearly have legitimate uses, by no means can we automatically hail them as inherently "brain-compatible." Just as it is handy for students to become familiar with operating a car, office copier, video cassette recorder and other machines now part of daily life and work, so it also seems desirable for students to know how to use electronic keyboards. But we should strongly guard against their superficial use and any mystique arising from "computer literacy" or "technology" as ends in themselves. How computers are used and for what purposes determine how well they will enhance learning.

Curriculum and Lesson Design. Many adults engaged in planning or carrying on instruction operate from a conviction that certain learning must occur before other learning. It seems apparent, for example, that numbers must be learned before any mathematics can be tackled. When carefully studied, however, truly mandatory sequences become hard to find.[14] Even this example of learning numbers before mathematics isn't so. Using modular blocks or counters (bottle caps will serve nicely) and without numbers, children beginning mathematics can acquire some major, fundamental concepts such as *square, equation, reversibility, and conservation* without numbers. Yet routine teaching may fail to give them such concepts in nine years of elementary school study. In fact, if the numbers are learned in rote fashion as the names of symbols not clearly understood, the numbers can easily get in the way of the more basic concepts!

In reading, many children learn a number of words before they master the alphabet; such words, especially their own names, are an excellent way to begin mastery of their letters. Since words in print are neatly spaced apart, unlike spoken language where the pause within a word may be greater than between words, grasping the convention of evenly spaced words may be one of the earliest needs for a sound start in reading.

A NEW VIEW OF LEARNING

Since the brain is indisputably a multipath, multimodal apparatus, the notion of mandatory sequences, or even of *any* fixed sequences, is unsupportable. Each of us learns in a personal, highly individual, mainly random way, always adding to, sorting out, and revising all the input—from teachers or elsewhere—that we have had up to that point. That being the case, *any group instruction that has been tightly, logically planned is wrongly planned for most of the group and will inevitably inhibit, prevent, or distort learning.*

Let me hasten to say that this does not imply that instruction should be haphazard and uncontrolled, or that the students should do the planning—which would likely be worse than that of the school's. Rather it suggests that instructional planning should:

- Have broad clearly-defined objectives accompanied by specific descriptions of expected learning *achievements* (as distinguished by descriptions of the lessons or units to be taught);

- Be for long periods of time rather than a few hours, days, or weeks

- Not try to move large groups of students along in lockstep but instead be highly flexible and *designed to accept individual progress over a wide range.*

Perhaps there is no idea about human learning harder to accept for people familiar with classroom schools than this: That the ideal of neat, orderly, closely planned, sequentially logical teaching will in practice, with young students, *guarantee severe learning failure for most.*[15]

Having been led to believe, as they believe day will follow night, that students should learn from logical, sequential presentation, teachers in conventional classrooms commonly present lessons logically and sequentially. Not surprisingly, they find that extremely little learning occurs, as revealed by recitation, tests, or homework. Yet teachers cling to such an approach, often feeling inadequate, guilty, and deeply discouraged, suffering what has been fashionable to call "burnout."

For most teachers, school, from early childhood, has meant above all an institutional building composed of classrooms in which active, aggressive teaching goes on. It is a specialized place to teach just as a tennis court is a specialized place to play tennis. Many teachers feel that they have been hired *to teach,* that they must control all that goes on in the room, that it is almost wicked and reprehensible not to "drive" the class, and that their status with coworkers will rest mainly on their aggressive teaching and management efforts. Not to *teach* in a school is seen, or felt, as a breach of behavior, something like going to church in a bathing suit or eating popcorn at a symphony concert. School does not signify a place where continual study goes forward on how best to educate children for the world they are in. Rather it is a building dedicated to certain old, little-changing activities. One enters the building as an employee to perpetuate these rituals; otherwise, one goes elsewhere. As Katz has said,

> Education has not suffered from any freedom granted teachers to run school as they see fit; it has suffered from the suffocating atmosphere in which teachers have to work.[16]

Slavin maintains:

> The problem is not with teachers, who I find to be overwhelmingly dedicated and hard-working but with the

classroom system they are trained to use that guarantees failure for so many.[17]

A disconnection, indeed a head-on contradiction, exists between the aggressive behavior forced on teachers and what they have observed about learning. They know that students in today's information-rich world learn a great deal, though not necessarily what fits the official curriculum, and that both youngsters and adults "pick up" learning in quite random, happenstance fashion from all sorts of exposure. Such useful competencies as money management, cooking, home maintenance and repair, games and sports, crafts and hobbies, health care, and social skills are plainly acquired this way rather than through course work. Even where courses are taken (Chinese cooking, home electrical wiring, bridge), they often have defined limits and can account for only a fraction of all that is learned. Again and again, teachers find that their students know something because of a family trip, the mother's political activities, the father's occupation, or from television or reading, or some chance event.

Administrators, too, know how ineffective logical instruction can be. Yet even those who would like to make change may dread the task of challenging the logic myth, either with their public or with their teachers. They, too, are caught in the system's trap. Few have had the experience of bringing about anything more than marginal student-learning gains, except where exceptional failure has been rectified to usual failure—and even that is rare. But as public pressures for learning increase, the logic myth will become intolerable.

The conventional, outworn system supports the logic myth and the myth supports the system. The brain approach offers at least the hope of cutting this Gordian knot by changing the question from "How should schools be run?" to "What does the bodybrain require for best learning to occur?"

NEW TRUTHS ABOUT LEARNING

To summarize:

1. The information substances of the bodybrain took shape tens of thousands of years before Greek-type, sequential logic was invented. *No part of the brain is naturally logical.*

2. While a logical arrangement or presentation may serve the needs of transfer of information between people with good knowledge of the material, it consistently produces very poor learning results with students not already familiar with the material. Prior to learning something, students cannot perceive the logic that may seem apparent to the instructor or once the learning has occurred.

3. Since we learn individually in different, multipath sequences—with previous *individual* experience as the foundation to which more learning is added—logical group instruction inevitably produces a large degree of failure.

4. Examination of the *useful* learning we have acquired as adults shows that the great bulk has been acquired at random, from random experience.

5. The tremendous acceleration of learning and human capabilities attributable to science resulted from breaking away from old-style logic, especially world theories. Most scientific and technical discovery has occurred fortuitously, in the course of persistent effort and high input.

6. We can point to little in our world that has been accomplished by old-style, sequential logic, especially *word* logic.

7. Our view of logic as respectable, high achievement rests on a surviving tradition that has been little examined.

8. Sequential logic plays a large part in the building of curriculum. Furthermore, the conventional classroom school system has become a specialized place for this kind of aggressive teaching. Alternatives are seldom considered as both teachers and administrators are caught in the trap. Considering the learning requirements of the bodybrain may suggest new and fruitful paths.

NOTES

1 Steve Rose, *The Conscious Brain* (New York: Alfred A. Knopf, 1973), p. 173.

2 For a brief, fairly technical discussion, see C. U. M. Smith, *The Brain* (New York: G. P. Putnam, 1970), Chapter 10. This excellent book by an English neuroscientist is a standard work. It gives a very complete overview of knowledge of the brain.

Editor's Note: For a recent source, see *How Brains Think: Evolving Intelligence, Then and Now* by William H. Calvin (New York: Basic Books, 1996).

3 See John E. Pfeiffer, *The Emergence of Man* (New York: Harper & Row, 1969) for an outstanding, readable, and broad-ranging discussion. The same author's *The Emergence of Society* (New York: McGraw-Hill, 1977) deals with prehistory in remarkable detail.

4 See *Science News*, March 31, 1979, p. 196, for pictures of the "Leakey footprints" found in northern Tanzania.

5 For a comparison of brain sizes, see Richard E. Leakey and Roger Lewin, *Origins* (New York: E. P. Dutton, 1977) pp. 198-199 and accompanying text.

6 See Hugh Kearney, *Science and Change 1500-1700* (New York: McGraw-Hill, 1971). John Maynard Keynes, the economist and student of Newton, is quoted on p. 190.

7 "There is no sign of further brain development . . . if changes have occurred they have been very small." Steven Rose, *The Conscious Brain* (New York: Knopf, 1973), pp. 139-140. See also *How the Mind Works* by Steven Pinker (New York: W. W. Norton & Co., 1997).

8 Morton Hunt, *The Universe Within* (New York: Simon and Schuster, 1982), p. 121.

9 Editor's Note: One of the most disturbing and challenging issues confronting educators today is the logical, sequential layout of traditional curriculum, with its tidy progression of logically sequenced bits of content, and mythical spiral from year to year.

10 Editor's Note: Richard Bergland in, *The Fabric of Mind*, refers to just long-standing mental mistakes as "mismemes." Like physical genes,

they are passed from generation to generation. The field of education is rife with mismemes. (Australia: Penguin Books, 1988.)

11 See William H. Calvin, *How Brains Think: Evolving Intelligence, Then and Now* (New York: Basic Books, 1997), Chapter 8.

12 "The initial stages of processing are largely parallel rather than serial, and feature analysis results from patterns matching rather than from feature detection." See Karl H. Pribram, in *Cognition and Brain Theory,* Spring 1981, p. 110.

13 The listing of reading subskills that appeared in the 1970s exploded into the hundreds; one large city school system reportedly identified over 800 subskills, until the teachers rebelled! A list of 250-300 is typical.

14 Recent discoveries about how young children learn mathematics have uncovered some startling facts. For instance, young children can add before they can count, even before they develop the capacity for speech. See "A Head for Numbers" by Robert Kunzig, *Discover,* July, 1997, pp. 108-117.

15 According to Benjamin S. Bloom, "Group instruction, as presently used in most countries of the world, may approach optimal qualities of instruction for only a small proportion of students in a given class. Even when this is the case, it is likely that the majority of students in the class are paying a heavy price for the ways in which the different qualities of instruction serve the special needs of a few members of the class." *Human Characteristics and School Learning* (New York: McGraw-Hill, 1976), p. 136. Bloom echoes a complaint common ever since there were classrooms, but perhaps too seldom made today.

16 Michael B. Katz, *Class, Bureaucracy, and Schools* (New York: Praeger, 1971), p. 131.

17 Robert Slavin, in *Character,* March 1981, p. 12. Dr. Slavin, a professor at Johns Hopkins University, is widely known as a leader in cooperative learning approaches which permit students to aid one another, rather than always compete. See also *Renewing America's Schools: A Guide for School-Based Action* by Carl D. Glickman (San Francisco: Jossey-Bass Publishers, 1993), pp. 95-96.

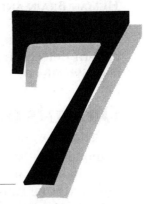

FIRST FUNDAMENTAL OF LEARNING: THE DETECTION OF PATTERNS

> Pattern-matching is inherently pleasing because that is what our minds are designed (or programmed) for . . . Quite apart from anything the teacher does. . .the student, being human, is a pattern-finder and a pattern-maker. Possibly the greatest obstacle to our making use of this not very startling principle is our ingrained notion that education is the acquisition and mastery of new material. What we "teach" and they do not "learn" is the "material."
>
> —David B. Bronson[1]

Let me suggest that there is no concept, no fact in education, more directly important than this: The brain is, by nature's design, an amazingly subtle and sensitive pattern-detecting apparatus.

The brain detects, constructs, and elaborates patterns as a basic, built-in, natural function. It does not have to be taught or motivated to do so, any more than the heart needs to be instructed or coaxed to pump blood. In fact, efforts to teach or motivate the pattern detection, however well meant, may have inhibiting and negative effects.

ORIGINS OF THE FIRST FUNDAMENTAL[2]

This key aspect of learning—patterns, and the related concept of modeling—has scarcely penetrated education at all, as a glance at the index of almost any major work on learning will show. Yet it can hardly be called a new idea in psychological, ethological, or behavioral contexts.

Sixty Years of Research

Over 60 years ago, for example, Aldous Huxley remarked:

> What emerges most strikingly from recent scientific developments is that perception is not a passive reception of material from the outside world; it is an active process of selection and imposing of patterns.[3]

The findings Huxley referred to were well known in fields more scientifically oriented than education then and that are thoroughly established now. Brain researchers of the 1990s accept this as a given.[4] We do not have to look far for confirmation—our own daily experience tells us most convincingly that the brain has this ability and has it to an astounding degree.

Examples from Personal Experience

Imagine that you are attending a sporting event. People by the thousands stream by as you find your seats. The merest glance tells you they are all strangers. But now you see two figures that immediately seem familiar and in a moment you have identified them as former neighbors, Francine and Peter. Somehow, your brain has picked them out of this vast crowd; somehow it has separated them from all the other people you know so that you can identify them and greet them warmly by name. There is no question that our human brain can do this—usually effortlessly. (If we simply look at what we all can do, we begin to glimpse the enormous powers of the brain.)

The feat is even more impressive because you haven't seen these friends for three years, didn't expect to run into them here.

Both are wearing clothes you have never seen them in. Francine has a new hairstyle, Peter wears sunglasses that partly hide his features. Yet, you recognized them as familiar while they were still 50 feet away.

Clearly, the recognition does not stem from any logical process. You did not check Francine's height in inches or Peter's weight in kilos. You put no measure to their middle finger bones, Bertillon fashion,[5] nor did you use a color-comparison guide to determine the shade of skin and hair. While Peter has a distinctive walking movement and Francine an animated manner, trying to measure or describe these exactly would be an impossible task. Let us grasp firmly the clear fact that your brain does not work that way but that it did quickly and accurately accomplish recognition and identification by some other means.

Nor was this an isolated, unusual phenomenon. If I were to display a teakettle, a paint brush, a handsaw, a necklace, a bunch of carrots, a pencil sharpener, a violin, a telephone, a sweater, a microscope, a toothbrush, a slice of Swiss cheese . . . you would recognize and name each in the same effortless way. You were plainly not born knowing these objects, so this recognition has been learned at some time between birth and the present.

We are so used to looking at something and immediately knowing what it is that we come to think of the process as automatic. Comparisons of eye and camera may also mislead us. A camera can't recognize anything; our brain can, using not only vision but also hearing, smell, touch, and other aspects of our senses.

When we are exposed to something quite unfamiliar, we simply do not see it in any meaningful way. To look inside some complex machine, for example, we may see only a confusion of forms. In a museum, observing some fossilized remains of various ancient animals, we may see only vague shapes, in contrast to what the curator sees. I often dramatize this in workshops by showing a newspaper in Arabic or Chinese. The participants see only squiggles that a moment later they are hopelessly unable to reproduce—although a person knowing the language would see headlines and news, information at a glance.

If we place a teakettle before a month-old infant, the baby will regard it with momentary interest but plainly have no notion of what it is. As adults we can see a vessel, a handle, and a spout; the baby can see none of this arrangement, only edges, shapes, and surfaces.

Even if the teakettle were made of unfamiliar materials or shaped like an elephant, we would recognize it as a teakettle. Any familiar item, from a paint brush to a necklace,would be identifiable. Moderate differences do not bother us a bit.

Examples from Classroom Life

Consider, for instance, the 20 different forms of the letter *a* that appear in Figure 5. Despite the range of shapes they cover, we have no difficulty seeing any one as *a*. We could, of course, carry this recognition much further, to letters of many larger sizes, in different colors, formed of lights or dots, put into three-dimensional materials, tilted, laid on the floor, or seen on the side of a moving vehicle. Even holding just to typefaces available for printing, there are literally thousands of alphabets; handwritten, drawn, or printed forms add thousands more. There is no *letter a*, only a pattern we conventionally call "a."

In the same sense, teakettle, paintbrush, carrots, violin, and the rest are patterns. Our knowledge of the pattern is what enables us to say what object is what. But we are by no means

Figure 7.

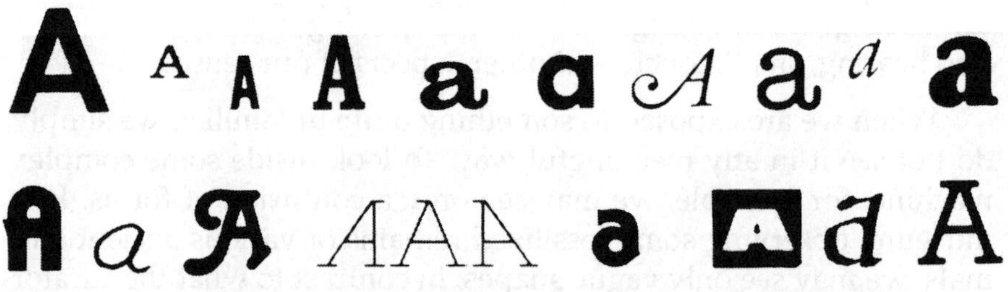

limited to hard, visual patterns. We can detect and learn patterns far more subtle or complex. In time, adults normally become quite familiar with such patterns as cat, city park, affection, boss, fraction, racial bigotry, jealousy, or adventurousness.

Just how the brain detects and recognizes patterns cannot be easily or quickly explained. Yet, it is an astoundingly powerful, subtle, living computer with billions of neurons at its command.

We do know in a general way that *the brain detects characteristics or features and also relationships among these features.*

The lower-case letter *a*, for example, may consist of a hook facing left which may take a variety of forms,

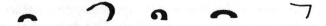

connected to a more or less round enclosure form.

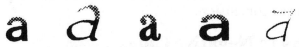

The relationship between these shapes has a key role. If the hook were 20 centimeters tall and the enclosure only a millimeter high, one might have much difficulty seeing it as an *a*. On the other hand, there is a different pattern for small *a* that lacks the hook altogether, one that we can

$$a \quad \mathbf{a} \quad \mathbf{\alpha} \quad \mathbf{\sigma}$$

readily learn to accept as an alternate. It is illogical to have two forms but, as we have seen, logic is the least of the human brain's concerns.

KEY FACTORS IN PATTERN-SEEKING

When looking at the brain as a seeker of patterns, consider five key factors: Use of clues and cues, use of multiple sensory input and prior experience, sensitivity to negative clues, categorizing down through patterns within patterns, and using probability.

Use of Clues and Cues

Our brain's ability to detect and identify patterns is impressive for its flexibility. We can be certain about our identification of something without needing to perceive most or even many of its features and relationships. With experience, in fact, we normally become extremely expert in using *clues* (sometimes the term *cues* is used in the same sense) to make very rapid judgments. We would not be able to read at all if we had to study all the features of letters. The capable reader goes much further and uses clues for whole words and even phrases.[6]

Use of Multiple Sensory Input and Prior Experience

In practice our pattern-detecting ability depends on clues from vision, hearing, touch, or other senses, on behavior and relationships, and/or on the situation. In short, *the ability to detect and recognize patterns depends heavily on our experience, on what we bring to the act of pattern detection and recognition.* The more that experience tells us what we are likely to be looking at, or dealing with, the less detailed, feature-type information we need to jump to a probably correct conclusion.

Sensitivity to Negative Clues

One reason we can rely on little information is the sensitivity of the brain to *negative* clues. When clues do not fit together rapidly within a pattern, or when one or more are jarringly strange or contradictory, our pattern-detecting apparatus quickly senses something wrong. Suppose that I am going to the house of people I have visited a couple of times before, on a dark suburban street where house numbers are hard to find. As I walk toward what seems to be the house, I come to a flagstone walk. It "doesn't feel right," prompting me to retreat and try the house next door. Or, perhaps another day I identify an all-black bird as a Brewer's blackbird. When I see a flash of color on the wing, I must revise my identification to "red-winged blackbird."

Patterns Within Patterns: Categorizing Down

In the example of recognizing friends Francine and Peter, only a yes/no kind of decision was involved — they were or were not those individuals. But more common is the detection and recognition of patterns *within* patterns, which leads to finer and finer discriminations, a process called *categorizing down,* a most important aspect of learning. For example, we can detect the pattern "animal," then categorize it down to "dog," and then to "Afghan hound." Or, observing a number of people at a gathering, we may categorize further by noting that the people are festively dressed, a "party," and then on seeing a cake with candles, conclude it's a "birthday party."

But we must note that a person from a country where birthday cakes are not a custom would not be prepared to interpret that clue the way we so easily do. Again, what the observer *brings* to the recognition act—in terms of prior relevant experience and previously acquired knowledge—plays a critical part. (It is startling to observe that in conventional teaching this absolutely fundamental principle is largely ignored.)

In small children, the process of enlarging pattern detection and extending and refining categorizing-down chains is often clearly observable. A girl just starting to talk may say "Daddy!" while pointing to any man who comes into sight—we gather she is using *daddy* in the sense of *man*. A little later, guided by such feedback as "No, that is not Daddy—Daddy is at his office," the child may point to any man who comes into the home, whether young cousin or elderly grandfather, as *daddy*. With further feedback, categories gradually get straightened out and *daddy* is used to mean only one person. It may take much longer for the child to become clear on the fact that her friend also has a daddy (and some years to grasp the relationship). It may take still more time to be able to categorize surely from people to males, to relatives and friends, neighbors, policeman, mailman, Mr. Jackson (who lives next door), as well as boys, girls, and many other subtle relationships.[7]

It seems apparent that the brain must have some kind of organizational process that enables humans to rapidly categorize down patterns as they are detected, so that they can be identified quickly.

Matching. The principle of *matching* is well understood. In simplest terms, one receives an input from outside the brain—for example, visual input that comes from a door. Inside the brain, stored, is a pattern, *door*.[8] If the current input and the stored pattern pretty well match, recognition occurs. Looking in the night sky, one may see any one of several patterns that match up with stored patterns for *moon*. Hearing some sound waves that compose a certain pattern, we recognize it as the word *scarecrow,* since it fairly well fits our stored pattern for scarecrow. The matches do not have to be precise—another principle, *probability*, applies. This permits us to recognize "scarecrow" whether spoken by a child in a thin, high voice or by a man or woman in other pitches, and despite various pronunciations. *The brain searches for a probable match.* (If this were not so, we would all have a terrible time trying to read English, with its frequently weird spellings!)

Parallel Processing. But to operate effectively, the brain cannot afford to search sequentially through tens of thousands of stored patterns to find the match. It seems likely that patterns are grouped in categories within hierarchies, or layers, much as mail is addressed (reading from the bottom up and right to left):

The country (USA).

The state (Connecticut).

The city or town (Bethel).

The street (Maple Avenue).

The house number (628).

The person in that house (Mr. or Mrs.)

This method, we know, quite efficiently makes a match between the letter and one out of more than 250 million inhabitants. If the address (the input) is a little wrong, the letter may still be delivered but if the error is large, no match can be made, no delivery can occur.

Experimental studies suggest that the brain does not usually need as many as six steps to categorize down. (That investigation is beyond the scope of this book.) Nor is the brain limited to one linear chain of categorizing down (such as that illustrated above in addressing a letter). It can employ many such chains simultaneously, as we have noted. This "parallel processing" enormously speeds recognition. It's like having 1,000 clerks sorting the mail rather than just one.

Using Probability . . . Jumping to Conclusions

A variety of studies indicate that the brain naturally works on a *probabilistic* basis. The brain skillfully jumps to conclusions! It isn't an adding machine that must reach a correct total. For example, seeing a creature that has four legs, a tail, fur, and barks at a friend's home, we jump to the conclusion that the pattern "dog" applies. Why not "cat"? Because we pick up negative clues: Cats don't bark and ordinarily don't come aggressively to the door when a stranger enters. Why isn't it a monkey? Because the relationship of limbs is different. The situation also gives clues; we expect to find a dog in a home. If we visited a zoo, however, and found this same animal exhibited in a cage, we would assume it was not a dog but some similar creature. Our experience tells us that dogs are not displayed this way.

THE BRAIN—A MASTER AT HANDLING SERENDIPITOUS INPUT

This is the process of learning that Frank Smith and others aptly call "making sense of the world."[9] The ability that even infants have to gradually sort out an extremely complex, changing world is nothing short of astounding. And it's natural. But even more surprising still is that we learn *from input presented in a completely random, fortuitous fashion* — unplanned, accidental, unordered, uncontrolled, the polar opposite of didactic classroom teaching.

Consider, for example, the sorting-out problem a child has to grasp for such patterns as *dessert, pie,* and *cake*. Since a great variety of dishes may constitute dessert, the child must extract the idea that meals have a sequence (program) and dessert is the last course. He or she must also learn that *dessert* does *not* mean a particular dish, or even a tight group or class of dishes. *Pie* presents few problems to an adult with years of experience to draw on but, to a toddler, an open pumpkin pie, a crusted blueberry pie, and a lemon pie heaped with meringue topping present little in common. Or does pie mean *round,* the most obvious feature? Unfortunately many desserts are round, particularly cakes — which vary from pie-like cheesecake, to coffee cake, to layered birthday cake elaborately iced and decorated.

While adults and older siblings may provide gentle, casual, and almost incidental corrective feedback when the child calls a pie a cake or doesn't regard a fruit dish as dessert and cries in frustration, it would be most unusual for anything resembling teaching or instruction to deal with dessert, pie, and cake as subjects. Yet in a few years, from this confused, random exposure and experience, the child has extracted the patterns, gradually coming to see which features and relationships have significance in which settings, and which can be ignored. Frequently, however, the child extracts a pattern that sooner or later has to be revised in the light of new information. For example, everything if let go falls — until someone presents a gas-filled balloon. Children often find the need to revise something disturbing. The world keeps proving

more complicated, with more exceptions, than they had previously thought. Adults have a similar problem; in time, they may
become less flexible, cling to old ideas, refuse to revise, and even
try to avoid the input that forces the contradiction. "Nonsense . . .
that's crazy . . . I won't listen . . . don't bother me!"

Even more amazing is the obvious ability of preschool children to extract rules about language from the quite random
speech they hear about them and engage in. We hear such expres-
sions as *sheeps* and *deers*, plurals plainly not picked up from adults
or older children. The added *s* makes unmistakably clear that the
small child has extracted a general rule for plurals—end with the *s*
sound—and is applying it even to what will later be learned as
special exceptions. In the same way, most youngsters will use such
constructions as "Tommy hitted me," or "I falled down," showing
that they have extracted the pattern of past tense and the use of
the *-ed* sound, again even where there are common exceptions. Yet
it would be absurd to expect a three- or four-year-old to explain
plural or *past tense*.[10]

These familiar experiences and others like them are so preva-
lent that we cannot reasonably doubt that all of us, at whatever
age, *do extract patterns from the quite random, confused mass of input we
are exposed to in the course of normal living. Nor can it be easily denied
that the great bulk of practical knowledge we have and use to get along in
the world is acquired in this way.*

CONFLICT: EDUCATIONAL BELIEFS VERSUS CURRENT BRAIN RESEARCH

When I've presented these ideas to educators, I've encountered heavy resistance. That's understandable. From our earliest
exposure to school, as noted in the last chapter, we have relied on
the opposite approach. The notion has been drummed into our
heads that we learn by being taught and, conversely, if we aren't
taught, we won't learn.

Educators in particular are endlessly told that teaching must
be planned, tightly organized, sequential, and logical. Instructors
are considered skillful if they perform well in this area.
Prospective teachers may even be hired if "competency tests" suggest they'll perform in this manner and if they've taken the courses
that promote such a process.

The concept of discipline, the old notion that the child is inherently evil, lazy, disinclined to learn, or incompetent, is another factor. It is tied with the notion that the child must constantly be pushed ("motivated"), threatened, held in check, and often reprimanded or punished. In most conventional school systems, for example, the most admired teachers are those who most effectively *control* their students, regardless of how much the students learn or however deep the distaste they acquire for schooling and the subjects studied.

Further, many teachers will attest that many parents agree with these ideas and want the school to punish and discipline their offspring to make them "toe the line." Today's parents, often frustrated by efforts to exercise control from the home, may wishfully turn the task over to the school.[11] They exert pressures on teachers, stated or unstated, to apply a repressive approach.

Nevertheless, our observations about how children really learn can not be wished away, nor can the learning failures that have brought our schools and colleges into increasing disrepute.

The real nature of learning may be startling and disturbing. But once it is seen, it cannot be denied.

New Definition of Learning

The nature of natural learning leads to the Proster Theory definition of learning:[12]

Part one : Input— The process of learning is the extraction, from confusion, of meaningful patterns

and

Part two: Output— Learning is the acquisition of useful programs

Part One: The Extraction of Meaningful Patterns

Part one of the process of learning is the input stage: *Learning is the extraction, from confusion, of meaningful patterns.* In my view, the great bulk of general learning occurs in this way. The only other important method is via rote memory. But while "pure" rote learning—straight memorization—appears to suffice, as in the case of learning the alphabet in sequence, even rote learning is greatly helped by detecting the patterns involved where patterns clearly exist, as in the multiplication tables. Or consider the marching band, very much a rote activity. If the patterns in the music and in the maneuvers are understood, learning can be far faster and surer.

As the educational literature reveals, attempts to define the process of learning have been rare, indeed. The one that emerges from Proster Theory can, I submit, be immediately useful in guiding educators to effective, brain-compatible approaches.

Unfortunately, pressures of tradition have blinded educators to what seems obvious once it is brought to our attention:

- The brain is by nature a magnificent pattern-detecting apparatus, even in the early years.

- Pattern detection and identification involve both features and relationships, processes that are greatly speeded up by the use of clues and a categorizing down procedure.

- Negative clues play an essential role.

- The brain uses clues in a probabilistic fashion, not by digital "adding up" of clues.

- Pattern recognition depends heavily on the experience one *brings* to a situation.

- Children must often revise the patterns they have extracted, to accommodate new experience.

This learning process, being natural, appears effortless, but (as we will soon see) it requires much random, fortuitous exposure and experience—input.

We need only look around us to see people learning well and easily using this brain-compatible way: Preschool children rapidly making sense of their home world; middle school youngsters racing ahead as they follow their enthusiasm for electronics, animal care, music, some form of collecting, an aspect of science or history; teenagers successful in an apprentice situation or adults in on-the-job training; middle-aged and older people evolving a specialization.

In contrast, we see people in formal, classroom-type, aggressive teaching producing boredom, conflict, misbehavior, apathy, cheating, confrontations, acceptance of minimal standards, and every variety of learning inadequacy.

NOTES

1 David B. Brown, "Towards a Communication Theory," *Teachers College Record,* May 1977, p. 453.

2 Editor's Note: With each succeeding book he wrote about how the brain learns, Leslie Hart continued synthesizing his conceptualization of the two fundamental brain concepts: pattern detection, addressed in this chapter, and program building, described in Chapter 9. This revised edition takes yet another step forward, defining learning as a two-step process—one involves input, the other output. Each step is divided into two stages.

> **Pattern detection**, the input stage, consists of first identifying or recognizing the pattern and, then, making meaning of the pattern, including its relationship to other patterns.
>
> **Program building**, the output stage, consists of learning to apply what is learned, at first experimentally and conscious of each step, and then, after practice and wiring it up into long-term memory, applying what is learned with the almost automatic ease and skill.

This conceptualization of learning is an extremely important contribution to the field of learning because it is comprehensive enough to cover the wide range of practicalities that teachers, administrators, and parents face on a daily basis—from establishing curriculum to instruction to assessment.

For example, if we use Hart's two-step definition of learning when we examine current standardized testing instruments, we see that the ubiquitous multiple choice and true-false items call for no more than identification of a pattern (this choice *sounds* more familiar than that choice). *Understanding* the pattern is not necessary. Knowing how to use the information is well beyond the scope of the test and long-term memory of how to use it isn't even an issue.

This fuller, more comprehensive view of learning provides a set of lenses for examining all issues of curriculum, instruction, and assessment. It also provides a useful perspective when considering resource allocation and the success of improvement efforts.

3 See *The Human Situation* (Lectures at Santa Barbara, 1959), Pierro Ferrucci, ed. (New York: Harper & Row), p. 173. Also compare George A. Kelley, *A Theory of Personality* (New York: W. W. Norton, 1963): "Man looks at his world through transparent patterns or templates which he creates and then attempts to fit over the realities of which the world is composed." (p. 17)

4 Editor's Note: That the brain learns by detecting patterns among incoming sensory data has been amply confirmed by numerous brain researchers since the first edition of this book in 1983. See *The Growth of the Mind and the Endangered Origins of Intelligence* by Stanley I. Greenspan with Beryl Lieff Benderly (New York: Addison-Wesley Publishing Company, 1997), p. 114 and *Molecules of Emotion: Why You Feel the Way You Feel* by Candace B. Pert (New York: Scribner, 1997), p. 147.

5 Alphonse Bertillon (1853-1914) devised an elaborate system for positively identifying individuals in spite of their variety. It was intended primarily for criminal justice purposes. Later, fingerprinting proved far simpler but the system is still used by physical anthropologists.

6 John B. Carroll, speaking of the mature reader, suggests that it may be true, "astounding as it may seem, that reading is based upon a capability of instantly recognizing thousands or even tens of thousands of individual word patterns, almost as if words were Chinese characters not structured by an alphabetic principle." See *Theories of Learning and Instruction, 63d Yearbook of the National Society for the Study of Education* (Chicago: University of Chicago Press, 1964), p. 341. For actual use of Chinese, see "American Children with Reading Problems Can Easily Learn to Read English Represented by Chinese Characters," by Paul Rozin and others, in *Psycholinguistics and Reading*, Frank Smith, ed. (New York: Holt, Rinehart and Winston, 1973), Chapter 9.

7 Editor's Note: Much can be learned about the process of learning by observing how young children build their vocabulary and the knowledge of the world that that vocabulary represents. In going about this prodigious feat, children make great use of categorizing down. If something is at first not understandable, children, if unguided, rarely resort to repeated attempts at memorization of the original input or memorization

of a definition. Instead, they move on, gulping in massive amounts of new input until they hit upon a kind of input that finally provides a recognizable pattern, triggering the "aha" response.

8 Editor's Note: Just because the brain has stored a pattern for "door" does not mean that it has stored all of the attributes of the pattern called door in a single location. A truly startling quality of the brain is that it can access bits of information stored in different locations and array it to make sense, and do so with astonishing speed.

9 See Frank Smith, *Comprehension and Learning* (New York: Holt, Rinehart and Winston, 1975), p. 1. The "make sense" concept has been widely discussed by many brain researchers. Harry J. Jerison, for example, suggests that reality is "a creation of the brain, a model of a possible world that makes sense of the mass of information that reaches us through our various sensory (including motor feedback) systems." See *The Human Brain* (Englewood Cliffs, N. J.: Prentice Hall, 1977), p. 54.

10 This stage of language acquisition is familiar to many parents, teachers, and others who have contact with children. It has been discussed by many psycholinguists. See, for example, James Britton in *The Teaching of English, 76th Yearbook of the National Society for the Study of Education* (Chicago: University of Chicago Press, 1977), p. 11.

11 The George H. Gallup poll of the public's attitudes toward its schools has consistently shown "lack of discipline" as the number one problem. This view, however, is not shared by teachers or administrators. Just what it means is unclear. Possibly some racism may play a part. Recent polls suggest, however, that schools are seen as lax, don't demand homework or themes, and lack high standards of performance and behavior. Perhaps a general uneasiness finds expression this way. The annual polls are reported in *Phi Delta Kappan* each fall. As in previous years, the 1997 poll shows lack of discipline as the "biggest problem facing local schools."

12 Editor's Note: Hart's two-part definition of learning is the first attempt to define learning based on brain research findings from the latter part of the 20th century:

Part one: **Input**— "The process of learning is the extraction, from confusion, of meaningful patterns."

and

Part two: **Output**— "Learning is the acquisition of useful programs."

This definition of learning fundamentally changes our sense of teaching and evaluation. A 90 percent score on a pop quiz or a 90th percentile score on a standardized test is possible even in the early stages of Part One of learning—recognition of answer B as being more familiar than A, C, or D. But learning that can be used and that will become part of long-term memory is yet to come.

Thus, how we teach, how long we teach a concept or skill, and the kinds of engagement with the concept or skill we orchestrate must change. And, the tools teachers need must go beyond reliance on a textbook.

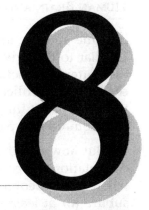

INPUT: ESSENTIAL FOR PATTERN DEVELOPMENT

> Man is no longer viewed as a passive sponge soaking up a flood of information. Instead, he is seen as an active seeker of information which he then filters, processes, encodes, and organizes into complex hierarchical schemes.
>
> —David L. Horton and Thomas W. Turnage[1]

Again, let me emphasize an idea that has received little attention in education, at least in the special sense I use it here.

The concept of *input* is a key factor in Proster Theory. Like some other aspects of natural, brain-compatible learning, it becomes obvious enough once we take the time to reflect on its role in our own learning. Input is critically important in any kind of learning situation, whoever the learner and whatever is to be learned.

The process of learning, defined in the preceding chapter, is the extraction, from confusion, of meaningful patterns. Input is *the raw material* of that confusion, what is perceived through the senses by the individual that bears on that particular pattern in any way.

Think of a 13-year-old suburban male who as yet has no clear concept of what is meant by *city*, although his teachers, his texts, and other sources have often presented that term. It easily can seem incredible to adults that children or adults less experienced in some specific area do not grasp a pattern that is already so familiar to those who already understand it. Once we have done the pattern extraction—a gradual process—and melded the concept into our collection of patterns, it seems so obvious that we have trouble putting ourselves into the brain of someone who has not acquired that pattern!

But how could this 13-year-old come to understand the main connotations of *city*? If he is told in school that a city is a place where many people live close together, he may fail to see why his suburb (or at least those denser parts of it) is not a city. If he has contact with commuters, he may assume that *city* means Boston or St. Louis or Los Angeles, or whatever city his community is near. If he visits that city occasionally, he may be impressed by traffic, noise, many stores, busy sidewalks, bridges, tall buildings, apartments, or development houses—yet a visit to another city may present quite different features, such as zoo, museum, or historic places. A trip to a downtown part of a nearby suburb may impress him as being to a city, since he experiences crowded sidewalks, many stores, movie houses, considerable dirt, and apparent crowding—yet if he refers to this place, technically a village, as *city* he may be corrected or receive some negative feedback, such as being tolerantly laughed at.

WHY "TELLING" IS INSUFFICIENT

It seems simple enough to *tell* him what city means. But it isn't simple, when we get down to trying it. A dictionary may say something like "a closely settled place of significant size," or "a chartered, incorporated municipality," but such definitions simply introduce new questions. With little effort, the boy can learn by rote a "right answer" to give in school but that hardly amounts to pattern extraction. It may function more as a cover-up answer to conceal uncertainty or lack of insight. The distress of teachers who by accident discover that students able to give "correct" answers actually don't understand the topic at all has long been familiar. Most adults, too, experience chastening moments when by some circumstance they discover that conventional right answers are like thin ice over a deep lake of ignorance or misconception. From personal and professional experience, educators have long been aware that "telling" methods can prove extremely ineffective in instruction.[2] Despite much evidence to the contrary, they are heavily used in conventional teaching.

Words Only Convey Limited Meaning

For one thing, words fail to convey much meaning *except as the hearer already has experience and extracted patterns* that give meaning to the words. Consider a stockbroker saying: "If you sell a security to establish a loss, you must wait 30 days to buy it back or it will be viewed as a wash sale but the waiting period doesn't apply to gains." Or an engineer: "If you put the recorder in the record mode, the erase head will wipe the tape before the new signal is encoded." Or a musician: "Since the B-flat clarinet is a transposing instrument, the note you play from the written music will actually sound a full tone lower." All of these are perfectly clear, simple statements, provided of course, that the listener brings an understanding of what is being talked about; otherwise the listener can be quite baffled. Telling and lecturing works somewhat better with older students and adults, as noted earlier, simply because the chances of having the experience necessary to comprehend what is said increase with age. The inexpert or insensitive lecturer assumes that if he or she uses correct language, the meaning will be conveyed; he or she is often astonished to discover that the audience grasped very little and much of that got twisted.[3]

Nonverbal Aspects

Communication, we must remember, also depends heavily on *nonverbal* aspects. The speaker's tone of voice, gestures, expression, and muscular tensions greatly enhance the listener's ability to properly receive what is intended. In most instances, the *setting* also contributes heavily. If two cars collide, the conversation that follows between the drivers is likely to illustrate both points. Inquire in a kitchen, "How do I light the oven?" and the query will probably be heard and understood. Ask the same question in the same way while strolling through a meadow, and the response will likely be some form of "Huh?" A question or remark out of context is often heard incorrectly *because even hearing speech intelligibly demands bringing information to the situation.*[4]

Confusion of Possibilities

While input via telling or lecture may be the most common and usually the easiest to provide in the classroom, it can prove ludicrously ineffective, even in supposedly simple situations. For example, a primary-grade teacher tells the students to "leave an inch margin at the top, put your name at the left and the date on the right." Such instructions are full of booby traps. How much is an inch? Adults know fairly well, young children may not. What does *margin* mean? One does not automatically know — it calls for extracting a pattern of blank space around written matter, a sort of frame. To some children, leaving space may seem rather wicked, especially if they have been urged not to waste paper. In any case, does the inch refer to space above one's name and date or only to space above the main text or answers? What is the date and how does one write it — is the first figure the month or day? Since the name of the day seems most familiar and important to the child, should *Tuesday* be put down? Which should go left and which right? What does *name* mean — first name or full name? (I have seen a child baffled by the term *first name* and insist that it is the only name she ever had!) A child's given name is intimately important and so may be put first, in huge capital letters.

I discovered how hard it can be even for perfectly competent adults to follow simple but unfamiliar directions when my wife and I taught folk dancing. "Start with your left foot" would appear clear enough, yet normally solid citizens would stand immobile, leap forward madly, or start with the right. As we shall discuss shortly, people may lack the program necessary for doing what somebody asks, directs, or recommends. In such cases, purely verbal input may prove, at best, only slightly helpful; at worst, devastatingly confusing.

THE REALITY PRINCIPLE

What may be called the *reality principle* (with no reference to uses of that term in other fields) is a neglected but critically important aspect of input. It focuses our attention on several aspects of input in conventional classrooms, particularly on the nature, kinds, and amount of input.

Shooting at a basketball hoop offers a sharp example. One shoots; the ball either goes in or it does not. If it misses, the shooter doesn't need a second party to tell him whether or not the shot was successful. That information, which we can loosely call feedback, comes directly, and usually instantly, from the reality. Take another example. On a playground, some children climb to the top of a pipe structure or fort while others stop short out of caution or difficulty. None of them need to be told whether they went all the way or not—they clearly see for themselves. And, if an adult making a repair tries to remove a stubborn screw, either it comes out or it doesn't. The real outcome is apparent.

Dependence on a Second Party

In a teaching situation, however, the second party often plays a dominant role. The student performs a task but the degree of success is usually not evident from the outcome, from reality. Rather, the student must wait for the teacher to evaluate and provide verbal feedback. For example, the student who writes an essay or report or answers a verbal question on science or history becomes *dependent on a teacher telling whether it is right*. Normally, "right" means conforming to authority—that of the teacher or some more distant source such as the author of the workbook—rather than based on real world criteria inherent in the task itself.

Similarly, if a letter is written to the mayor as a homework assignment but not intended to be sent, it is essentially a fake, though it may more kindly be called simulation or practice. Again, the feedback comes from the teacher. The great bulk of what students write throughout the 12 grades usually has this fake quality. It is not communication in the sense of producing real outcomes and a result that learners can judge for themselves.

Under these conditions, a new, distorted form of reality enters—leasing the teacher, getting a good mark, passing an exam. The material or skills supposedly being learned become simply a means to those distorted ends rather than learning itself being the desired end. Clever students figure out what kind of response the teacher or instructor is looking for and try to provide it. Even very young students expertly read the nonverbal signals a teacher may emit regarding what answer or behavior is wanted.

Feedback Based on Who the Learner Is

Perhaps the most serious problem with feedback, especially for younger children, occurs when the authority's (the teacher's) comments are colored by how well he or she likes the student overall, rather than on the quality of the student's work. The student whose work is frequently criticized soon feels that the teacher doesn't like him personally. We can hardly pretend that the child may not have good reason to feel so when social class or minority factors enter in or when the student is perceived as smart-aleck, contrary, annoying, frequently misbehaving, or withdrawn because of boredom. Teachers, being human, tend to view their personal standards and values as, in broad terms, those to which students should aspire. And since teachers usually work under stressful conditions within an antique and brain-antagonistic structure that creates constant difficulties, they *quite naturally seek the "right" answer that fits most neatly into their plans and rituals for conducting the class.*

Mistaken Belief: Praise Is Helpful

Another widespread but harmful belief about feedback is that praise is helpful to learners. The rationale most used for this belief stems directly from behaviorist psychology: The praise is intended as a reward and rewards motivate—two ideas that couldn't be more obviously wrong, yet persist.[5]

We need merely watch the youth endlessly shooting baskets, or the girl who pursues anything to do with horses beyond her parents' patience, or the high school student (including one of my acquaintance) who becomes an expert on snakes despite the opposition and revulsion of family and friends. Strongly "motivated" people seem largely disinterested in casual, superficial praise. Teacher praise often takes the form of "Very good," or "Fine, Thomas, you are really trying!"—remarks that appear to applaud effort and behavior rather than outcomes. As teachers have become more conscious of criticism of racial, class, and ethnic prejudice or bias, the use of praise with such students appears to have increased. In at least some cases, the consequence has been serious: students have been led to believe that they were doing well when, in fact, actually they were doing very poorly.

Paucity of Input

In addition to all the problems discussed, perhaps the most universal is that, *overall, the total amount of input tends to be extremely low.* As many observers have found,[6] the conventional classroom characteristically has low input due to incessant interruptions for control, discipline, announcements, etc., plus a great deal of time allotted to noninstructional activities (settling down, distributing materials, record keeping, changing classes, organizing, and the like). A good part of the time, there is nothing that an observer could call input, even by the most generous definition, is being presented. When asked "What'd you learn today?", the typical response of "Nothing" shouldn't surprise us. Students aren't being difficult, they are telling us the truth. Little input, little learning . . . nothing.

Oversimplification of Input

But we are still not at the end of the classroom's input deficiencies. From a Proster Theory viewpoint, the worst aspect of classroom input is oversimplification. By tradition and logic, teachers try hard to organize their presentation and reduce its apparent difficulty, in the firm belief that the simpler, more restricted, and clearer the input, the more easily and certainly it will be grasped. Such is the power of logic and common sense that the constant failure of this belief to produce the hoped-for results may be given little heed. When I show educators, from their own familiar experience, that *the process of learning is the extraction of patterns from confusion – not from clarity and simplicity –* they usually find that view at first hard to credit. After all, it is a distressing overturning of previous assumptions. At one session, an experienced teacher was moved to burst out, "That's crazy!" – a thought I'm sure others shared but were able to suppress.

The history of science, of course, is one of "crazy" ideas: Galileo maintaining that light objects would fall as fast as heavy ones of the same shape; Pasteur insisting that microbes could cause many diseases; Einstein submitting that atoms could be converted into an enormous amount of energy. Good scientific ideas are not correct because they sound crazy – but they often do sound crazy until they become familiar.

To clarify the process of extracting patterns from input, let's return to our 13-year-old youth and his problems in grasping the pattern of *city*. Over a period of time, let's say, he receives these inputs:

- Traveling by car into the nearby city, he observes a sign, "City Limits." He also notices that the pavement changes at that point from concrete to blacktop.

- Looking at a road map before a trip to the circus, he notices "City Limits" borders for the first time.

- He hears in a news broadcast that the city population has fallen and exact figures are given. He has never had a clear idea of what population meant but gets a hint that a city has a finite number of inhabitants.

- A family friend, in the city fire department, talks about fearing for his job because the city is short of money. The boy gathers that the city must be an entity, if it can be short of funds like a person.

- He sees a documentary on television about the excavation of an ancient city.

- His mother asks a friend who has returned from a European trip what cities she visited.

- After a heavy snow storm, the news on television shows several views of residential streets and reports that citizens are angrily complaining to city hall about delay in plowing.

- His brother, attending college in a distant city, mentions on a visit that the city is holding a celebration, having become a city 150 years before.

- His father remarks that a local milk strike will not stop supplies "in the city"; if necessary, he will bring some milk home.

- He hears a remark that only a few American cities are large enough to support a symphony orchestra.

From such bits of input, random and unorganized, over a long time period, our youth gradually extracts a fairly accurate and complete pattern of city. The concept may continue to sharpen and deepen. He may come to understand why early cities fostered craftsmen and specialists and were essential in bringing about various cultural gains; that there can be "twin cities" such as Minneapolis and St. Paul; and that the word *city* is related to the ideas in *citizen* and

civilization. The features and clues in time add up to permit recognition and discrimination.

This is the process of learning that leads an individual to possess an inventory or collection of patterns, eventually in great number—possible in humans because of the huge size of the brain and its more than 100 billion specialized cells.[7] To repeat, the brain was designed by evolution to deal with *natural complexity*, not neat, "logical" simplicities such as found in lesson plans. Should that surprise us?

In educational institutions of almost any kind, we find virtually an obsession with *levels*: The curriculum and the work must be exactly tailored to the age and supposed competence of the students. The goal is unrealistic and reflects neither brain research nor common sense based on our own experiences. But let us shift once more to what we can commonly see children achieving and then let's be guided by realities, not word-systems.

CHILDREN LEARN BEST IN REAL-WORLD ENVIRONMENTS

In the typical home, young children have some toys and playthings and a few pieces of furniture such as crib, highchair, and perhaps low tables or scaled-down chairs. But by and large *our children grow up in adult homes.* Most of the furnishings, the bathrooms, the kitchen, the stairs, the windows, the light switches, the utensils, plates and cutlery, the car, the appliances, the tools, and much more are all on adult scale. The conversation that goes on, most of the programs on television and radio, the newspapers and magazines, the entertainment, the sports, games, and fitness activities are heavily adult dominated. In short, while the presence of children certainly is evident, and markedly affects family lifestyle, there is little question that children are brought up in adult environments. Even the fortunate child who has a good supply of children's books, records, and playthings will still be overwhelmingly exposed to adult input. And as we have noted, learning in this environment—language, daily activities, operation and use of physical facilities, extraction of interpersonal relationship patterns, acquisition of traditions and development of many skills—usually proceeds so rapidly and well that we scarcely give heed to how successful it is.

However, the moment the astonishingly competent five-year-old enters the environment of formal education, he or she will likely be treated as essentially incompetent. The child who has explored the neighborhood must now get into a line to move to another room. The girl who has acquired a vocabulary of thousands of words, covering a great range of length and complexity, must now work with a basal reader that uses 400 selected, short, "regular" or high frequency words. The real world outside is banished in favor of whimsy and talking animals. The boy who has learned to ride his bike around his home, with frequent spills and minor injuries, must now use blunted scissors; the girl who is a daring, confident, aggressive athlete must now be protected (the school might be sued). At every turn, the rich, random input of the real world is choked off and the sparse, anemic, filtered, highly contrived input of the school is substituted.

When I visit classrooms, I make a habit of observing the entire room to see what I can find that is real world, rather than "school stuff." In many cases, I have found almost nothing in the room that can be put under the first heading. The world of reality, the world of rich, random input, has been totally shut out.

Does my stress on random input suggest that instruction must be muddled, unplanned, even unfocused? Of course not. But the recommendations from brain research may surprise you.

THOUGHTS FROM BRAIN RESEARCH

The key thoughts from brain research are these.

1. In real life, the extraction of patterns is from confusion, because real life input is fortuitous and random. The brain copes readily with such input. In contrast, logically sequential curriculum taught for a short number of minutes a day, over an extended period of time makes learning difficult.

2. The learning process, by which patterns are sorted out to make sense of a complex world, goes on incessantly and each individual, in a purely individual way, gathers features and clues that gradually mount up. Progressively, the pattern is grasped more sharply and greater discrimination, and thus greater learning, becomes possible.

3. Verbal presentation of direct, orderly, lesson plans ignores the fact that the learner must bring information *to* the words to understand what is being said.

4. Feedback is essential to the learner. Feedback from reality is usually clearer and more acceptable than second-person feedback from authority, which introduces complicating, distorting aspects.

5. Schools and schooling put strong emphasis on trying to adjust the level of input to the students' supposed level. To so simplify content enough, to make it low enough, the real world is excluded.

6. The classroom—the walled-off, closed-door cell in which a fixed group of students is "taught" by one teacher—seriously reduces the amount of input that students get and thus the amount of raw material from which they can extract patterns. In such a flagrantly brain-antagonistic setting, the variety of activities is severely restricted.

RECOMMENDATIONS ABOUT INPUT

Turning from criticism to constructive recommendations, the principles of Proster Theory and bodybrain-compatible instruction provide a lot of guidance when planning the amount and kind of input provided for students.

Amount of Input

As a starting goal, I suggest that input from the world outside the school should be increased by at least ten times[8] that which the typical classroom provides.

Random Rather Than Orderly Input

The input should be random rather than orderly—youngsters simply do not learn from a logical presentation. For one thing, what is logical to one person often makes little sense to another. For another, people need to come at a pattern from many directions, in many contexts to flesh it out as in the example of learning about *city*.

Ongoing Input

Repetition within the input can be valuable, however, because what a particular brain is not ready for at one time will be welcomed and utilized at another.

Suppose we give 25 jigsaw puzzles, all the same, to 25 students, whether children or adults. Each will put the pieces together in a different sequence and at varying speeds; but given time, all will likely complete it. Any learning of patterns, as we have seen, involves just this kind of jigsaw assembly. But it is more complex because the pieces must be separated from the many other pieces which are not part of this particular puzzle. Each learner will have different assortments of pieces.

Once we grasp the individual way that human brains extract patterns, we can begin to see the futility of offering a standardized, limited input.

THE BRAIN AS AN ACTIVE CONSTRUCTOR OF MEANING

Among those investigating and substantiating this approach, M. C. Wittrock, a professor of educational psychology in the Graduate School of Education at the University of California, Los Angeles, ranks as a highly influential pioneer and leader—the more so for present purposes since he works on the learning of school-age children. He writes:

> The brain does not usually learn in the sense of accepting or recording information from teachers. The brain is not a passive consumer of information. Instead, it actively constructs its own interpretations of information and draws inferences from it. The brain ignores some information and selectively attends to other information.[9]

In short, a teacher aggressively instructing a class of 25 is actually not addressing a group at all but rather 25 individual brains, each of whom will attend to what *it* chooses, then process that input in an individual way, relating it (if at all) only to previous individual input or experience. "The basic implication for teaching," Wittrock adds, is that teachers need "to understand and to facilitate the constructive processes of the learner," who is given "a new, more important active role and responsibility in learning from instruction and teaching."[10]

NOTES

1 *Human Learning*: (Englewood Cliffs, N.J. Prentice Hall, 1976), p. 223.

2 Editor's Note: The Kovalik ITI model expresses this concept by contrasting the typical input of the traditional classroom life (*second hand* and *symbolic*) and the input needed for fully brain-compatible learning (primarily *being there* and *immersion* when used as follow up to *being there*). The difference in the amount of sensory input, and thus learning, is enormous. Sensory input from *being there* and *immersion* experiences are especially important when learning something new.

3 This point has been made by many writers on instruction. For instance, see David R. Olson and Jerome S. Bruner in *Media and Symbols, 73d Yearbook of the National Society for the Study of Education* (Chicago: University of Chicago Press, 1974), p. 141: "If the information intended by the speaker falls outside the listener's 'competence,' the listener will interpret that sentence in terms of the knowledge he already possesses."

4 Scientists investigating speech and listening to language have produced an impressive body of knowledge, much of it long established. Yet, apparently, it is all but unknown to most educators, who commonly refer to "auditory" and "listening" skills and similar ideas far off the mark. For an excellent discussion, see George A. Miller, *Language and Speech* (San Francisco: W. H. Freeman and Co., 1981), especially Chapter 6.

Editor's Note: See also the work of Pat Lindamood and Nanci Bell of the Lindamood-Bell Learning Processes Center (416 Higuera Street, San Luis Obispo, CA 93401; 800/233-1819). This center, and satellite centers around the country, work with hundreds of people—ages 5 to 85—each year. Their primary work is in the area of creating neural wiring for decoding and for comprehension of language (from both the spoken and written word).

5 Editor's Note: Alfie Kohn has compiled some startling research data about the long-term damage of external rewards and how to avoid them. See *Punished by Rewards: The Trouble with Gold Stars, Incentive Plans, A's, Praise, and Other Bribes* (Boston: Houghton

Mifflin, 1993) and *Beyond Discipline: From Compliance to Community.* (Alexandria, Virginia: ASCD, 1996.)

6 See Philip W. Jackson, *Life in Classrooms* (New York: Holt, Rinehart and Winston, 1968) for a well-known and colorful account. He notes, "It is surprising to see how much of the students' time is spent in waiting" (p. 14). Since the concept of input has not engaged researchers, to my knowledge, there is no direct measure of it. There seems little doubt, however, from observation alone, that input typically is low, often nearing the zero point. Time on task does not equate to input; input involves raw material from which patterns can be extracted, not the amount of time devoted to something. See also John Goodlad's milestone work, *A Place Called School.*

7 The figure is far understated. In addition to neurons themselves, the glial cells alone, which appear to nourish and assist neurons, number near this total.

8 Editor's Note: As brain research continues to explode old paradigms, we should not be surprised to discover that humans have more senses at work than the traditional five—sight, hearing, smell, taste, and touch. Even as early as 1987, Bob Samples began to report 19 senses. (See *Open Mind, Whole Mind.* San Diego, California: Jalmar Press, 1987.) A recent surfing on the internet turned up lists of 21. In addition, many of the information substances discussed in Chapter 5 are generated as a result of the bodybrain "sensing" data from both outside and inside the body. Look for major scientific breakthroughs in this area in the next five years. Sight, hearing, smell, taste, and touch are not *the* five sense; they are five of many ways the bodybrain partnership has for making sense of the world around it. For more information about these senses and their implications for curriculum and instruction, see the Kovalik ITI materials appropriate to your grade level in Appendix C.

Also see the graphic on the following page illustrating the kinds of input which promote learning. The top two, which are infrequently used in traditional classrooms are the most effective. However, the bottom two, which are most frequently used in traditional classrooms, are the least effective.

Kinds of Input

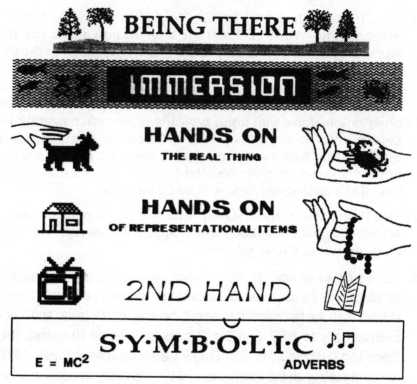

© 1992 Susan Kovalik & Associates

Figure 8

9 See *Education and the Brain, 77th Yearbook of the National Society for the Study of Education,* Part II, Jeanne S. Chall and Allan F. Mirsky, eds. (Chicago: University of Chicago Press, 1978), p. 101. See also *Molecules of Emotion: Why You Feel the Way You Feel* by Candace B. Pert (New York: Scribner, 1997), pp. 146-148.

10 Ibid.

9

SECOND FUNDAMENTAL OF LEARNING: WE LIVE BY PROGRAMS

> [Man] creates intentions, forms plans and programs of his actions, inspects their performance, and regulates his behavior so that it conforms to these plans and programs; finally he verifies his conscious activity, comparing the effects of his actions with the original intentions and correcting any mistakes he has made.
>
> —A. R. Luria[1]

Extraction of patterns—identifying and making meaning of them—as discussed in Chapters 7 and 8, constitutes the first of two steps in learning. But plainly enough, we do not live by sitting in an armchair and detecting patterns. We live by doing, by action. Thus, the second step in learning is the development of mental programs to use what we know, i.e., the patterns we have come to understand. Step two in learning is defined as "the acquisition of useful programs."[2]

THE MYSTERY OF BEHAVIOR

For thousands of years, back to the dim origins of humans, behavior has seemed largely a mystery. What people did seemed utterly haphazard, unpredictable, and unexplainable.

Teachers have long struggled with the behavior of their charges, often to the degree that class management threatens to push instruction into a secondary function. Even corporate personnel specialists confess to being frequently surprised and baffled by the behavior of workers, for all the "motivation" that pay and prospects of advancement would seem to offer. More than half of marriages in the United States go astray; the inability of spouses to understand each other, even after years of intimacy, stands out. At any gathering of parents, the difficulties of comprehending the strange worlds children inhabit take a prominent place in the discussions.

However, in the last four decades and more, researchers studying the brain and several other disciplines have made progress on many fronts. When their findings are brought together and unified, our understanding of human behavior can take a great leap. This opens the door to revolutionary advances in education and gives us the chance to catch up, at least somewhat, with the discoveries resulting from the dazzling and often upsetting advances in technology.

Two Approaches: Behaviorist Versus Ethologists

Before today's extraordinary breakthroughs in research technology, there were basically two approaches to studying the way creatures behave, approaches representing opposite poles. One way, the stock-in-trade of the behaviorist psychologists, was to put an isolated creature in captivity, do things to it, and try to make sense of what the animal does as a consequence. The subject animal is regarded as passive, inert, a "sample" that must be stimulated from outside to take action.

The opposite approach is that of ethologists, who primarily observe creatures who are, as far as possible, free and in their natural setting, to see what they do on their own. These researchers recognize from the outset that these animals are not samples, but individual, social, living animals, far from passive, in no need of contrived outside stimuli to become active.

It can hardly be surprising that the manipulators, even after a century, have produced little that illuminates human (or even lab animal) behavior. To this day, they have not really sought to observe the natural way various creatures behave in their natural environment. Real world examples of this can strike us as ridiculous. For example, if a teacher takes students to visit an old-fashioned zoo with cages, students will likely report that "tigers are large, striped animals that pace back and forth all the time." While this is what tigers may do *in a cage*, it doesn't help understand what tigers really do in their natural environment, their normal behavior.

Captivity has a profound effect on most animals. We can suspect that for millions of years loss of freedom to move was a prelude to early death, probably by being eaten. Humans, too, are put into captivity, commonly in three settings: prisons, mental hospitals, and schools. It seems unreasonable to expect behavior more normal than that of the caged tiger in any of those places. Yet, when it comes to the classroom, because we are so used to it, it seems to become invisible to those who work in it or deal with it.[3]

Although the classroom is a grossly arbitrary, artificial setting and form of captivity, the behavior of inmates is somehow expected to be normal and compliant. Such is the power of wishful thinking that resistance, rebellion, and withdrawal are regarded officially as misbehavior rather than as the perfectly natural, to-be-expected consequences of their environment. Elaborate studies are conducted of "how students learn" in this oppressive setting—the exact equivalent of observing "how tigers behave" in a zoo cage.

Instead, we should follow the lead of ethologists by beginning to observe humans in ordinary, free settings, and apply modern understandings of the brain; much of the old mystery surrounding behavior would then evaporate.

THE BASIS OF BEHAVIOR: PROGRAMS

The key to understanding human behavior is the realization that we act very largely by programs. The word *programs* need not alarm us with visions of robots. It means simply a fixed sequence for accomplishing some *intended objective*. In other words, we act to carry out some purpose, some personal, individual, and usually self-selected purpose—the exact opposite of robot behavior.

Suppose, for example, that I wish to telephone my dentist. I pick up the phone, push the buttons in a certain order, and put the receiver to my ear to wait for the call to go through. I have executed a program for making a phone call. Should I call him again tomorrow, I will go through just about the same procedure.

Should I wish to phone a local store, I may have to use an additional program to find the number. I get the phone book, look up the listing, then dial—a variation of the program I used to call my dentist.

If now I want to visit the store, I must implement a longer program. I go to my car, take out my keys, find the right one, unlock the door, open it, get in, put the key in the ignition switch, fasten the seat belt, turn the switch and start the engine, release the parking brake, put the car in gear, press the accelerator pedal—just to start on my trip. To get there in my accustomed way I go through a series of dozens of steps, including the right choices of turns at street intersections. Yet I can "reel off" this program with the greatest of ease, hardly giving any attention to what comes next, much as I can put a cassette in a player and have the tape reel off a musical or other program.

Clearly, one of the reasons for our huge brain is that as humans we need and use a great number of programs to carry on our complex activities—thousands of times as many as the most intelligent of other animals. The programs we learn are stored in the brain.[4] Exactly how that is achieved remains unknown, although the progress of researchers in the neurosciences suggests that we may have a good start toward understanding the neuronal, chemical, and molecular mechanisms involved within another few years.

The Source of Programs

Present knowledge makes clear that programs can be acquired in two distinct ways: *transmitted with the genes* or *learned after birth*. As a general rule, the more brainpower an animal has, the more it learns after birth. The more neocortex or new brain it possesses, the greater the relative reliance on after-birth learning. We see once more why the laboratory rat and other small experimental animals can shed so little light on human learning: Their programs are largely species wisdom, transmitted genetically, while humans use the splendid new brain to do most learning after birth, over many years.

No aspect of being human appears more dominant than this incessant accumulation of programs. The process, of course, is most rapid in the earlier years then gradually tapers off. But since we live in a world that changes constantly, we are under far greater pressure than our forebears to continue to learn, to continue acquiring new programs. The man of 75 who is given a video tape recorder to honor that birthday must master some new programs to operate his new machine. A few centuries ago the programs acquired by age 25 would pretty well see one through a full life; today much of what is learned by age 25 will become obsolete. Failure to keep on learning can prove restrictive, costly, or embarrassing.

Programs As Building Blocks

As we become more familiar and at ease with the concept of *programs as the building blocks or units of behavior,* we must wonder why many brilliant psychologists and other investigators did not see this rather simple explanation long ago. A partial answer, I think, is that the present knowledge of DNA molecules and their ability to hold an enormous amount of information—the instructions for building the next generation—lets us readily believe that the storage of elaborate programs is biologically possible. Also, we are familiar with phonograph records, magnetic tape, photographic film, holograms, computers, and other means of storing information, a miraculous innovation in their day.

The earlier investigators did see programs in action, as their writing reveals, but did not know how directly to make sense of them as we so easily can now. They turned to far more complicated and unsatisfactory explanations, such as stimulus-response sequences, habit chains, "superstitious" behaviors, and the like.

Today, however, leading brain researchers accept the concept of stored programs as a basic of brain function.[5] It is also a powerfully useful concept for anyone engaged in any kind of instruction.

How Programs Work

To carry on activities, one must constantly *select* a program from those that are stored in the brain and *implement* it—put it into use. Even to walk across the room, one must use an extremely complex program involving many of the body's 600-plus muscles and the shifting of weight from one side to the other as the feet alternate in moving forward. The program has to be repeated every two paces, with continual fine adjustments to change direction or to pick up and carry articles. To walk, one program is used; to go up stairs, another; to go down stairs, a third. To take a stroll outside one may have to use programs for going uphill, downhill, crossing rough ground, jumping over a puddle, or running a few steps to avoid traffic. *Each time, the program in use has to be switched off and another selected and switched on.* The brain does this so smoothly that we ordinarily are not aware of the switches being thrown, but this is the main key to our present insight into behavior.

If I am getting dressed in the morning and open a drawer full of shirts, I must make a conscious selection of which I will wear. After I have made that choice, opening up the shirt, putting it on, and buttoning it up "runs off" as a kind of automatic program to which I don't have to give any conscious attention unless something goes wrong — I find a button missing — and interferes.

Which shirt will I select? It depends on a perception of the *pattern* I will be dealing with. If I am going to a business meeting, I select a dress shirt; if I plan to make some repairs, I choose a work shirt; if I plan to exercise, I choose another type of shirt. Even more subtle patterns may influence me: I may want a conservative dress shirt for the meeting or a brighter one if the meeting will become a celebration with old friends. Though the decision may be trivial, I cannot act until some decision is made. (Following fixed habits or rituals, where possible, avoids decisions and so may seem more "comfortable.")

In much the same way, we select the most appropriate program from those stored in the brain to deal with what is happening at the time. For example, seeing stairs ahead, I select a going-up-stairs program. Having accidentally jostled somebody, I choose an offering-apology program. Facing an arithmetical problem, I tap my division program. Meeting a neighbor, I select a greeting program, complete with smile, nod, and suitable words.[6]

THE PROGRAM IMPLEMENTATION CYCLE

In each of the above examples, a basic cycle is plainly in use. One must:

1. *Evaluate* the situation or need (detect and identify the pattern or patterns being dealt with).

2. *Select* the most appropriate program from those stored.

3. *Implement* the program selected.

Human behavior looked at in these terms may hardly seem simple but such a perspective provides more penetrating insight.

Key Observations

For educators, viewing behavior as a function of the program implementation cycle significantly expands our ability to observe and analyze student behavior during the learning process. Key observations include:

1. Unless the learner can reasonably accurately evaluate the need or problem at hand (that is, detect and identify the patterns involved), the cycle goes astray at the outset. The student simply does not know what to do.

   A familiar example is a student trying to cope with an arithmetic problem couched in words. Unable to detect the pertinent pattern, the student flounders, wondering whether to add, or divide, or give up entirely. Another example is spelling of longer words. Lacking any sense of the structure or pattern of the word, the student tries to simply remember the order of the letters—perhaps producing some weird versions.[7]

2. People can access and use only those programs they already possess. However much one may be coerced or urged, or motivated or rewarded, there is no way to perform the program *unless it has already been stored*. He or she does not know how to do it. No program, no ability to perform the needed action.

   There is no way to force a person to ride a bicycle, or play Chopin on the piano, or write a scientific paper, if those programs have not previously been acquired. That many other people can do these things has no bearing. Yet in almost any classroom, at any level, this principle is ignored. On the playground, one may hear a child being called "clumsy" or "poorly coordinated" when the real difficulty is that the child has not yet learned certain programs. In homes, parents scold children; in businesses, bosses scold employees—all in the same futile way for the same futile reason. *If the program has not been acquired, the solution is to acquire it,* not in criticizing, labeling, or giving a poor mark, practices that prove devastating to learners.

3. A student cannot implement a program unless given the chance to do so.

A test question might ask, "How can you verify the correct spelling of a word?" The answer intended is, "Look it up in a dictionary." A student who gives that answer, we must note, is not using that program. Rather, he or she is *using a program for answering a question on a test.* So commonly are tests used in instruction that this all-important difference may be overlooked; students may pass tests yet often be unable to carry out the programs themselves—a complaint loudly uttered today. Similarly, if students are always *directed* to use certain programs, there is no way to know whether they can detect the pattern, have a program to select, and can implement it. Rather, they are implementing programs *for following directions.* Such "learning" may prove fictitious.

As I indicated earlier, a program always has a goal, an objective—it is an activity to achieve some intended outcome. What happens if the program selected and implemented does not work?

WHEN PROGRAMS DON'T WORK

During the program implementation cycle, the brain asks, "What *pattern* am I dealing with; what *program* should I choose to deal with it?" The most appropriate program is then implemented. Usually it will work. If it aborts, the brain must recycle—pattern detection, program selection, implementation.) Let's say that I have taken out my keys to open the car door. I insert the key but it won't turn—the program *aborts.* I must now go through the three-step cycle again: reevaluate the situation, select another program that seems appropriate, and implement that. Perhaps I have the wrong key, in which case I recycle to find the right one and try again. Perhaps the lock has jammed, so I recycle to the unusual program of going around to the opposite door.

Aborting Programs Is Disturbing

Aborting a program *always causes some degree of emotional shift* because the failure of a program to work is in general disturbing and *threatening,* especially when no workable alternative program can be found. The degree to which programs usually work when implemented to achieve the intended goal serves as a direct, continuous measure of how well one has "made sense of the world," how competent we generally are. Programs *should* work. When they do, confidence in oneself increases; when too often they don't, confidence diminishes.[8]

Impact on Self-Confidence. Teachers have long sensed that self-image and the belief that one can successfully learn is important to self-concept and, in turn, to learning. Brain research now concurs. An individual's confidence rises or falls when programs do or do not work. We can see, too, that children whose parents or teachers have over-directed their activities and over-stressed second-person estimates of achievement, may mistrust their own ability to evaluate situations and select appropriate programs.[9]

This program view of behavior, I submit, is consistent both with present scientific understandings of the brain, and with what we can clearly see—once we know where to look—in the normal functioning of children, other adults, and ourselves. True, we cannot see into another person's brain to observe what pattern-detecting abilities and programs have been established there. However, we can see with new insights what happens when that person is allowed to use what he or she considers the most appropriate program—or when the individual has none to apply, or can't identify the pertinent pattern to begin with.

LEARNING AS A TWO-STEP PROCESS

In Chapters 7 and 8, we explored the first step of learning: The extraction, from confusion, of meaningful patterns. The second step of learning is *the acquisition of useful programs.*[10]

Learning = Stored Programs

Educators are accustomed to thinking in terms of knowledge. But we can now see that certainly the great bulk of knowledge, if not all, takes the form of stored programs.[11] One learns a mathematical, mechanical, artistic, or horticultural *procedure*, not how to answer a question. It has long been observed, by philosophers and those in behavioral fields alike, that however splendid or intense our private thoughts may be they do not have an impact or effect until we act in some way. While we commonly tend to think of motor and intellectual activity as being in different categories, observation reveals that mental activity involves motor activity: speaking, writing, operating machines or equipment, doing something with the hands, *performing* in some fashion. Even *to accept input* demands acting—to see, we use elaborate muscle control to orient body, head, and eyes, which move millions of times an hour. To feel, we extend arms and fingers; to listen, we orient the ears; to smell, we sniff.[12]

We also talk to ourselves—within our heads or sometimes aloud, more often subvocalizing—a process that appears often to involve very small muscular movements. The distinction between motor and intellectual programs does not seem to have much practical value, I suggest. Arguments about whether action is "externalized thought" or thought is "internalized action" seem to show only that the two are closely linked.

Experience with in-school applications of Proster Theory has convinced me (and many others) that when teachers shift to using this *pattern and program* concept of the brain, they almost immediately see student learning and behavior both take a quite startling jump. It is as if a curtain has parted, letting instructors see where the students are having trouble and how to remove it, by constantly attending to the cycle: (1) detect and identify the key pattern being dealt with; (2) select the most appropriate stored program to deal with it; and, (3) implement it. Hammering at the student without this insight merely produces unpleasantness and frustrations.

Useful Programs: What Students Can Do With What They Learn. Anywhere we look at conventional brain-antagonistic schools we see an obsession with *information*. The effort seems to be to stuff the student's head with discrete "facts," the "right answers" to questions. Teachers (doing what they feel is expected of them) spend much time asking questions and more time is invested in the kinds of testing that is typically concerned with bits of information rather than with patterns or programs. Even the best scores and grades tell us little about what students have learned, which may be very little indeed. When we see a classroom where students are being asked for right answers to informational questions, we are witnessing a form of futility that goes back centuries, one from which many instructors, administrators, boards of education and parents seem unable to break away, however much the actual learning outcomes are bemoaned.

Behavioral Objectives and Proster Theory. When we define learning as the acquisition of useful programs, we plainly move in the directions of "behavioral objectives," a much-abused term in schooling. Its main idea is to focus, at the outset, on *what the student will be able to do after instruction.* In practice, however, teachers may simply continue their old approach, "covering the material," merely giving lip-service to behavioral objectives or stated outcomes. Too often in the past, the objectives were seen in test terms — what students will be able to *do* is pass some kind of examination, as directed, when directed! I suggest this behavior tells us little about what the student can and will do when not ordered to perform in a prescribed way.

Although also focusing on behavioral outcomes, Proster Theory would have us ask different questions. Will the student detect the key patterns involved, without help? Will he or she select an appropriate program from those stored in the individual's brain? Will it prove, in use, an adequate program that achieves the intended goal and does not abort?

When behavioral outcomes are interpreted in these sharp Proster Theory terms, they help pinpoint, and list,[13] what goals are sought over a flexible period of time: several weeks, or months, or perhaps a year or two in some cases. Similarly, assessment of individual learning can be precise if focused on examining what programs a student now has compared to those not previously evident. In what order these programs are acquired rarely matters much. Nor do students need to progress in lockstep — they never will.

Subskills Versus Programs. One caution about the "subskills." *Subskills and programs are emphatically not identical and may have little in common.*

During the 1970s, the subskill approach to basic skills went wild. Reading, for example, was broken down into literally many hundreds of subskills. The poor teacher was expected to keep full records of which each student had mastered, on the dubious assumption that this is how one learns to read. In contrast, a program, as defined in Proster Theory, is a sequence for attaining a goal preselected by the individual; we may doubt that subskills often represent such a goal for the learner.

Even if selected by the student, subskills often fail to "add up" for students and fail to become part of a complete program for doing a real world task. For example, one does not learn to ride a bicycle by separately learning (1) steering, (2) pedaling, (3) balancing, and (4) leaning into a turn. The coordination of these makes easy riding possible, and that is the essential learning.

The Proster Theory version of behavioral outcomes also leads to *scrapping,* to great extent, the use of tests, quizzes, and examinations that call for "right answers" and so direct the student's behavior. To reiterate, *we almost never can find out from directed behavior what a student would do if not directed.* This might seem apparent, yet billions of man-hours and huge amounts of money are expended on testing futilities.

In schools, contrived, simplistic testing is an ingrained bad habit that tends to distort learning. It is axiomatic that as testing is emphasized, "teaching to the test" increases; and testing may become a regressive screen behind which administrators seek shelter from criticism. Standardized testing also represents a large vested interest, with ample funds to sell and lobby. Because formats that can be scored by machine cost far less to process, the multiple-choice type has largely driven out what little nondirective testing used to be done by teachers.

Until very recently, only the scantiest attention has gone to nondirective assessment strategies, a far more informative technique. It remains to be seen, however, whether funding will be adequate for creating the tools necessary to assess student ability to apply conceptual understandings and related skills in real-world settings.

ACQUISITION OF USEFUL PROGRAMS

The word *useful* in "acquisition of useful programs" deserves attention. Primarily, it means useful to the individual who will possess the program—in that person's view, rather than in someone else's view or to satisfy some supposed social or other standard. While it is true that one can be coerced into acquiring a program and may use it under duress, such programs are likely to become unused as soon as the duress ceases, if good mental health prevails. If use of the forced program does continue, it usually will signify either superstitious ritual, with anxiety that something dreadful will occur if it is not used, or the inappropriate behavior that goes under the common name of neurosis. *Inherently, the use of a freely learned program satisfies; that of a coerced program brings back the old fears under which it was built.* We see this in mild form when people do arithmetic with obvious pain and reluctance and, in more serious degree, when individuals who have been forced to learn a musical instrument well cannot bear to play before an audience in later life.

Transfer of Learning

In a far wider sense, *useful* conveys the possibilities of *transfer* of learning, which can greatly increase the speed of new learning. For example, a program for roller skating can readily transfer to ice skating; one for using a typewriter keyboard can easily be extended to using a computer keyboard which then can serve as a mental anchor for learning new information about the computer. *The ability to transfer some of these behavioral building blocks, adapting and adjusting them to new needs, explains why some individuals can master a new task far more rapidly than others* who lack the programs to transfer, or who in some cases may not yet have recognized the similarity of pattern involved which leads to and permits transfer.

Source of Creativity

The capacity to use old programs in fresh combinations seems to underlie what we call creativity. Greater sensitivity to pattern similarities facilitates the transfer. While I would doubt that sensitivity can be directly taught, it seems probable that it can be facilitated.

THE POWER OF PROGRAMS

The implications for education of the program concept of behavior—*evaluate, select, implement* program cycle—are stupendous, bringing not only fresh insights into human behavior but also generating some major guidelines for improving learning achievement.

To summarize:

1. We live by programs, switching on one after another, selecting from those that have been acquired and stored in the brain.

2. As humans, we are far more dependent on programs acquired by the tens of thousands after birth, in contrast to animals that rely more on programs genetically transmitted.

3. A program is a fixed sequence for accomplishing some end—a goal, objective, or outcome. Our human nature makes the working of a program pleasurable; the concept of some after-the-event "reward" is neither necessary or valid. However, feedback is essential to establish that the program did work more or less as intended.

4. We can use only those programs that have already been built and stored. What programs another person has, or many people have, has no bearing. If a person does not possess a program, efforts to force its use are absurd.

5. We routinely use a three-step cycle: evaluate the situation (involving pattern detection and recognition), select the program that seems most appropriate from our store, and implement it.

6. The abortion of a program—upon its failure to work—calls for recycling. When a high proportion of self-selected programs work well, confidence rises; when too many programs are aborted, confidence is reduced and the learner may become far less able to self-select programs.

7. Although laboriously built, fully acquired programs have an automatic quality that can easily lead one to forget that other individuals may not have acquired these programs.

8. Learning can be defined as the acquisition of useful programs.

9. Learning progress can be properly evaluated only by observing *undirected* behavior.[14] Questioning and testing dealing primarily with *information* can reveal little. It shows only poorly what individuals can *do*.

10. Effective transfer of learning depends on using established programs in new applications and combinations. (Skill in putting together new combinations may equal "creativity.") The learner who can adapt established programs to new tasks, by seeing similarities of patterns involved, learns much more rapidly than one who cannot.

11. In general, if we regard human learning and behavior in terms of continually asking, "What program is being used?" sharp new insights can be gained, and many confusions avoided.

When extracting patterns and building programs, specific information may be helpful to the task or even required. But, this does not imply that there is necessarily any great virtue in "stuffing the head with facts."

It can be handy to carry in memory certain information that will be frequently used. For example, we may store the phone numbers of a dozen people we often contact so we don't have to look them up each time. If patterns are involved, such information is much more easily remembered as when one knows that Tim, Linda, and Vance all work in the same office, and can be reached though its main number, at hours when that office will be open.

In our real world today, there exists vastly more information than can be memorized and it tends to change or obsolete rapidly, so that trusting memory can be treacherous.

A better strategy than trying to collect facts is to possess programs for finding various information—knowing what reference books are available and how to use them, or where to obtain help. But until specific information is linked to need for pattern or program, it serves little purpose. When such needs exist, learners typically "gobble up" information at an astonishing rate because they see it has immediate and meaningful application.

NOTES

1 A.R. Luria, *The Working Brain* (New York: Basic Books, 1975), pp. 79-80.

2 Editor's Note: To grasp the significance of Hart's conceptualization and definition of learning as a two-part process, consider for a moment what is required of a student taking a typical standardized test with its multiple choice and true-false items. With both kinds of test items, the right answer is present. The student has only to detect the answer (pattern) that is most familiar (a process usually accompanied by a small niggling in the back of the brain that says, "Hey, we've heard of that one before!") "Familiar" doesn't represent understanding of the concept inherent in the test question; ability to apply in a real-life setting is clearly light years away. Thus, in essence, the multi-billion dollar testing juggernaut assesses only the first half of the first stage of learning. To push this realization further, consider the Friday quiz, also typically weighted heavily toward multiple choice and true-false items. Sometimes 80% is accepted as indication of mastery; sometimes it is considered sufficient to just record the letter grades, A-F, and then the whole class moves on to the next topic.

If America is disappointed in the student outcomes of its public schools, it must examine what definition of "learning" is serving as the basis for the design and implementation of its curriculum and instructional practices. If Hart's two-part definition of learning were adopted, outcomes would—and do—soar because it forces profound and radical change at the very core of the business of teaching-learning.

3 See for instance Leslie A. Hart, "Is the Classroom Door Your Enemy?", *K-Eight*, September-October, 1972, and "The Case Against Organizing Schools into Classrooms," *The American School Board Journal*, June 1974.

4 Editor's Note: Recent research suggests that memory storage is not restricted to the brain only but is a bodybrain function (see Chapter 5). However, until researchers can provide a clear, detailed picture of how this functions, we will continue to refer to the brain as the location for storing programs.

5 For example, see such dominant books as A. R. Luria, *The Working Brain* (New York: Basic Books, 1975), and Karl H.

Pribram, *Languages of the Brain* (Monterey, California: Brooks/Cole, 1971). A famous and influential presentation of the program concept appeared in 1960, *Plans and the Structure of Behavior* by George A. Miller, Eugene Galanter, and Karl H. Pribram (New York: Holt, Rinehart, and Winston.) Plans here is interchangeable with programs. See also J. Z. Young, *Programs of the Brain* (Oxford: Oxford University Press, 1978).

For recent discussions of programs, see David Perkins *Outsmarting IQ: The Emerging Science of Learnable Intelligence* (New York: The Free Press/Simon and Schuster, 1995), especially pp. 249-265; *The Growth of the Mind and the Endangered Origins of Intelligence* by Stanley I. Greenspan, M.D., with Beryl Lieff Benderly (New York: Addison-Wesley Publishing Company, 1997); and *How Brains Think: Evolving Intelligence, Then and Now* by William H. Calvin (New York: Basic Books, 1996).

6   Dr. Jose M. R. Delgad has stated this as: "To act is to choose one motor pattern from among the many available possibilities and inhibitions are continually acting to suppress inappropriate or socially unacceptable activities." See "Intracerebral Mechanisms and Future Education," *New York State Education,* February 1968, p. 17.

7   James Doran, director of Algonquin Reading Camp, Rhinelander, Wisconsin, has demonstrated to me a simple, quick technique for giving students a sense of pattern that produces startling gains in their competency in spelling. His brain-compatible methods also produce large, rapid gains in reading.

Editor's Note: For truly surprising gains in reading, see *The Auditory Discrimination in Depth* (ADD) and the Visualizing and Verbalizing for Improved Comprehension programs by Lindamood- Bell. For information, contact the Lindamood-Bell Reading Processes Center, San Luis Obispo, California 1/800-233-8756.

8   Editor's Note: Self-esteem or self-concept programs have long had a questionable base, primarily a "touchy-feely" approach aimed at "feeling good about yourself" as a result of others telling you that you are a "good person" (sometimes in the face of evidence to the contrary). Current brain research tells a different story about the brain producing

and receiving its own opiate-like molecules as a response to mental programs that work, to a sense of competence in handling the world. See *Molecules of Emotion: Why You Feel the Way You Feel* by Candace B. Pert, Ph.D. (New York: Scribner, 1997); *The Growth of the Mind and the Endangered Origins of Intelligence* by Stanley I. Greenspan, M.D., with Beryl Lieff Benderly (New York: Addison-Wesley Publishing Company, 1997), p. 104; and "The Neurobiology of Self-Esteem and Aggression" by Robert Sylwester *(Educational Leadership,* February, 1997, Volume 54, No. 5), pp. 75-78.

9 Editor's Note: Parents might well ask if this over-emphasis on valuing of performance by a second person might not also contribute to the extraordinary power of peer groups and peer pressure during the teen years (and beyond). See Alfie Kohn, *Punished by Rewards: The Trouble with Gold Stars, Incentive Plans, A's, Praise, and Other Bribes* (Boston: Houghton Mifflin, 1993) and *Beyond Discipline: From Compliance to Community* (Alexandria, Virginia: ASCD, 1996).

10 Millions of teachers and other instructors have been taught that learning is something that causes a change in student behavior — unless, of course, that change is due to something else. Hilgard has offered a well-known version: "Learning is the process by which an activity originates or is changed through reacting to an encountered situation, provided that the characteristics of the change in activity cannot be explained on the basis of native response tendencies, maturation, or temporary states of the organism (e.g., fatigue, drugs, etc)." This effort, while perhaps better than some, seems manifestly useless and almost double-talk. In using the terms reacting and response Hilgard clearly suggests that learners are passive, rather than the active, aggressive creatures humans obviously are. Hilgard adds: "The definition is not formally satisfactory because of the many unde-fined terms in it but it will do to call attention to the problems involved in any definition of learning." With that estimate few will disagree. The problems, of course, arise from trying to use bits of rat-based theory rather than comprehensive, human, brain-based theory. Ernest R. Hilgard and Gordon H. Bower, *Theories of Learning, 3d ed.* (New York: Appleton-Century-Crofts, 1966), p. 2.

11 To quote Luria: "According to these concepts, any animal or human activity, complex in its organization, is determined by a program that ensures, not only that the subject reacts to actual stimuli, but within certain limits foresees the future, foretells the probability that a particular event may happen, will be prepared if it does happen and, as a result, prepares a program of behavior." See *Human Brain and Psychological Processes* (New York: Harper & Row, 1966), p. 531.

For a recent discussion of programs, see David Perkins' discussion of "realms" in *Outsmarting IQ: The Emerging Science of Learnable Intelligence* (New York: The Free Press/Simon and Schuster, 1995), especially pp. 249-265.

12 The notion that perception is largely a passive process, and that stimuli impinge on the brain or senses freely, prevails widely but conflicts with a large, solid body of literature on perception that shows, in fact, that the brain selects what stimuli it will attend to and usually seeks out the input it desires, which is then elaborately processed. Reading and watching television often are described as passive activities but actually involve intense mental, and some motor, operations. (To see at all, the eyes must constantly quiver rapidly!)

13 Editor's Note: To pinpoint what we want at the end of a lesson or unit of study is a much more difficult task than it would seem. Two major reform efforts, behavioral objectives in the 1970s and outcomes education in the 1980s, have come and gone, leaving little if any change in the curriculum-testing cycle. As for portfolio assessment, the jury is still out.

Oddly enough, parents seem to have a better intuitive grasp of what constitutes learning than we educators. Perhaps the most common criteria of learning by parents is "Because he talks about it all the time. . . because she does something with it, often using it in ways that surprise us." As Hart says, "most useful information is embedded in programs."

The Kovalik ITI model identifies the challenge with two questions: What do you want students to understand? And, what do you want them to <u>do</u> with what they understand? ("Do" in this case means applying what is understood in real-world applications.)

14 Teachers "driving" a conventional class and initiating most activity have little chance to observe what students do on their own. In good "open," Montessori, or similar settings, teachers can readily become observers because they have time and can be more detached. Students feel relaxed, absorbed in their work rather than on guard against criticism or a bad mark.

10

PROSTERS: STORING AND SELECTING PROGRAMS

> Our perceptions do not come simply from the objects
> around us but from our past experience as functioning,
> purposive organisms. We take a large number of clues,
> none of which is reliable, add them together and make
> what we can of them. All that this gives us is an estimate
> of our surroundings. It is never exactly right. It is never
> the same for different individuals.
>
> — Earl C. Kelley[1]

Much that I present in this book represents synthesis. When
dealing with the awesome human brain[2] and all its complexity,
one is well advised to "stand on the shoulders of giants" whenever
possible. The concept of *proster*, however, is original, at least in
simplifying and visualizing the complex function of our brain. It
is useful in obtaining a fresh look at the issues of curriculum and
instruction.[3]

As we observe human behavior in terms of program, it quickly
becomes evident that we must deal with a huge number of programs, any of which may have many variations. And they cover an
enormous range of complexity, from the relatively simple one of
nodding the head to signify approval, to the thousands of gross

steps required to play a Chopin etude on the piano. These gross movements in turn utilize smaller, finer programs that bend fingers and wrists to the exact degree, for example, to press the keys so as to achieve the intended emotional effect.

Similarly, language requires a tremendous number of programs. One must develop not only the complex muscular sequences for *uttering* each word but also many variations for giving it the loudness, tone, and emotional color needed to convey the desired message.[4] To *write* the word, separate programs are needed for cursive writing, printing, and typewriting or keyboarding. Lettering the word with a brush or felt marker calls for still more variations. We also need *recognition* programs to understand what we hear or see.

DEALING WITH COMPLEXITY: THE NEED FOR COLLECTIONS OF PROGRAMS

As we deal with the real, and therefore complex, world, we find we need a *collection* of programs for almost any sort of action. For instance, we constantly deal with *doors* which we variously operate by pushing, pulling, pressing a latch, turning a knob, pressing a bar, pushing in a button, pulling on a handle, or sliding to one side or up. We do not ordinarily give much attention to the variety of doors and ways of operating them; since we have learned a good deal about doors, there is no need as a rule to do so unless one of our acquired "door" programs aborts, obliging us to consciously think about it.

We go though a day implementing a great variety of programs, drawing from the huge stock we have stored. As a rule we have no more need to think about this process than we do about breathing (another very complex process). Once we have a few years' experience of the world, we get so used to complexity that we usually ignore it. If we look at a handyman's shop, the array of tools suggests the many ways of dealing with wood and metal. An inspection of a kitchen reveals hundreds of tools, utensils, devices, machines, and materials for the production of meals. Look about your own home; it's no wonder "Simplify your life!" has become the rallying cry of the 90s. Complexity is everywhere and relentlessly increasing.

THE PROSTER THEORY

The term proster is a neologism, from a compression of the words *program structure* (pronounced "prosster").

Proster Theory Defined

A proster is *a collection of programs, all for the same general purpose.* A proster for locomotion would provide programs for walking, running, going uphill or down, hopping, jogging, skipping, and so forth. All relate to the pattern of advancing by repeated steps of some kind. All the programs have the common purpose of getting to some other place on foot. The programs are represented in Figure 10 on page 177 as loops because a program can be "run off" much the way a loop of magnetic tape can be run off on a tape player. And, like a tape player, *only one program at a time can be selected and put into use.*

A music proster provides programs for singing, beating time, playing the piano or guitar, or whatever one can do. (If you know nothing about playing the trumpet, there is no such program in the proster and no way you can select it. Note again that we can only select a program if it is there because we built it previously or acquired it genetically before birth.)

A car-driving proster would include programs for starting, steering, controlling speed, making left or right turns, braking, etc. The proster of a beginning driver would be far less elaborate than that of an old hand. In general, a person we would term an "expert" on a particular subject will have built, stored, and refined a much greater number and assortment of applicable patterns and programs for that subject than most people. This concept gives us, I believe, a much sharper image of "expert" than the usual definitions and helps show why the expert can often quickly solve a problem that baffles others or can quickly and seemingly effortlessly learn large amounts of new information related to their area of expertise.

In simplest terms, a proster is a conceptual diagram of how the brain is organized to take action on the world. It is based on the physical structure of the brain. When the neurons in the cortex are studied, they are seen to be arranged in columns and layers, with some major connections of columns.[5]

Figure 9.

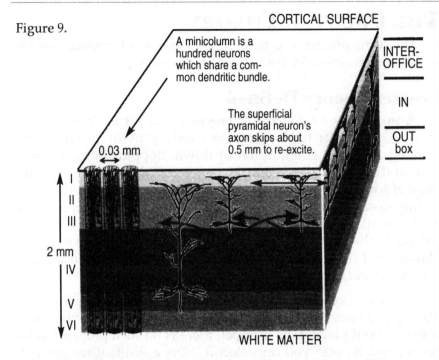

Source: *How Brains Think: Evolving Intelligence, Then and Now*
by William Calvin

The brain does not randomly scatter information about, storing information higgledy piggledy, but rather establishes an "address," or column, and stores related data in that column.[6] These columns specialize, so to speak, in an area of operation such as driving a car or working on a computer. In Proster Theory terms these columns in the brain are seen as prosters containing programs related to that area of operation.

Figure 10 illustrates how prosters contain a set or group of programs (shown as loops). The diagram also illustrates layers of subordinate prosters developed to handled related but more specialized tasks. For example, a locomotion proster (for climbing stairs) with its subordinate program (selected) for climbing a ladder—a modification or refinement of general "climbing stairs"; and the third layer of subordinate programs provides a still more detailed program for climbing a ladder with a large bucket of paint in one's hand! This structure illustrates one of the most striking (and valuable) aspects of human attributes: the ability to endlessly refine programs to more and more specific functions.

Prosters in Action

In Chapters 7-9, I suggested that we select a program by first *detecting and recognizing the pattern*. When still relatively unfamiliar with the pattern or when needing to take action (by selecting a program) as a result of it, we "categorize down" to finer consider-ations. For example, we identify an object as a door; the sign "push" or the door's construction tells us which way it opens; we identify the knob as the type that twists. We perceive all this so easily that we ordinarily pay no attention to the process. Also, in the cerebellum, the "little brain," we have built muscular coordi-nation programs that we now call upon to know approximately how hard to push or pull the door and how much to twist the knob. (Observe a child of three trying to do these same things and it is apparent how much learning is required.)

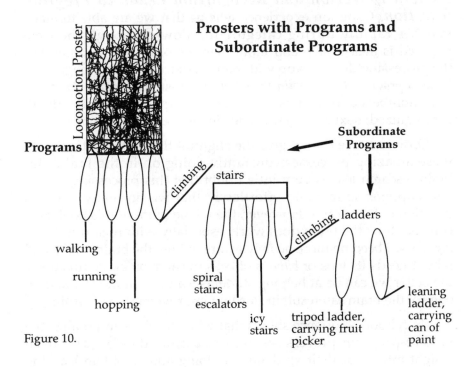

Figure 10.

The Role of Prior Experience. As we enter a dark room in our own home, one arm reaches out for the unseen light switch, our fingers locate the lever or button and apply just the needed pressure — all "automatically." In a strange house, however, it is not as easy. We must pay attention to look and feel for the switch — our grasp of the *patterns* of light switch locations gives us a good idea of where to hunt for it. Because we have to explore various possibilities and do not know just what kind of switch we are seeking (lever, button, twist, pull-chain), an observer might call us clumsy or dull-witted for taking fifteen seconds, rather than one, to turn on the lights. However, a visitor from an Arabian desert, say, ignorant of our wiring patterns, might have even more trouble — illustrating again the often overlooked fact that *one's stock of patterns and programs reflects* **experience** *much more than something called intelligence.*

Pattern Detection and Recognition Leads to Program Selection. Common experience tells us that we are able to make matches rapidly during categorizing down — though the time required is measurable and more than we ordinarily assume. But the processing doesn't stop with pattern detection and recognition. Next, *a program to deal with the situation* must be selected from the huge numbers of programs stored. For example, the pattern "door" is recognized; next a program is needed to *operate* that door.

Ordinarily we do not give the slightest thought or attention to these amazing processes constantly going on in the brain. But brain research leaves very little doubt that this processing occurs and happens so fast and effortlessly that we normally have no occasion to focus on it. However, the whole point of this book is to consider how the brain does work, especially with regard to *learning.* As we become more acutely aware of how the brain works and why it needs its tens of *billions* of cells to carry on all its functions, the better we can be at helping students learn. Even modest knowledge of the brain can result in startling improvements in learning.

(In-school experience shows that when teachers internalize the pattern-program process we are discussing, they acquire fresh insight into what their students are doing and so obtain learning jumps that can be astonishingly rapid . . . and that, of course, makes the work of teaching far more rewarding. "It's as if I can now see the process going on!" a teacher may say.)

The Brain Is Not Passive; We Act Upon the World. We must also become more aware of one other principle, perhaps obvious enough once we consider it: In life *we act upon the world.* We do not doze like a cat until a "stimulus" happens by and then "react" to it. As humans, we take the initiative almost moment by moment, constantly deciding what to do next, from turning a page or eating a cookie to starting a course of study or beginning a long-term political project, all through the pattern-program cycle.

THE PATTERN-PROGRAM CYCLE

Moment by moment we have to go through the cycle of

1. Evaluating and recognizing the PATTERN we are dealing with

2. Selecting the most appropriate PROGRAM(S) from those we have stored

3. Implementing that program

This, I submit, is one of the constants of human behavior. Every possessor of a human brain uses this procedure, although few indeed currently are aware of that fact. Support for this broad concept is found throughout much of the modern scientific literature. My particular phrasing helps clarify the work of teachers in producing student learning and, even more, to throw light on what *learning* means. (Other phraseology may be acceptable; the constant applies in all situations, not only instructional.)

A New View of Learning

We can also see here that *building programs, enriching the proster, refining the subordinate programs, are fundamental aspects of learning.*[7] Teachers can obtain a clear image of what they are trying to do by direct instruction or arranging the instructional situation. Clearly it is not "transmitting knowledge" except incidentally. *The new focus of instruction is to increase the student's ability to act upon the world in a useful and appropriate way, by being able to recognize more patterns and to learn and implement more appropriate programs.*

The Complexities Behind Selecting a Program

The selection of a program to implement is anything but mechanical or simple. First, the input comes from other parts of the brain which have detected and recognized patterns within current sensory input and/or prior experience and arrives at the proster which contains a collection (we might say "inventory") of programs, any one of which might be selected if judged appropriate for implementation. Second, when faced with the need to act or, more precisely, to select a program, the brain finds a pertinent proster by categorizing down. The problem then becomes one of *selecting the program in the proster that promises to be most appropriate for the purpose.* Only one program can be switched on at a time — but which one (trying to turn on a program for going upstairs and at the same time one for going down wouldn't work at all!).[8]

Here we come to a fundamental aspect of the nature of the brain. Neurons connect richly to other neurons, via the tiny gap junctions called *synapses* (as well as from various information substances from throughout the bodybrain), with two quite opposite effects: to help *excite* the next neuron into firing or to *inhibit* it from firing. Obviously, at any given moment, the great majority of the programs stored in the brain are inhibited or switched "off," much as most of the dozens of switches in our household are normally in the off position. *In the brain, a program will be implemented only when the total of excitatory impulses ("on" or "go") exceeds the total of inhibitory impulses ("off" or "wait").*

For a familiar analogy we need look no further than the nearest state legislature. Some of the legislators strongly favor a bill, which others vigorously oppose; the reasons for support or opposition scatter. But if the total *for* (excitatory or "go") exceeds the total *against* (inhibitory or "wait"), the bill passes.

This process is anything but neat or "logical" but a decision is reached. Even in a legislature of only a few hundred members, the influences can be too complex to analyze; in the brain we are dealing with millions or billions of influences, particularly when we add in the hundreds of "information substances" which include the classical neurotransmitters as well as steroids and peptides.

I call the cumulative effect of these vast numbers of influences *biases*.

Biases: Why We Select the Program (Behavior) We Do

Bias is both a common term and an engineering term. In common speech we may say that we consider some opinion or criticism or attitude "biased" rather than equitable or fair — probably reflecting some sort of previous experience or relationship.

The engineering term *bias* may be less familiar but we can grasp the essential meaning if we think of the wall thermostat in our home that controls the furnace. By moving a little lever, the thermostat can be set, or biased, to turn on the furnace at 68^0 or it can be biased so that heat will not come on until the room gets down to 65^0.

The biasing affecting a proster is very complex, reflecting not only current incoming biasing but also the sum of what is stored in the brain relating to this proster that results from experience; from plans, aims, and fears; older brain influences; and from information substances produced by the body and brain. In Figure 11 on page 183, biases are shown as side influences that determine how readily any particular program in the proster will turn on and be used.[9] The plus and minus signs shown next to each program suggest, in very simplified fashion, the total of "go" and "wait" influences on each one. In the graphic, Program M is the program selected, the "winner" of the most excitatory responses.

This is simply to say that the decision within the proster will be based on the huge amount of experience stored in the brain (*that particular* brain!) as it emerges from the "legislative" process boiled down to a simple for-or-against or plus-or-minus value. To be more precise, we have to go beyond experience to include in the biases plans and hopes for the future plus current conditions and emotions that apply.

If Biases Don't Change, Behavior Doesn't Change. Let's look at Figure 11 on page 183 again and ask another question: "If Program M was selected the first time, what program will be selected next week or two months from now?" The answer — a very important one to teachers, both in terms of subject content and behavior/misbehavior — is Program M. Here we see a crucial aspect of this whole mechanism: *If the biases do not change, the program selection will not change, whether it be a day later or ten years later. The decision the proster makes always reflects the total influences of all the biases as of the moment.*[10]

Ordinarily, we do not probe much into why other people behave (make their decisions) as they do; we may find it hard enough to understand our own. Teachers in conventional classrooms, busy "teaching" and not focused on the brain, only occasionally hazard guesses which may be far off the mark even if they could ever find out. However, as we begin to apply brain-compatible approaches, we enter a new and surprising world, one that will likely feel strange for a while. Proster Theory, experience shows, ordinarily requires some months to learn—although some of the benefits of applying it in any instructional situation usually become apparent in a few weeks.

In reality, of course, our biases are constantly being modified by the world we are experiencing, sometimes subtly and marginally, and on rare occasion, more significantly. As has been noted, the decision-making in prosters tends to be enormously complex, routinely involving millions of influences. Human decisions, even on a conscious level, usually involve a pro and con balancing of many factors. For example, a student may feel it wise to study for tomorrow's classes yet be reluctant to miss a favorite television show. An adult may consider purchasing a pair of shoes, weighing how much he needs them and the inviting price against other things he needs. a lack of time to try on the shoes properly, and some previous problems with this kind of footwear. A job offer may call for a decision much more complex, with many factors on one side and a list of negatives and uncertainties on the other. These go/wait decisions rest on fairly evident biasing, the sum of pro and of con reasons, many of them from "feelings," others much more complex and subtle.

IMPLICATIONS OF THE PROSTER THEORY

While the proster concept leaves many unanswered questions about brain functioning, it does seem to advance understanding to a degree. For the educator, especially, some quite sharp conclusions emerge.

Conclusion #1: No Program, No Behavior

A program *not* in the proster cannot be used. The needed program may never have been built. *Or it may be stored but at another "address" in the brain in another proster.*

"No program, no behavior" is a key factor in instruction. First the learner must acquire the program; next, *it must also be addressed*

Figure 11.

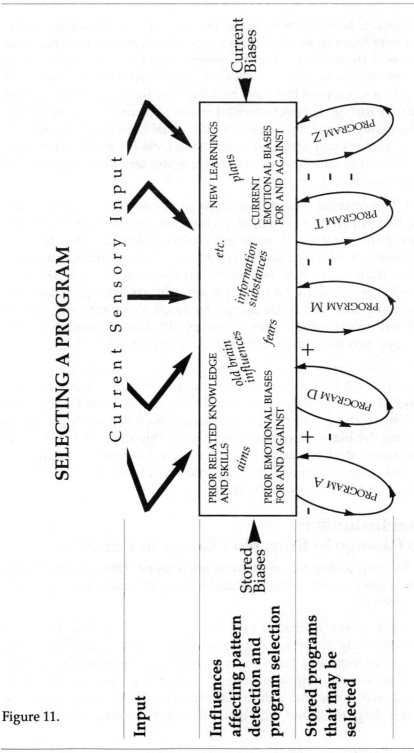

SELECTING A PROGRAM

Input

Current Sensory Input

Current Biases

Influences affecting pattern detection and program selection

Stored Biases

PRIOR RELATED KNOWLEDGE AND SKILLS

aims

old brain influences

fears

information substances

etc.

NEW LEARNINGS

plans

PRIOR EMOTIONAL BIASES FOR AND AGAINST

CURRENT EMOTIONAL BIASES FOR AND AGAINST

Stored programs that may be selected

PROGRAM A   PROGRAM D   PROGRAM M   PROGRAM T   PROGRAM Z

so it remains available for use in the proper context. For example, a student may learn to work percentage problems in mathematics class but never think of applying the program to figuring a sales tax or the cost of a bank loan. In civics, one can learn the organization of the city government but have no idea how to obtain some needed information on a governmental matter. Youngsters commonly make heavy use of the telephone for social conversations but—as many parents can testify—fail to make calls for many other purposes, such as announcing late arrival at dinner or canceling dental appointments.

When conventional instruction is dominated by student awareness that impending examinations must be passed, the normal uses of programs *in the real world* get pushed aside or subordinated. Both instructor and student may focus on the test-taking procedure rather than on useful, real-world applications of the skills or knowledge. Asked to write a paragraph, for example, students may make sure that it has a topic sentence at the start; in real life they will worry about what to convey. (In most professional writing, topic sentences more often than not can't be found.)

In many cases the instructional setting provides strong biasing, especially when the content or skill is new to the learner. If the biases of the instructional setting differ sharply from those in the real-life setting, the program learned may not be transferred because the biases don't transfer. We see this demonstrated when a language student can't converse with a foreigner or the person who has prepared and practiced a speech at home has to deliver it to an actual audience of 200 people.

Conclusion #2:
No Change in Bias, No Change in Behavior

So long as the biases remain unchanged, the selection function in the proster will *repeat* and exactly the same program will be selected.

While many instructors believe that varied approaches bring more learning success, nothing is more common in classrooms than reiteration and "review" which seem to express the conviction that the student who did not "get it" the third or fifth time around will somehow gain insight the seventh or tenth time. The proster diagram shows why this is not likely. *To change behavior, the biases must be changed,* not the behavior directly. This is equally true with student misbehavior as with staff failure to implement the skills presented during an inservice training. We may regard this as an earth-shaking rule, the more so because biases are not easily changed—just saying the opposite, by either teacher or learner, does not "re-wire" the brain. Biases prove to be very robust and "tend to disappear only when individuals have gained a great deal of firsthand experience with situations that run counter to the bias or stereotype."[11]

Two critical areas of experience in schools that must be changed are: the *setting* (the small world that a learner inhabits, such as the school-home combination) and the *situation* (the specific circumstances or ambiance immediately surrounding the individual). The student, or teacher, who day after day enters the same room, with the same furnishings, people, and routines, is subjected to many unchanged biases that produce unchanged behavior.[12] Once the influence of such biasing on selection of programs is understood, the often baffling resistance of learners becomes less of a mystery. We can see, too, why our own habits can be so difficult to change. The biases affecting the proster that is selecting the program don't change, so the same choice of program is made. Again, *"to change behavior, change the biases."*

As we consider school reform or "restructuring," the magnitude of this factor becomes evident. To put a teacher in a conventional "cell" classroom and ask for a very different style of instruction and "class management" is obviously futile. The biases, unchanged, will push the teacher right back to the earlier ways of behavior even though the teacher may be enthusiastic about the proposed changes. On the other hand, if the old biases are deliberately and significantly altered (different rooms, changed furnishings, new procedures, and support instead of isolation, to name a few), the opportunity for real change is greatly enhanced.

Fortunately, such changes of setting and situation require little financial resources, just commitment and mindfulness.

Conclusion #3: Current Learning Is Heavily Influenced by Previous Learning

The proster diagram, I believe, can help to remind everyone concerned with instruction that:

All current learning is heavily influenced by previous learning (pattern recognition and programs acquired) and by a vast array of stored biases.

"Now, class," a teacher may say, "we are going to take up a new subject, logarithms" (or mechanical drawing, subatomic particles, baking, Shakespeare's plays, or computer terminal operation). But the students are not passive empty vessels into which new knowledge can be poured. Rather, each learns by aggressively *processing* the new input.[13]And each learner will do that, inescapably, in relation to what that learner *brings* to the new effort.[14]

To illustrate, let us consider three children getting instruction in first-grade reading. One may have had thousands of highly pleasurable hours of experiences with books the second may have had only a few hundred hours of any such exposure; and the third virtually no experience in being read to or handling books but a good deal of being told stories and being sung to. The relevant prosters and biases to these three students differ enormously, yet they will likely be offered substantially uniform instruction. Similarly, of three army recruits being taught to fire a rifle, one may have been brought up with firearms, the second may have never handled a gun and rarely seen one, and the third may be terrified of weapons as a result of an early, traumatic experience. They, too, will likely be given identical instruction.

Though *diagnosis* is a word popular among educators, a candid observer may regard it with some suspicion. Teachers generally lack the time and resources that the medical term implies. In any case, some grasp of the intricacies of brain functioning makes clear the difficulty of "seeing inside someone's head." To offer uniform instruction, and *then* try to diagnose why good learning did not result, seems to me to compound absurdities. The effort to "patch" appears doomed to failure, all the more so when it becomes a sort of ritual cover-up and the diagnosis, even if made by a specialist, gets recorded but not acted upon—an elaborate and expensive way of blaming the victim for the institution's shortcomings.[15]

IN SUMMARY

Only a few dozen years ago, most educators, and the public, regarded the human brain as almost a total mystery. Now, however, as Proster Theory shows, a knowledge base with impressive scientific underpinnings exists in quite accessible form. It can guide both daily and long-term applications in any setting where the prime objective is to produce learning.

Aspects of Proster Theory that have proved in practice to be immediately valuable to teachers in planning and effecting gains in learning include:

1. The brain uses the categorizing-down process extensively, greatly speeded by simultaneous processing along many paths.

2. The brain uses the principle of "the match" by which incoming pattern information matches, more or less exactly, the pattern stored in the brain, or else it is not recognized.

3. The brain seems to be organized as if programs are grouped in prosters of alternative programs for a common purpose. Only one of these programs can be used at one time.

4. Prosters are arranged in hierarchical layers, so that gross programs may be further and further refined or modified to meet slightly differing needs.

5. Neurons influence other neurons either by exciting them (go) or inhibiting them (wait). The total of such influences determines whether a neuron does or does not fire.[16]

6. Similarly, which program in a proster will be selected depends on the total go/wait influences on that program as determined by biases affecting that proster.

7. Biasing involves all that is stored in the brain relevant to a program decision. Biasing arises from experience; from plans, aims, and fears; and from body and older brain influences; and from the current, situational input.

8. If the biases remain unchanged, the program selection will remain unchanged.

9. To effect a change of behavior, or "open a new door" to learning, we must try to change biases, rather than try to change behavior directly.

10. How programs are "addressed" determines where they are stored in prosters and whether they will be utilized in real-world situations.

11. Present learning depends heavily on previous learning and biases stored in the brain of each individual. Giving individuals uniform instruction without regard to what they *bring to* the learning effort virtually guarantees a high incidence of failure.[17]

NOTES

1   Earl C. Kelley, *Education for What Is Real* (New York: Harper and Brothers, 1947), p. 34.

2   Editor's Note: As mentioned earlier, research about the operation of the brainbody partnership is in its early stages and less is known about how the "information substances" carry out their roles as part of the brainbody learning process. Thus, as in preceding chapters, the term "brain" is used as an anchor for our discussions about learning. Clearly, the information substances that travel the intracellular fluids of the body have much to do with biasing as discussed in this chapter. Educators should look forward to the upcoming research on this topic to refine their pictures of how learning takes place and how best to nurture it.

3   Editor's Note: Hart's Proster Theory is a vital contribution to education because it allows a brain-based, rather than a tradition-based, perspective from which to analyze why traditional curriculum fails so many of our students. It also changes our focus when rethinking curriculum—from viewing curriculum as a compilation of "the right stuff" to looking at curriculum development as a pattern-enhancing activity.

4   Stephen D. Krashen points out that the brain must also put the ideas and words in proper order: "What is essentially involved in language production is the programming of an idea, itself containing no intrinsic temporal order, into a sequence of linguistic units, which are also intrinsically unordered." See *The Human Brain* (Englewood Cliffs, New Jersey: Prentice-Hall, 1977), p. 117.

5   Editor's Note: According to William H. Calvin, "Neurons with similar interests tend to be vertically arrayed there, forming cylinders known as cortical columns, which cut through most of the layers. It's almost like a club that self-organizes out of a crowd at a party, where people of similar interests tend to cluster together. We have naturally given names to these cortical clubs. Some of the names reflect their size, some their seeming specialties (so far as we know them). The thin cylinders, or *minicolumns*, are only about 0.03 mm in diameter (that's a very thin hair, closer to the threads of a spider web). The best-known examples of these are the visual cortex's orientation columns, whose neurons seem to like visual objects with a line or border tilted at a particular angle. The neurons in one minicolumn will respond best to boundaries titled at 35º, those in another will like horizontals or verticals, and so forth." (*How Brains Think: Evolving Intelligence, Then and Now.* New York: Basic Books, 1996, p. 118).

6   To further study the complexities of the brain's incredibly intricate structure, my earlier book, *How the Brain Works* (New York: Basic Books, 1975), is a useful next step before plunging into more technical treatments.

Editor's Note: This astounding book reveals how resistant the field of education has been to utilizing the results of brain research. The research upon which Hart based *How the Brain Works* occurred more than 25 years ago! Surprisingly, the research during the past quarter of a century has not invalidated the findings Hart discussed in significant ways. Instead, the concepts described have been expanded (what was thought to be "the" story is now know to be but part of the story,) fine-tuned, and shown to be more complex. The reader can rest assured the brain described in this book is not a fad nor will it go away.

For a more recent reader-friendly publication, see *Magic Trees of the Mind: How to Nurture Your Child's Intelligence, Creativity, and Health Emotions from Birth Through Adolescence* by Marian Diamond and Janet Hopson (New York: A Dutton Book, 1998). See also the bibliography at the back of this book.

7   Editor's Note: Once we adopt the development of programs (Proster Theory) as our new goal for learning, true-false and multiple choice tests begin to look like the pale, inadequate substitutes for learning that they are. We must look for assessment tools that match this new definition of learning.

8   Editor's Note: While this example—simultaneous selection of a program for going upstairs and for downstairs—may sound ridiculous, rapid switching from near-opposite programs often occurs during times of near-panic during which a person tries one response to the situation, fears it won't work, and in a split second abandons it in favor of another, then another, and another. Comedy routines often include such examples of Proster Theory in action.

9   Editor's Note: William Calvin captures a similar idea with his analogy of "competing choruses"; groups of neurons fire simultaneously in response to a set of input, attempting to get others to join their song. The winning song is the response selected among the competing possibilities. See *How Brains Think: Evolving Intelligence, Then and Now* (New York: Basic Books, 1996).

10 Editor's Note: This is a critical issue. In the case of curriculum content, students do not come to us as blank slates. What we might think is "new" to students is unlikely to be responded to free of biasing. Nor can we be assured that an "old" topic will be remembered as it was last taught. For example, in the wonderfully

revealing video *Private Universe,* graduating Harvard students are asked the question, "What makes the seasons?" The overwhelming majority respond with a version of the sun is closer to the earth during the summer and thus hotter. Whether the responder had taken lots of science, including advanced planetary motion, or none, the proster that fired was a version of "Hot, baby, hot," learned as an infant, i.e., the closer to the source of heat, the hotter it is. Subsequent information about the near-perfect circular orbit of the earth around the sun had insufficient excitatory power and the childhood version won out. While very common and frustrating in the field of science, this issue occurs across all subjects. Likewise, English teachers can attest to how hard it is for students to learn to suppress "ain't" or "Me and (Joe). . . ."

Application of the Proster Theory to the area of behavior/misbehavior is equally fascinating. Pat Belvel, educational consultant from San Jose, California, encourages teachers to examine persistent misbehavior not as a deliberate attempt to get the teacher's goat but as a teaching opportunity: Either the student doesn't know (have a program for) the correct behavior or knows too many of the wrong behaviors (the proster is loaded with inappropriate responses that are loaded to fire with little excitatory push).

11 Gardner, Howard. *The Unschooled Mind: How Children Think and How Schools Should Teach* (New York: BasicBooks, 1991), p. 172

12 See Leslie A. Hart, "Necessary Ingredients for Retraining Teachers," *Bulletin,* National Association of Secondary School Principals, December, 1973.

13 Editor's Note: Although developed outside the fields of brain research, the constructivist theory of curriculum is consistent with Proster Theory in its core belief that students must construct their own version of a concept, that information cannot be poured into students' brains in a uniform way with uniform result .

14 Jerome Kagan has stated this succinctly: "When we say that a new entity is learned, we mean that an element is connected with a second element that already has been learned. No act, idea, image or word is learned in isolation or ever becomes completely isolated. Every mind consists

of nests of interconnected elements that are continually being reorganized with use. Practice of a skill has the inevitable consequence of making that skill more autonomous and more likely to operate as one unit, rather than a sequence of separate elements" (in Proster Theory terms, one program). "Psychologists Advance Efforts to Probe the Mind," *The New York Times,* January 12, 1970, Education section, p. 72.

15 See a pilot study on reading, for example: A. Weinshank, *The Relationship Between Diagnosis and Remediation in Reading* (East Lansing, MI: The Institute for Research on Teaching, 1979). It found that the clinicians gave four times as many diagnostic as treatment statements, with only moderate relationship of problem to treatment, and used a core set of five treatments to blanket almost all cases. Other studies and observations have shown only a faint connection between diagnosis and subsequent effective treatment.

16 To be technically correct, it should be noted that individual neurons may spontaneously fire. What one or a few neurons do in the brain has no significance among the billions active.

17 In passing, we should also note that uniform instruction may also result in teaching students what they already know. Their subsequent success on an examination may then be taken as outcome of this unneeded, wasteful, and boring reinstruction. For example, a study recently conducted in six Long Island, New York, school districts by Educational Products Exchange Institute, funded by the National Institute of Education, tested fourth graders on the contents of a mathematics text before they used it. Sixty percent scored 80 or above.

11

THE ROLE OF EMOTIONS IN LEARNING

When a person does an intrinsically disliked task because he fears not to do it, it is always necessary to confine him. This is what happens to animals in many psychological experiments. . . . Under such circumstances the creature is likely to seem more stupid than it really is, and to learn much less efficiently than it would in its natural habitat, where it is positively motivated.

Exactly the same is often true of children in school. Parents, teachers, and everyone else concerned are so used to the idea that children will not go to school unless they are made to go, will not stay there unless they must, will not behave "properly" unless compelled to, and will not attend to lessons if there is a chance to do anything else, that they take it all for granted. . . . But human nature is only that way under certain conditions, and particularly under conditions of negative motivation.

—James C. Murselli[1]

Editor's Note: Our first window into the role of emotion and learning came through the triune brain theory proposed by Dr. Paul MacLean in the mid-1950s (see Chapter 5). Twenty years later, Leslie Hart put the triune brain theory to practical use. Coining the term "downshifting," to describe how emotions of the faster-moving limbic system overshadowed the slower moving cerebral cortex, Hart effectively argued for the need to create absence of threat in order to prevent downshifting or, more accurately today, "emotional override," and thus nurture academic learning, a task of the cerebral cortex. His discussion of the importance of creating and maintaining absence of threat is retained here as it is as relevant as ever.

Another 20 years later and brain research has expanded our knowledge of the role of emotions. With technology allowing us to "see" molecules in action, we now know the very molecules that convey emotion as they travel throughout the body. Thus, creating absence of threat is just the beginning of designing an environment that most enhances learning. The second part of this chapter therefore outlines some of those additional elements.

When this chapter first appeared, it was entitled "The Triune Brain: Emotions, Downshifting." With minor editing, including a slight title change and substitution of the term "emotional override" for "downshifting," the content of the chapter is useful and is presented here to again illustrate the point that brain research of the 1990s has expanded our pictures of how the brain works rather than invalidated them. Much that Hart recommended 15 years ago may surprise you with its relevance for the 21st century. The latter part of the chapter, in the same font style as is this editor's note, brings the reader up to date and offers suggestions for applying recent discoveries about the role of emotions in learning.

LEARNING AND EMOTION

Learning involves emotions. Biasing (a key concept in Proster Theory), the triune brain concept, and some human history throw light on emotions that appear to be of great potential value in education.

Learning and Emotion Are Inseparable

It has long been recognized that in practice emotion cannot be separated from cognitive thinking.[2] One feels fear *because* a situation has been recognized as calling for fear. To be angry at an insult, we must first recognize that we have been insulted. To mourn a lost friend, we must grasp the pattern of death and its consequences. Most of the emotion we feel *follows* pattern recognition that often can be very subtle, as when a new wife feels that her husband's family is gradually warming to her, or an employee gathers that changes in the business are reducing his influence and value. A student may "read" tiny signals from a teacher that convey developing hostility, and so feel growing alarm.[3]

The Role of Emotion in Resetting Physical Biases.

Emotion as a word may lead us to think of love, sorrow, poetic ideas, and the arts but understanding its less ethereal aspects leads to consideration of blood pressure, oxygen use, and homeostasis or balancing of body systems. The oldest function of emotional shifts, it is now clear, was to change the biasing of these systems.

Imagine a wild rabbit quietly feeding in an open patch of grass. Its internal systems are biased at a low setting. But now the rabbit catches a glimpse of — possibly — a fox in a nearby group of bushes. Cognitively, the rabbit's highest level of brain decides "that could be a predator in there" and, in effect, sounds a general alarm. This is done, in all mammals, primarily by means of chemical messengers, moving through the bloodstream. The brain signals various glands to release the appropriate alarm hormones into the blood and these lead to the resetting of a group of biases. The rabbit's heartbeat increases, as does the breathing rate; muscles tense for action; digestion stops. The new biases ready the animal for action. (Editor's Note: Fear mechanisms are centered in the amygdala. Most episodes of fear are triggered within the limbic area. Some, however, as in this example, are the result of the cortex recognizing a previously learned pattern resulting in the—"Hmm . . . oh . . . oh oh, look out!" response.)

Now the fox charges. The biases, influenced by further hormonal signals (the term hormone derives from the Greek for "urge on"), push over to extreme settings. What happens in the next few seconds will determine whether the rabbit survives or dies, so a supreme effort must be made — energy will be used at a rate that can be sustained only for a few minutes. The rabbit bounds off in an all-out effort to escape.

The same resetting of biases, of course, occurs in the fox. As its brain interprets the pattern to mean "that could be my next meal," its glands pour out the messengers to prepare the entire body for the extreme effort of attack.

The Role of Emotions in Resetting Mental Biases. As humans, we have largely escaped this kind of drama, a daily event for less complicated creatures. Although as a pedestrian one may leap for the safety of the sidewalk when surprised by an approaching car, or as a skier desperately swerve to avoid a rock while coming down a slope, most of us live such relatively safe lives that this violent resetting of biases seldom becomes necessary. Therefore, we commonly turn to active sports, travel, gambling, business risks, new ventures, and "taking a chance" quite voluntarily, to put more excitement into our lives. On any weekend, hundreds of stadiums fill with roaring spectators, obtaining at second hand the thrill of victory and the agony of defeat, as one broadcaster put it. On a still milder level, people engage in card and board games, nonhazardous activities such as tennis, bowling, or horseshoe pitching, where competing tends to move the biasing to a higher—but comfortable—level. Or we may challenge ourselves with puzzles, self-imposed tasks such as jogging five miles, or choose a game of golf which has been deliberately contrived to be full of trials and obstacles.

We must note here the difference between voluntarily accepted and chosen risks, and *externally imposed hazards.* Being mugged on the street, or sent into armed combat in war, brings one back to the rabbit and the fox. In children, we can observe readily the gleefully *selected* risk—climb this tree, wade this puddle, walk this wall, jump off this high place—that involves physical challenge, and equivalent more cognitive challenges (that of course involve physical activities) such as putting together a model, learning to operate a computer, or building a tree house. *What risks a person will want to take, to what degree, clearly is a highly individual matter,* with children as well as adults. *That there exists a deep human need to select and take risks seems hardly arguable;* but when in instructional situations students are directed and coerced *to take risks not of their choosing,* the need is little met. Risk becomes threat.

Emotions and Body Language

Emotions are physically expressed, and readily detectable. If spouses meet for dinner at a restaurant, one may quickly become aware that something is bothering the other, though nothing specific has been said. Joining a social group, one can realize a slight hostility exists—perhaps some remark has just been made, or an interruption has been inadvertently caused. Parents will often sense emotion in a child returning to the home. As previously noted, students usually show great sensitivity to teacher emotions.

When we remind ourselves that humans have long been highly social animals used to living in close quarters all the way back to caves, small tents, and earliest buildings, we can see the value of this. To get along in such circumstances, *it is essential to give and receive signals.* A cat approached by a dog may raise its fur, assume a tall stance that facilitates a sudden swipe of claws, and put mouth and ears in warning position. The signals given can hardly be missed. Human signals most often are subtle, so much so that we may have difficulty describing them in words. Extremely slight changes in posture, in muscle tension, in breathing, in eye movement and pupil size can be detected. (As in all human matters, individuals differ. We neither emit signals in the same fashion nor interpret them uniformly.) While probably the old mammalian brain still has charge of emitting the signal, only the new, great neocortex has the resources to detect fine pattern changes and interpret their message.

BEING HUMAN: BUILT-IN DRIVE TO RESET BIASES

All of this points to one major characteristic of being human that often is not seen, or is lost in layers of confusion: we are creatures that have a deeply built-in drive to *frequently reset body biases*—to exercise rebiasing rather than lead a placid, cow-like existence. If our work and daily routine does not provide enough shifting of bias, we actively seek out risk, competition, art, music, theatre, and other activities that cause shifts. Sad, thrilling, romantic, and horrifying theatrical entertainments all draw audiences (but again, with strong individual preferences.)

Volatility of Biases and Students

What we may call *volatility of biases* is associated with youth. Children can move from anger to laughter in seconds. People strike us as old, whatever their actual years, if their biases seem fixed in a narrow range, while a person of 90 who displays much volatility strikes us as remarkably youthful even if immobilized in a wheel chair.

Though the volatility of children decreases rapidly and steadily from eight months to 18 years, the high volatility of youth relates importantly to instruction. *The teacher or school or system that attempts to suppress or routinize emotion in students, or take a group rather than an individual approach, is flying in the face of deep human needs.* Many who teach suspect this intuitively; not all know what to do about it, especially within the rigid class-and-grade structure. Suppression of emotional content makes classes boring and "flat" — as students often complain.

But emotions have even larger implications for instruction. We must consider the effect of *threat.*

THE POWER OF THREAT

A student brings into the classroom not only personal but also species history — millions of years of evolution, very much present in the nature of the brain. The reptilian brain,[4] by virtue of being relatively small and capable of only crude decisions, can make its decisions quickly. Our species exists because over great periods of time such brains made decisions well enough and fast enough to survive when life or death hung on the next second or two of activity, as with our rabbit. The much larger old mammalian brain introduced a compromise: a brain far more complex and therefore slower to make decisions but on the other hand much better able to detect and interpret situations (patterns) and to store and execute many more programs. But the huge neocortex that developed became impossibly too big and intricate, I submit, to make quick action decisions. So there arose another compromise: the newest brain was superb for pattern discrimination and the storage of a vast collection of programs and was therefore a brain that enabled humans to adapt to and innovate living conditions as no creature on earth ever had before. But it had to rely on the older brain structures, especially the limbic area with its rich concentrations of receptors to receive information from the information substances flowing throughout the body (see Chapter 5), when speed survival decisions were needed.

Emotional Override

Thus we have the phenomenon, readily observable in ourselves and others, including students, that I have called "downshifting" or emotional override. When the individual detects *threat* in an immediate situation, *full use of the great new cerebral brain is suspended and faster-acting, simpler brain resources take larger roles.*

In at least a rough way, the degree of emotional override will reflect the degree of threat—always, of course, in individual terms. A severe threat to one person may be of little consequence to another.

One of the most familiar examples of violent emotional override occurs in automobile collisions, an experience few of us escape. We are driving along in comfort; suddenly an impact brings the crunch of metal and screech of brakes. Let us say no one has been hurt. But a half hour later the participants realize how much of our memory of the event has been "washed out." What was the color and make of the other vehicle? How many people were in it? Who was driving? What other cars were around? What was the sequence of events? Detail may be very hard to recall—witnesses to violent happenings notoriously differ widely in their reports of what happened, what people did or looked like, and what was said.

What occurred under the threat of violence, I suggest, was a quick emotional override. Passengers in the car that was hit probably "ducked," using a program from the reptilian brain to pull in the head to the chest, throw up the arms to protect the face, and raise the knees to defend the vulnerable belly area. The old mammalian brain ordered hormones into the blood stream causing, a few minutes later, a knot in the pit of the stomach and trembling legs. The limbic system took charge, but since this brain has no interest in makes and models of cars and rules of traffic, and lacks the pattern discrimination ability of the neocortex, it cannot provide the detail the police officer or an insurance company may request.

Sources of Threat

The sources of threat are many; some are triggered by instinct, others learned. Threat is a result of individual perception. What one person perceives as a threat may seem of little consequence to the next person.

Physical Attack and Confinement. The fundamental basis of threat, as that term is used in Proster Theory, is fear of physical harm. Deep in our DNA is the ancient fear of predators who could quickly kill or of death from natural forces such as a landslide, earthquake, volcano eruption, flood, storm. Equally strong is fear of any kind of captivity that could mean impending death. For many tens of millions of years of our evolutionary line, inability to move freely has implied just that, and confinement threatens right down to the reptilian level. *The confinement of the school, of the classroom, of having to stay in a small area or in a specific seat stands as no exception.*

Separation. Another source of threat to humans is separation from parents in childhood, especially the mother, and then later, as some independence is gained, from the home group. For perspective here we must go back to the long ages of hunting and gathering in small bands; to lose contact with the band would usually mean great anxiety, suffering, and probably unpleasant death. Status within the band, we can feel reasonably sure, became an elaboration of being in or being out, and observation shows loss of status within what the individual regards as a home group to be a serious, sometimes devastating threat. (A home group is one the individual perceives in that light, not merely a group into which he or she is thrust, as for example the classroom, a military company, or an enforced work team.) Finally, since humans characteristically acquire possessions which may have both practical usefulness as well as status value, the threat of loss of possessions can be substantial in some circumstances.

The Impact of Threat on Learning

If we now remind ourselves that virtually all academic and vocational learning heavily involves the neocortex, it becomes plain that *absence of threat is utterly essential to effective instruction.* Under threat, emotions override the cerebrum; in effect, to greater or lesser extent, it operates in snatches if at all. To experienced teachers, this shutting down of the newest brain is an old story and a familiar frustration. The threatened child (threatened in the Proster Theory sense) "freezes," seems unable to think, stabs wildly at possible answers, breaks into tears, vomits, or acts up, perhaps to the point of violence.

Since language exists almost wholly in the new brain, emotional override leaves us speechless, quite literally. An unexpected insult, accident, piece of bad news, or other cause of sudden biasing produces even in adults temporary inability to talk, and quite possibly even to grasp what others are saying. Stage fright is similar.

Another manifestation of a sudden emotional override is "being rooted to the spot," often reported by people exposed to an explosion, train wreck, or similar disaster. In war, trained soldiers may fail to fire their weapons or use the tactics long rehearsed. Programs developed in the neocortex simply become unavailable because of the emotional override; the individual does nothing unless the older structures of the brain take charge and the person flees wildly or holes up in some hiding place for shelter.

While rote learning can be accomplished under a good deal of threat, although the threat may impede learning, pattern discrimination and the more subtle choices of programs from prosters suffer severe inhibition. So does the use of oral or written language and any form of symbol manipulation. The valuable learning that is built through any kind of play, of course, comes to a full halt; threat forestalls play — play implies absence of threat! *The inescapable point emerges: cerebral learning and threat conflict directly and completely.*

Threat Is Built Into the Conventional Classroom. In the conventional classroom, threat to the student stands ever present through the basic setting of captivity; the power of the instructor to punish, demean, embarrass, reject, or cause loss of status; and the "fishbowl" effect of being forced to perform in constant danger of ridicule or public failure. The same factors may apply, though often to a lesser degree, in training settings. Even in graduate-level work in colleges the threat of incurring a powerful person's displeasure, or failing to get over the next hurdle on the way to a degree that represents much desire, time, and money, can have an almost paralyzing effect.

Threat pervades most educational settings, as a holdover from times not long past when teachers were invariably portrayed with a cane, switch, or other implement of torture in hand. A surprising number of public school teachers still favor corporal punishment as an ultimate resource of management and control.[5] Grading, the issuing of marks and report cards, is widely abused, by common knowledge, for punitive or threat purposes.

Pressure or Challenge Do Not Constitute Threat. Threat, we should note, means not so much what is happening as what reasonably can be expected to occur in the very near future. It is the sword hanging by a thread over one's head. Threat is not the same as pressure — one may rush to catch a train or plane with worry and fear about missing it, but without threat. Nor is threat the result of challenge that one believes can be met through effort and application of one's personal best. *Threat arises from the perception that some power, usually a person or group, can and very well may harm us.*

Threat also gives us a profoundly revealing clue to the muddled area of "learning disabilities." It is only necessary to read a score of full case histories of victims of this vague condition to observe a glaring, common factor: these students have long been subjected to acute, continued threat by a parent (often the father) or other dominating adults in their lives. One must wonder why this explanation, so obvious once examined, has been so little remarked until the 1990s.[6]

The concept of emotional override appears to fit with both what is now known about the nature of the human brain and what can continually be seen happening in instructional settings, as well as in our own daily living. In education and training we are concerned primarily with the superbly subtle and powerful newest brain. If we shut it down by threat, we must expect learning failure. One's neocortex functions fully only when one feels secure. Yet schools commonly create and tolerate threat, perhaps because they feel it contributes to control of students. Ironically, experience in brain-compatible (low threat) schools shows strikingly that students protected from threat and encouraged to learn behave marvelously well.

THE BODYBRAIN PARTNERSHIP

The discovery of the molecules of emotion—the "information substances" of the bodybrain learning partnership described in Chapter 5—has radically expanded our awareness of the role the body plays in the learning process. Our early although partial views—thanks to the triune brain theory—made it clear that absence of threat was an essential quality of an effective learning environment. Now, we must come to grips with the fact that the body can no longer be considered a necessary but uninvolved vehicle to carry the brain back and forth to school. Instead, the body is as much a "student" in our classrooms as the brain—Siamese twins so to speak. One cannot be dealt with in isolation from the other. With their body-soul concept, the Greeks were ahead of their time. It is time that we stepped out of the intervening shadows and began to view the experience of school from the body's perspective. What conditions are affecting the body and what are the messages it is sending to the brain? Are these messages enhancing or hindering learning?

Learning is enhanced when, in addition to ensuring an absence of threat, the bodybrain partnership has a supportive physical environment and meaningful curriculum content.

Supportive Physical Environment

The physical environment—the milieu of the body—of our schools must create bodybrain messages that enhance rather than impede learning. The elements are many and not mysterious; a good guide to implementation is our own bodybrain system. For example, ask yourself what in your working environment at school hampers your ability to do your personal best. We owe students the respectful consideration that they, too, may react much the same as we adults do when faced with such conditions as bathrooms that become smelly by the end of the day and which frequently run without soap and paper towels; poorly cleaned classrooms and halls, dust balls in the corners, stains and smears left unattended for months, grimy desktops; paint either institutional "dullsville" or garishly bright; desks and chairs that cause one to squirm and slump (we complain bitterly about having an all-day inservice in them); temperature typically 5-10 degrees from comfortable with air that is stale and odorous; and moving from room to room so that one never seems to have the right tools at the right time.

If any of these fit your situation, you know the bodybrain interferences with learning that go with them. So, stated in the positive, the physical environment of our schools, for students and adults, needs to be:

- Healthful—free of toxins, clean, well-lighted (with full-spectrum lighting matching natural sunlight), well-ventilated with fresh air, pleasant smelling, ambient temperature, and safe

- Aesthetically pleasing—calming colors and music (primarily 60-beats a minute), living plants (those especially effective in absorbing toxins while providing a source of oxygen), and well-laid out for multiple uses (not institutional rows)

- Uncluttered yet reflective of what is being learned
- Supplied with multiple resources for topics currently under study.

Meaningful Curriculum Content

Of all the areas of school life, the content of our traditional curriculum is the most out of sync with the definition of learning as a bodybrain partnership. The constructivists are on the right track when they maintain that each learner must construct his or her own meaning based upon prior experience and knowledge and current experience. But it all goes much deeper than that. Given the role of emotion in determining what the brain will attend to and recall, we must accept that the challenge is not solely an instructional one—how to motivate Johnny to want to learn. The issue is much more serious. What we face is a content problem. We must have the courage to admit to ourselves that there is little in our traditional curriculum that is recognizable as useful or relevant to the brains of today's youth or emotionally and physically engaging at an intrinsic level. The curriculum of the 21st century must be conceptual in nature, based in the here and now, and experienced in the context of real life.[7]

A Curriculum of Concepts. Textbooks must give way to the study of concepts in the context of real life. In their watered-down, single point-of-view form, textbooks are a poor statement of curriculum—of what you want students to understand and be able to do with what they understand. What is needed is a continuum of concepts[8] which empowers students to generalize and apply what they know to new circumstances. Factoids, the typical fare of textbooks, do not empower the learner as they do not lend themselves to generalization or application to new contexts. They are essentially dead-ends. Teachers and students alike squander precious energy and time trying to make textbooks "come alive," to stretch for applications to reality. We should begin with reality.

Study Based in the Here and Now. The central focus of study in our schools must be on understanding the present. Students should study the science and mathematics used today in the fields of their interest, in the solution of problems faced by their community, and in the enrichment of their own lives. Study of the past—to help understand, predict, and shape the future—is only meaningful when one has a firm grip on the present. Curriculum should be based in the present informed by the past rather than beginning with the past and hoping to get to the present before the semester runs out.

With students, here and now means just that. Here where I stand and now while I'm standing here.

Curriculum Experienced in the Context of Real Life. Armed with the knowledge that input from the senses bursts into the nervous system on its way to the cerebral cortex through nodal points or hot spots of neuropeptides, we must make every effort to heighten the amount of input to those nodal points. Simply stated, we must take students outside the walls of the classroom on a regular basis, at least weekly, to that "slice of life" that illustrates the concept(s) being studied, a practice the Kovalik ITI program calls *being there.* We also need to make the school itself a living organism for study. There are, for example, few sociological concepts that can't be studied firsthand somewhere on campus.

As educators, not neuroscientists, the complexity of brain research may at times seem truly mind-boggling. But the overarching conclusions about how the brain functions are neither mysterious nor impossible to grasp. Viewing learning as a bodybrain partnership opens many doors.

NOTES

1 James C. Murselli, *Psychology for Modern Education* (New York: W. W. Norton, 1952), p. 95.

2 See the discussion of the point in D. O. Hebb, *Organization of Behavior* (New York: John Wiley and Sons, 1949), especially p. 147.

3 Emotions may arise, of course, from genetically transmitted sources, and become apparent with maturation. At around six months of age, the infant becomes distrustful of strangers — perhaps only partly due to limited ability previously to detect the pattern strangers. Young children have little fear of snakes as a rule; the fear grows with increasing age, even if no experience appears responsible. The horror and panic often shown may be strongly genetic.

4 Editor's Note: This description of the triune brain concepts of reptilian brain, old mammalian (limbic system), and neocortex are, we now know, oversimplifications that can no longer support the details of recent brain research. However, it is retained here for two reasons. One, because the triune brain theory is fairly well known in education, the discussion will help clarify what is still considered accurate and what must give way under the waves of current brain research findings. Two, a discussion of the brain's evolutionary process is important to an understanding of the interconnectedness and complexity of the brain. Throughout evolution, the supremacy of the brain has been maintained not in small part because its older processes and structures were not abandoned, resulting in duplication and redundancy much like our current space-age travel reliance on back-up systems which back up the back-up systems. Failure to operate in life and death circumstances is therefore made less likely.

5 Classroom teachers have always lived in fear of rebellion by the group or by older students. As youngsters have come to have larger physiques than teachers in many cases, and have largely lost the old privilege of dropping out of school without sanctions against them, real or potential attacks upon teachers have become an increasing problem. Threat affects both teachers and students.

6 See Leslie A. Hart, "Misconceptions about Learning Disabilities," *National Elementary Principal*, September-October 1976, pp. 54-57 and *Inside the Brain: Revolutionary Discoveries of How the Mind Works* by Ronald Kotulak (Kansas City: A Universal Press Syndicate Company, 1996) which is based on the Pulitzer Prize-winning series in *The Chicago Tribune*.

7 Editor's Notes: For a description of how to develop such curriculum, see the ITI (Integrated Thematic Instruction) model materials developed by Susan Kovalik & Associates described in Appendix A.

8 Editor's Notes: For an example of such a curriculum, see *A Science Continuum of Concepts for Grades K-6* by Karen D. Olsen (Kent, Washington: Center for the Future of Public Education, 1995). The continuum was developed for the Mid-California Science Improvement Program, funded by the David and Lucille Packard Foundation and based on the Kovalik ITI (Integrated Thematic Instruction) model.

12

Brain Development: Birth to Adulthood

The human way of life is essentially social. To get the things needed to keep alive we cooperate with other people. This requires special programs of the brain and the whole pattern of human lives is organized around social activities. The sequence of human development — early helplessness, long childhood, late adolescence, and long adult life — is designed to allow the brain to develop and to acquire and use a set of programs for the skills of a social life.

—I. Z. Young[1]

Anyone familiar with children knows the general scheme of physical development. The neonate has a huge head, a long trunk, short arms and legs. Within the first year, weight may triple. Next comes the chubby stage; then, around age four or five, growth stretches the body which may remain thin for a number of years. Early in the second decade of life, very rapid growth begins and the youngster "shoots up." Girls also show manifest sexual development. Around 15, boys are apt to be gangly and awkward, at least in appearance. At 17, a girl has usually filled out and shows maturity; the boy usually takes longer. At 20 or so growth slows almost to a stop.

PHYSICAL DEVELOPMENT OF THE BRAIN: A RELATIVELY NEW TOPIC

What has happened during this process in the brain? It is not hard to find people who have no idea and who, surprisingly, have given it hardly a thought. One does not ask a seven-year-old to reach something down from a high shelf—obviously she can't reach. But what are her brain capacities? A slender 12-year-old boy is **not** expected to lift a heavy barrel but what is he capable of mentally? Parents often may expect too much or too little and may be infuriated by the consequences. Those trained for education usually have given more attention to the idea of development. But, unfortunately, many ideas about mental development have been built into the school structure over generations and represent tradition and myths perhaps as often as sound studies. Only very recently has new knowledge of the human brain given the basis for much clearer, more factual understandings.

Historical Roots

Piaget, of course, has helped greatly (after being ignored in America for several decades) to give educators some sense of youngsters' progression in intellectual growth in terms of his famous "stages." His work was based on observation of human young, not laboratory animals, as they behaved in ordinary or gently contrived situations. It has considerable ethological content. But educators trying to apply Piaget tend to ignore the fact that he made no claim to having presented any theory of learning nor explanation of how the brain functions in terms of its physical structure or evolutionary history. He did drive home the tremendously important point that children always develop their understanding of the world *gradually*. But in dealing with individual students this is hardly a handy guide for teachers. We know that each student moves through the stages of development on a private schedule and is not necessarily consistent in one stage nor in the same stage in all matters simultaneously.

Updating Piaget. Although Piaget's concentration on learners' development and the necessity for their active involvement has had great impact and leads naturally to brain-based approaches, recent brain research findings conflict somewhat with his work. Most limiting, in my view, is the emphasis Piaget put on intellectual growth by which he seems to have meant pretty much our old friend, linear logic, to which he returns again and again as his main field of investigation. Piaget, I believe, should be read with the realization that he saw logical operations as the highest, and perhaps noblest, of mental goals—a concept one may seriously question today, especially in light of Howard Gardner's multiple intelligences.[2]

In addition, more recent study of the frontal lobes (forebrain) seem to fit less neatly with Piaget than earlier timetables of development seemed to suggest. Neo-Piagetians Kurt Fischer at Harvard University and colleague Samuel Rose have been matching Piagetian behaviors with brain changes.[3] Their work continues to confirm that brain growth and development follows a broad genetic program, just as body growth does, and that the physical brain growth and behavior are related. Recent research by Robert Thatcher, for example, theorizes a "traveling wave" of growth-stimulating hormone traveling through the brain in slow spiral waves starting in the left hemisphere, then the center, then the right hemisphere with each sweep taking approximately five years. If Thatcher's model proves to be accurate, it would give physical brain growth evidence for the language explosion period at 18 months to two and a half years and for a period of heightened imagination at ages four to five years old. It also appears that there are gender differences in these waves.[4]

In addition, Proster Theory conflicts with Piaget's conclusions—perhaps mostly on semantic grounds—on the ability of young children to extract abstract patterns. Pattern extraction, I have tried to show, is not a logical process but results in extraction of abstract patterns nonetheless. Also, psychologist Elizabeth Spelke of Cornell University has been discovering all sorts of built in "initial knowledge" in babies four and five months old. It appears they understand a form of physics: that objects move separately from each other, that they maintain their size and shape while moving, and that one object affects another's motion only if they touch.[5] Surprising? High school seniors flunking physics would likely think so!

Likewise, psychologist Karen Wynn, University of Arizona, Tucson, has discovered that five-month-old babies have a form of numerical reasoning, a kind of baby arithmetic for simple addition and subtraction. Although the whole idea of "initial knowledge" is very controversial (and a departure of Piaget as well as a complete rejection of basic tenets of the behaviorist movement), Karen Wynn feels that, even though the research is in its early stages, the findings "suggest the presence of innate baby physics, geometry, arithmetic, and psychology."[6]

As such research unfolds, it puts a wrinkle in Piaget's sense of tidy, gradual growth. While appearing to chip away at Piaget's work, we can honor this great pioneer without trying to apply his findings in ways he never intended. Again, rather than invalidating Piaget's work, such research merely puts it in context, shifting it from "the" message about development to being a contributing story about a much larger picture. Inaccurate details will fall away and educators will acquire a clearer picture of how the brain grows and works.

Physical Versus Brain Development

The essential picture we need may best be obtained by considering the neonate and then the same person 20 years later. If a baby can triple weight in a year, why cannot it achieve adult weight in three or four, growing at the same rate? If a one-pound puppy can become a 60-pound dog in little over a year, why does it take a human such a large share of lifetime to reach adulthood? The physical growth does not seem to be the problem.

But the mental development is another matter. At or shortly after the time of birth, we have about all the neurons we will ever have. In fact, the brain appears to have a winnowing-out period in which superfluous cells are discarded. Unlike most cells of the body, which die off rapidly and are replaced, neurons appear to serve us our entire lifetime. When they die, as many thousands do daily, we are left with fewer. But the supply we begin with is so fantastically large that we can sustain the loss: we start with 100 billion neurons.[7]

To hold this immense number, the head must be relatively large at birth; even so, children must be born while still in a state of general helplessness—far from "finished"—if that head is to pass through the birth canal. It seems clear that the reason we develop so slowly physically is to allow time for those billions of neurons to become organized. *The body waits on the brain.*

COMING OF AGE: GROWTH AND MATURITY

For educators, what enhances growth and maturity of the physical brain is a pivotal question. Actual growth—increase in size, density, and weight—occurs through complexity and myelination. Maturity—often measured by increased ability to plan ahead and control one's behavior—is a function of the development of the frontal lobes, a process that begins in year one and continues for roughly 20 years.

Growth Processes: By Complexity and Myelination

Without getting into the complexities of neurons,[8] we can appreciate that development takes place in two quite different ways: by increasing complexity and by myelination.

Growth by Increasing Complexity. Neurons (there are a number of types) grow by becoming more complex, much as the branches of a newly planted tree gradually divide and spread. Many neurons growing in this fashion come to have thousands of connections with other neurons. These are not actual joinings; the connections involve a tiny gap across which chemical neurotransmitters can move. This is the *synapse,* a mechanism that retains a good many secrets still, though much has been learned by persistent and often brilliant investigation. The maturing brain steadily increases the number and complexity of these interconnections which by adulthood total into numbers beyond meaning for most of us—as high as 1,000 trillion.[9]

Astonishing increases in complexity occur from birth to three months and then to six months. Such dramatic increases in complexity, of course, are not automatic or a function of time. It is in response to experiences in a rich environment. It has long been known that children deprived of a normal range of input, as was clearly the case in certain orphanages and foundling homes in the past, show greatly retarded development.[10]

The neonate of course has linkages or pathways already formed, particularly in the oldest structures of the brain, or it would not be able to survive. The general plan of the brain has been genetically laid down during gestation but adding new connections particularly in the gigantic cerebrum, the newest parts of the brain, goes on at a staggering rate. Much evidence indicates that input and experience strongly influence not only what connections are made but even how fast such growth proceeds.

While we may question how much input can be forced on a child, it seems probable that an ordinary home, where there is affection for and interest in the infant, provides a good supply. If we observe the motions of a baby's arms and hands over the first few weeks, the progress from random movements and jerks to controlled and purposeful actions shows the development in the brain going forward rapidly. However, more is involved than just muscular control; eye-hand coordination and interpretation relating to objects, people, and even situations is soon evident.

It is common to think of the baby's progress as very slow — the puppy gets organized a great deal faster and romps around long before the infant can sit up. If we could somehow see the neuronal connections being formed in vast numbers, however, we would credit the baby with far more rapid progress. In favorable circumstances, it will continue through all the years of childhood. Actual physical growth of neurons is involved throughout. Much as a tree sends out more and more branches and twigs, the neurons send out their dendrites. Increase in brain size and weight comes in part from this kind of physical development; however, by far the greatest increase results from myelination.

Growth by Myelination. The second kind of physical brain development involves *myelination.* A nerve is a conducting channel for electrical (more accurately, electrochemical) impulses that travel in one direction along it. Unlike a wire that conducts an electrical current from a battery in a smooth, continuous flow, the nerve can only conduct pulses of energy that make a succession of leaps along the fiber. But, like insulation on an electric wire, myelin helps keep the pulses confined and makes them move much faster. In the brain this insulation is provided by special myelin cells that form a fatty tissue which wraps around the nerve conduit many times.

At birth, the head is one-third its adult size and relatively few nerve pathways have this insulation. Much of the increase in size from birth to adult size is due to the build up of myelin, a process that continues for roughly 20 years. In this sense an adult brain is one in which the insulation has been formed.

A Word About Growth and Maturation. There can be large variations in the way neuronal growth and connections, and myelination, occur in any one individual. Again we must realize that *individual variations have great practical significance.* No child is average or typical nor should he or she be expected to be. Nor should he or she be treated as though defective or exceptional because of variations in ten or a hundred respects from a purely imaginary norm. *To be different is to be normal* — only within the artificial, bureaucratic structures of schools would clones be welcomed! It is the school structures that are abnormal, not the children within them. To send children to school on the basis of their birthdates, and then in large part treat them as alike is to ignore how real children develop. Even if we put them in chairs that are the right size for their average, more than half will be in chairs that are the wrong size for them! Mentally, we have every reason to believe, the variations range far more widely.

Maturation: The Importance of the Frontal Cortex

The frontal lobes, the cortex behind the forehead, are sometimes called "the brain's brain." This portion of the brain includes tissue structures that are exclusively human — *their equivalent does not seem to occur in any other animal.* The functions of the frontal cortex or forebrain are many and crucial to learning. Diamond and Hopson describe the frontal cortex as "playing a role in practically all thinking, reading, learning, and organizing."[11] In exploring how the mind learns mathematics, Stanislaus Dehaene describes the frontal cortex as "a region of the brain that enables us to select a strategy and to hold firm to it despite distractions"[12] and as the part of the brain used for "implementing and controlling nonroutine strategies."[13] Pinker describes the role of the frontal cortex as being "the seat of deliberate thought . . . the part of the brain that exercises will — forming and carrying out plans."[14] The frontal lobes are the part of the brain involved in inhibiting the natural reactions of other parts of the brain, giving opportunity for a second look, reconsideration, modulation of innate behavior, and so forth.

The frontal cortex does some maturing the first year, doesn't become fully prepared for action until age four to seven, and continues to develop for many years, even into the early 20s.[15] "This longer development allows abstract thought, language, reasoning, decision-making, and self-control to blossom—all linked to, and influenced by, other emotional brain structures."[16]

For a child, this three-year span from age four to seven makes an enormous difference. Not only does behavior (especially inhibition of impulsiveness) vary greatly as we have seen but also learning of the basic skills—reading, writing, and arithmetic. To throw students into first grade work with only lip-service provision for individualization may well be considered an invitation for trouble. Luria further describes these parts of the new brain as "a superstructure above all other parts of the cerebral cortex, so that they perform a far more universal function of general regulation of behavior"[17] than other parts of the neocortex. Elsewhere he adds: "It can thus be concluded that the frontal lobes of the brain are among the vital structures responsible for the orientation of an animal's behavior *not only to the present but also to the future*" (Luria's emphasis).[18] The frontal lobes, then, and especially the exclusively human prefrontal portions, provide the ability to look ahead further, to make longer plans, and to stick with them in spite of distractions. In an infant, up to a few months over age two, old brain structures dominate attention: the child *must* give heed to new sights or sounds; parents' verbal instructions to the contrary will be ignored. No amount of reproof or punishment will have effect.

As the newer brain areas develop their powers, these old survival programs or schema come under more control. As the prefrontal areas are brought into use, especially through age seven and even into adolescence, the child has enormously greater capacity to set more distant goals and carry through a chain of activity. *No amount of teacher coercion will substitute for natural development.* Subjecting a child to criticism or labeling him/her immature, impulsive, or learning disabled is to ignore the evidence plainly in front of us.

Particularly critical for success in early classrooms is a child's ability and willingness to follow verbal instructions, since teachers rely heavily on this kind of group direction. Conflict and frustrations inevitably result since the whole concept of the classroom is unrealistic and brain-incompatible. It typically *ignores* what is happening in the brain.

The surface area of the frontal cortex, Luria shows,[19] expands rapidly to around three-and-a-half years, then more slowly to around seven years, and from that point gradually until age 18 or more. Anyone who has raised children to adulthood has had opportunity to see the effect of frontal and prefrontal growth and myelination: lower-brain distractibility lessens, the concept of future time (later, tomorrow, next month, when you are 12) comes to have practical meaning, longer-term plans can be made and often completed, and in general self-governing capacity grows.

Applying What We Know About the Frontal Lobes. Observation suggests strongly, however, that parents and teachers alike tend to err far more often on the side of underestimating or misinterpreting what a youngster can do. A myth exists that children of a certain age have a certain "span of attention" — one more expression of the persistent idea that alikeness prevails, not differences. In actuality, a four-year old may spend hours during a day building an elaborate system of roads and bridges with blocks and toy cars, for example. The capacity of six-year-olds to carry on rope jumping, or fort building, or an expedition through meadow and woods, is readily observable. Often children will leave the activity briefly to return to it later — exactly what office workers do with coffee breaks, lunch, short social visits, trips to the washrooms or drinking fountain, or making phone calls. Span of attention will often be short and fragile for activities forced on the child by others, but many times longer and more persistent when self-selected. The term "span of attention," which in my view is more a mischief maker than useful, should not be confused with length and complexity of plans, reflecting prefrontal and frontal lobe development.

The most simple of approaches seems to work well to give adults a sound estimate of what individual children can handle: *provide the opportunity, stay out of the way, and then observe what the child chooses to do.* At a playground, for example, where children may freely climb, jump, or swing, self-caused accidents prove rare. Children know their own capabilities and "what comes next" in individual development. When even trained adults, such as physical education instructors, begin giving orders, injuries may skyrocket. When I was a youth, bicycles were thought suitable only for children at least ten years old; today one sees five- and six-year-old boys and girls who not only manage two-wheelers well but can rear up and ride on the back wheel alone. Yet other, well-endowed children may not get the knack of balancing a bicycle until two or three years later. *Differences are normal.*

Adult worry about financial liability may inhibit youngsters' achievement for fear of lawsuit or damaging equipment. Although young students can handle tools quite expertly with the briefest safety instruction and a little supervision, they are often denied them. I have seen junior high school students, supposedly the least reliable, use expensive photographic, television, laboratory, and computer equipment with faultless skill and care—provided they were carrying out activities they wanted to do, not those forced upon them. I have also seen severely retarded children do exquisite hand lettering and arrange and serve a meal at a beautiful, elaborately set table and have watched films of retarded, *blind* children doing daring, difficult tumbling!

The Range of Differences Is Huge. The key element that limits individual performance when following verbal instruction and doing or using long-term planning is frontal lobe development. Otherwise, ability to perform acquired programs can often be startlingly beyond conventional suppositions. The range of difference is huge and the rapidity of change of limits can be surprising. The idea that the adult in parental or instructional role "knows" the child must be distrusted—the adult judgment may be mistaken or influenced by what is seen as convenient, economical, or least risky. *Only when the child is asked, not by test or examination but by being given options and time, without threat, can the true current state of capabilities be assessed.*[20]

We cannot see inside the brain what neuron growth has taken place and how far myelination has gone in any particular area. But even if we could, normal variation can be so large as to make "average" guidelines more harmful than useful.

When we view the child as possessing at least 100 billion neurons that will be organized in individual fashion over some 20 years, we take a practical view. If we respect the mighty cerebrum and grasp what development is going forward, we may find it easier to respect the child and comprehend behavior.

IMPLICATIONS FOR EDUCATION

How the brain develops has profound implications for educators who deal with students at any age before adulthood. Here are a few key points that demand immediate attention:

1. The brain can be used only to the extent that it has become organized. This occurs over roughly a 20-year period. The time is required not for muscular and bone growth, which could be accomplished much faster, but because of the huge number of neurons involved.

2. At birth or within a short time after, a person has almost all the neurons he or she will ever have.[21]

3. Neurons literally grow, becoming larger and more complex, and a considerable amount of this growth is influenced by input and experience.

4. Myelination, or the insulation of nerve pathways, improves their functioning, and is a process that continues until adulthood. Individuals differ sharply in the specific progress of myelination.

5. The prefrontal portions of the cerebrum have a profound influence on human behavior, making possible longer-term programs. Individuals differ widely in terms of how soon these areas come into full use; these normal differences are not under parental or teacher control.

6. Children's abilities may often be underestimated by those adults who may claim to "know" them. Ability is best determined by providing opportunity, standing aside, and observing. Threat must be absent.

7. The class-and-grade or factory school system is unrelated to present understandings of brain development and, *in practice, ranges from severely to violently brain-antagonistic.* The school presses for alikeness, because that would be superficially more convenient, but brain development introduces a huge range of differences. *For "normal" children to differ greatly is normal; for children not to differ widely would be freakish and most unusual.*

NOTES

1 I. Z. Young, *Programs of the Brain* (Oxford: Oxford University Press, 1978), p. 25.

2 Editor's Note: Howard Gardner's work on the multiple intelligences is one such body of work that questions the broadness of the base of Piaget's foundation. Piaget's description of development appears to fit Gardner's logical-mathematical intelligence and perhaps also the naturalist intelligence but many believe that Gardner's other six intelligences (linguistic, spatial, musical, bodily-kinesthetic, and inter- and intra-personal intelligences) lie outside of Piaget's work. However, given the importance of logical-mathematical (and naturalist) intelligence for everyday living in our high tech world, Piaget's contribution remains valuable nevertheless.

3 Marian Diamond and Janet Hopson, *Magic Trees of the Mind: How to Nurture Your Child's Intelligence, Creativity, and Healthy Emotions from Birth to Adolescence* (New York: A Dutton Book, 1998), p. 113. See also *Human Development: From Conception Through Adolescence* by Kurt W. Fischer (1984) and *Human Behavior and the Developing Brain* edited by Geraldine Dawson and Kurt W. Fischer (1994).

4 Ibid, pp. 118-119.

5 Ibid, p. 121.

6 Ibid, p. 122.

7 Ibid, p. 23.

8 Editor's Notes: For the reader who would like to learn more about the functions of neurons without getting too deep technically, see *Magic Trees of the Mind: How to Nurture Your Child's Intelligence, Creativity, and Health Emotions from Birth Through Adolescence* by Marian Diamond and Janet Hopson (New York: A Dutton Book, 1998). For the more technically inclined, see *How Brains Think: Evolving Intelligence,Then and Now* by William H. Calvin (New York: Basic Books, 1996).

9 Diamond and Hopson, p. 37.

10 Lack of stimulation and normal cherishing can even result in reduced physical growth. See Lytt I. Gardner, "Deprivation Dwarfism," *Scientific American*, July 1972.

11 Diamond and Hopson, p. 221.

12 Stanislas Dehaene, *The Number Sense: How the Mind Creates Mathematics* (New York: Oxford University Press, 1997), p. 147.

13 Ibid, p. 138.

14 Steven Pinker, *How the Mind Works.* ((New York: W. W. Norton & Co, 1997), p. 144.

15 A. R. Luria, *The Working Brain* (New York: Basic Books, 1975), p. 87. Also, see Candace Pert, *Molecules of Emotion: Why You Feel the Way You Feel* (New York: Scribner, 1997), p. 288.

16 Diamond and Hopson, p. 126.

17 Luria, p. 89.

18 Luria, p. 91.

19 Luria, chart, p. 87. See also the current work of Kurt Fischer, Harvard University, "neo-Piagetian" and neuroscientist (refer to Note 3 on previous page).

20 Tests given children by neurologists, psychologists, school specialists, and others in their office can be extremely fallible, especially if a parent having difficulties with the child is present or nearby. The conditions of the test create threat—as indeed they do for the adult under similar circumstances. The adult, often pressed for time, relies on one, no-time-lost reading. It can happen, too, that the child gathers how he or she is expected to perform, and obliges. It is remarkable how adults who themselves are terrified by any examination by someone in a white coat still feel that a strange test by a strange person in a strange setting should not affect the child at all.

21 Editor's Note: Not until recently have we discovered that the brain regenerates neurons, especially in the hippocampus where short-term memories are created. Also, T-cells can become neurons under special conditions. Our best advice is treat your brain kindly: it does not fully regenerate on a regular basis as do the cells of the rest of the body. This is the most comelling reason for teens to avcoid drugs and all os us to practice a healthy lifestyle.

13

WORKING WITH THEORY: WHAT IT CAN TELL US

From the standpoint of the child, the great waste in the school comes from his inability to utilize the experiences he gets outside the school in any complete and free way within the school itself; while, on the other hand, he is unable to apply in daily life what he is learning at school. That is the isolation of the school — its isolation from life.

Nothing is more absurd than to suppose that there is no middle term between leaving a child to his own unguided fancies and likes or controlling his activities by a formal succession of dictated directions.

—John Dewey[1]

THE VALUE OF GOOD THEORY

One good test of a theory is its practicality. If on close examination it turns out to be little more than so many words — especially grandiose, sweeping words hard to pin down or "buzz words" that mean something different to each person — it may at best be entertaining or, at worst, boring and time wasting. But if, on the other hand, a theory touches base with reality and scientific findings, it may well have immediate utility, particularly if its language can easily be translated into specific, familiar examples that make the terms sharp, understandable, and not difficult to agree on.

That lucid philosopher, Whitehead, has observed:

> Success in practice depends on theorists who . . . by some
> good chance have hit on the relevant ideas. By a theorist I do not
> mean a man who is up in the clouds but a man whose motive for
> thought is the desire to formulate correctly the rules according to
> which events occur. A successful theorist should be excessively
> interested in immediate events, otherwise he is not at all likely to
> formulate correctly anything about them.[2]

Good theory for education should promptly suggest a bonanza of approaches, methods, techniques, materials, devices, and
practices that might be explored, tested, demonstrated, or experimented with. It is not at all necessary that the theory provide
wholly new ideas in these areas; in fact it is more than likely many
of the suggested applications will turn out to have elements of
familiarity. What will be new, however, is the formulation of rules
that permit us and help us to *see the old in quite a new way* and thus
allow us to move from tentative, personal intuitions that we can
scarcely express to sharply etched insights that we cannot only
state but agree on and *put into use.*

If indeed we reach back over the centuries and check the concepts and intuitions of such people as Confucius, Socrates,
Aristotle, Seneca, Quintilian, St. Augustine, St. Thomas Aquinas,
Luther, Erasmus, Comenius, Montaigne, Locke, Hecker, Rousseau,
Pestalozzi, Herbart, Froebel, Parker, and Dewey, we find ideas and
injunctions recurring again and again that fit neatly with some of
the main tenets of Proster Theory. They could not, of course, have
been expressed in brain-based terms before present insights into the
brain were available; nor could the truly new ideas that arise from a
brain approach have been advanced in prior times because they
would have seemed mad or bizarre. (Even today some of them may
induce a blink and swallow, especially among those who have not
been following the move toward brain-compatibility.)

THE LACK OF THEORY IN EDUCATION

Educators in general have lacked familiarity with the whole
idea of useful theory and its application. This is quite surprising
given that most are aware (sometimes painfully so) of the
astounding, science theory-based technology in most fields
throughout the 20th century. In a 1964 yearbook, for example,

Winfred Hill noted "an extremely incomplete background for dealing with the problems of teaching" and N. L. Gage observed: "As is well known, after more than a half-century of effort, no such unification of learning theory has materialized." Knowledge was "inadequate to tell us what we should do about teaching."[3] This absence of a "knowledge base" or foundation has been lamented almost to the present. We are only now entering an "age of theory" in education that—as we can already see—will radically change what we believe and what we do anywhere we try to train or educate. At last, we are expanding and putting to use a knowledge base that does in fact tell us what to do that will work and why—a strong indication of good theory.

Educational literature (as apart from general psychology) pays little attention to basic theory, even to the point of seeming to avoid the topic. Among teachers, principals, and other "working" educators, one finds overwhelmingly (as I noted in Chapter 3) the feeling that "theory" means the dreary lectures on long outdated psychologies they had to suffer through to get college credits. Having sampled mainly muddled, fragmentary, and often antique educational theory, they understandably do not realize the potentials of sound, modern, useful theory.

For many, educational research literature also carries with it the suspicion that much of the investigation is done by researchers who seem to prefer cozy grants with tidy studies to the messy realities of schools as they seek to find correlations: *this* was done in instruction and apparently resulted in *that* outcome. Unfortunately, despite their popularity, correlations do not necessarily involve causal relations at all, or even show what is cause and what is effect! Here again we see attempts to deal with complex, interactive systems with simple-minded linear logic. An advantage of a comprehensive theory of learning is that it can remind us of the danger of simplifying the complex, as well as help us to factor out elements that are truly causal.[4]

DEFINING "USEFUL" THEORY

It may then be proper to reiterate that useful theory does *not* mean a new, more fashionable collection of "what do I do Monday," cookbook-style recipes: do exactly this and the outcome will be pleasing. Rather, useful theory clarifies how and why events occur and suggests directions in which to move and areas in which to explore, invent, and develop techniques—*as well as those to avoid*. In my view a helpful image is that of a long corridor with many doors, some open and in use, and others long locked. Useful theory leads us to close some of the familiar doors that have led only to failure or poor results, year after year, and to begin using new doors that open onto fresh territories, resources, and opportunities. Good theory offers new freedom, incentives, stimulation . . . and rewards.

On the other side of those newly opened doors, educators will find innumerable choices, unlimited room to be creative. But they will not find a storehouse of mint-fresh texts waiting to be used, procedures ready to implement, or machines needing only to be switched on. Between good theory and its daily application lies a large region of development (in some cases, "engineering") that calls for a huge amount of work and effort. Theory is, after all, theoretical; it must be translated into the practical. It should also function like a well-powered machine that can clear the ground for new seeding.

OUTCOMES OF USEFUL THEORY: THE PROOF IS IN THE PUDDING

How large, exciting, and fast can we reasonably expect results to be when useful theory is applied and how quickly can they be looked for? Are we speaking of a generation or two, or of a few years? In-school experience with Proster Theory, while only a start, strongly suggests rapid results of startling depth and scope.

Results for All Students

A first question must be *the size of the potentials,* to the best of our estimate. Here what we can call incidence of success becomes a key. What the rare genius or very exceptional person accomplishes does not tell us too much, but when we find repeated examples of excellent achievement by individuals who seem to fall within more ordinary boundaries, we do not need great numbers to convince us of potentials.

Going Beyond "Normal" Outcomes

In both special and common settings there seem to be sufficient instances of success to demonstrate that learning can be far better and faster than "normal." Certainly many thousands of children learn to read before they enter school. Omar K. Moore and his associates established beyond doubt that children three and four years old who were well below genius level could learn to read and write (on typewriters) quite impressively, acquiring their skills easily and with apparent enjoyment. Later Moore showed that kindergarten and first-grade students in a school could consistently achieve reading abilities of sixth-grade and higher levels.[5]

In almost any school system, one can find instances of students whose learning in such fields as mathematics, science, or music runs years ahead of the norm, although they have to fight against the resistance of the class-and-grade system which operates to hold students back to "grade level," for bureaucratic convenience. Instances of success appear to show clearly that the potential for greatly superior learning exists.

WHAT HOLDS US BACK: THEORY AS LOOKING GLASS

Indisputably, learning depends on many factors—not only on what helps but also on elimination or reduction of those factors *that hurt*. Working educators commonly find it hard to think in these terms. For example, a reading teacher may simply refuse to consider that some of the instruction he or she is giving to students my actually *prevent* students from improving reading ability. After all, when people give instruction, as when they offer advice, the intent normally is to be helpful. Too often the negative possibilities may get little attention. As in medicine, medical doctors are traditionally warned, "above all, do no harm." Yet the side effects of medicines, unnecessary operations, and too hastily recommended procedures continue to contribute to problems for patients. Educators, however, are seldom even cautioned! Rather the assumption is made that education is good, better, or best. Possibly harmful effects tend to be ignored and those staff who do venture to mention them may be ostracized.[6]

A brain-compatible approach, however, suggests that *present schools and conventional formal instruction practices plainly can be brain-antagonistic and customarily contain seriously negative components*. If the plus and minus influences were to be factored out, and then the positives strengthened and negatives reduced or eliminated, the shift in learning outcomes could be dramatic. Despite the investment of hundreds of millions of dollars in research, this effort to factor for negative as well as positive influences has seldom been made. As noted, many teachers, and other practitioners, evince what appears to be genuine shock at the very idea that some of what they do as "teaching" may have an opposite effect, despite the fact that day by day they see students who lose interest, lessen effort, become confused and discouraged, and try to avoid certain topics and activities. We should not rush to conclude, of course, that the teaching is always at fault. The whole school setting is involved, or the source of the trouble may lie outside the school altogether, in the traditions we are about to consider.

USING THEORY TO TELL US WHAT TO STOP DOING

In application of theory, as we have noted, *what is stopped may be as important, or even more important, than what is introduced.*

Since humans live by familiar patterns and accumulated programs, stopping may be difficult to bring about, especially within large organizations with intricate social structures, such as public school systems. This helps explain why, despite all the emphasis on change over the past quarter century and particularly the last decade, the schools have, in fact, changed hardly at all and why so many efforts boldly and enthusiastically begun have tended to fade out over a period of time as old patterns and programs reassert their strength of persistence.

Why Traditions Die Hard

In addition to what is now frequently called the "structure" of our schools, we need to be aware of much broader and more complex *traditions* that affect the school, yet may get little attention and discussion. (It is tempting to explore them, rather than to barely mention them as here, but that could well call for a book in itself.) Since ordinarily even educational historians may pay only passing attention to these traditions, we might term them "invisible" but we should note that in sum they often exert strong—even fierce—brain-antagonistic effect.

Tradition #1: Children Are Bad. We can begin with a dominant attitude toward youth in the Western world over recent centuries:

that children tend, more often than not, to be badly behaved, sinful, disobedient, too little respectful of their parents and other powerful adults, given to trivial and foolish pursuits and squandering of time. The obvious remedy was punishment: "spare the rod and spoil the child" was among favored parental and religious injunctions. The school, as an institution designed for these probable malefactors, had to be stern, intolerant, tight-lipped, punishing, a place where many would fail and few succeed. That this tradition still applies can scarcely be doubted, even if, happily, it has moderated. "Do not smile until Christmas" is still proffered advice and many teachers continue to give much of their time to punishing—by penalties, low marks, detention, humiliation, reprimand, messages to the home, and verbal abuse, not to mention threats of corporal punishment. The many teachers who fight against the tradition at times find the going rough.

In Proster Theory terms, of course, the tradition is destructive: in conventional schools *threat* pervades, resulting in emotional override by virtually all students, thus preventing the fullest use of the neocortex and hindering the learning being sought. (See Chapter 2.)

Tradition #2: Roles of Teacher and Student—Active Versus Passive. Consider next the impact of a group of traditions concerning student achievement. One promotes the idea that learning is to be measured by a student's ability to give an approved *answer* to a specific *question*—a technique now commonly reduced to the absurdity of blackening a "balloon" for electronic scoring of a multiple-choice test. The passion for testing rests on a tradition going back centuries of having periodic *examinations*, so that in effect students progressed by getting over a series of hurdles, some of which became frozen and exalted as "promotion," "graduation," and "degree." However traditional, the concept conflicts head-on with the brain-compatible preference for learning that is continuous and natural rather than arbitrary, interrupted.

Other powerful traditions lie behind the conventional relationship between teacher and students—the teacher active and the students passive, doing what they are told to do, usually in great detail. By tradition the "good" students comply, the troublemakers and sluggards don't. Bound up with this view, which parents and school authorities tend to accept without question, is the somewhat newer tradition, stemming from the school as bureaucracy, that students should progress at the lockstep pace set, in denial of all kinds of individual factors. As a consequence, schools a century and more ago began to devote intense effort to *screening* students, ranking them across a continuum from shining example to dunce, dropout or pushout. For many years, students were physically moved: "go to the head of the class" is still part of our common language! Tracking, based on ability as indicated by a standard measure, flourishes today, despite protests about social, ethnic and racial inequities. Though lip-service is given to "all students can learn," in practice tracking expresses the screening concept.

Tradition #4: Control. Finally, in this sampling of traditions affecting our concepts of schooling, we can mention *control* and *evaluation.* The notion that educators should have a great say about how their pupils behave and what learning they may be exposed to goes far back, drawing both from religious sources and the doctrine of the school standing *in loco parentis,* acting in place of absent parents (but too often operating with pompous and meddling bureaucratic self-indulgence). For centuries control extended even to what students might read — college students could go to the library only to consult pre-approved sources, for example; and schools were expected to protect students from impure, worldly or perhaps controversial input. While one might laugh at such examples, who can forget the absurd "hair" battles or the blood spilled over measuring a boy's locks. Or, more recently, suspending students under a zero drug policy for taking an Advil for a headache. Such skirmishes still occur but on the whole the silly conflicts merely demonstrate how tattered the control tradition has become.

As formal school input into learning is dwarfed by radio, television, print, and other media beyond educators' influence, control represents a tradition in disrepair.

Tradition #5: Evaluation. If control appears to be fading, *evaluation* via standardized tests has intensified its corrupting influence. Recently realization has grown that standardized tests and such monsters as the SAT leave much to be desired, prompting a massive hunt for better methods and procedures. So far the search has produced more furor than useful results. Powerful voices within and outside education scream for more defensible evaluation, citing the high cost of schooling and international competition as sources of pressure to demonstrate results.

But the idea that each student's progress must be continually evaluated in some reportable form reflects just how invisible the tradition is that continues to see such evaluation as essential or even helpful. To the contrary, there is much evidence to support the realization that such continued press from on-going standardized evaluation in fact brain-antagonistic and actually harmful to the learning process for most students. A common experience of brain-compatible schools is that students will perform better without the overhanging threat of "being marked"; as a result, such schools sharply downplay continual, moment-to-moment evaluation and increase student participation in assessing the accuracy, comprehensiveness, and completeness of their own work.

In Proster Theory, the form of evaluation that proves most valuable is immediate feedback during pattern-seeking and program-building. This is most effective when it is inherent in the materials or activity itself. Third party feedback is far less effective.

Brain-Antagonistic Traditions: The Roots of School Ineffectiveness and Failure of Reform

Even this brief excursion into school-related traditions may serve to suggest brain-antagonistic features that underlie the abysmal ineffectiveness of most conventional schools. It may also help clarify why "restructuring" efforts flounder and fizzle. What may seem to be a mere modification of a school practice turns out to be a call to defy a tradition that has century-old roots.

Those who can adduce a coherent, successful theory as reason for the change may bring it about while those who seem just to be challenging the tradition can expect to be buried under protests.

It can be helpful to approach the problems of theory application on three fairly distinct levels: *settings, situations, and activities.* Chapter 14 discusses theory applied to settings; Chapter 15 explores theory applied to situations, particularly the convention of the classroom; and Chapter 16 examines theory applied to activities.

NOTES

1 *The Child and the Curriculum* (Chicago: University of Chicago Press, Phoenix Books, 1902), pp. 75, 130.

2 Alfred North Whitehead, *The Aims of Education* (New York: New American Library-Mentor, 1929), p. 102.

3 *Theories of Learning and Instruction, 63rd Yearbook of the National Society for the Study of Education* (Chicago: University of Chicago Press, 1964), p. 53; and (Gage), pp. 272, 274.

4 See John I. Goodlad, "Can Our Schools Get Better?" in *Phi Delta Kappan,* January 1979, p. 343: "How many researchers are moving from those studies of single variables in the learning process that have yielded no significant findings to those much more complex inquiries required for understanding school and classroom environments so that we might understand, also, how to improve them?"

5 Moore's work is described in part in Maya Pines, *Revolution in Learning* (New York: Harper and Row, 1966), Chapter 5, and many articles and reports have been published on what he and associates have demonstrated, particularly in reading. Moore is currently professor of sociology at the University of Pittsburgh, and continues work directly with children in inner-city areas. Perhaps because of his innovative (and brain-compatible) techniques, his striking successes have been largely ignored in educational literature. I have met with him, examined independent reports and other evidence, and found no reason to doubt that remarkable results were achieved. See also Omar K. Moore, "The Responsive Environments Laboratory," in Beatrice and Ronald Gross, *Radical School Reform* (New York: Simon and Schuster, 1969), p. 205.

6 Despite the enormous volume of criticism that regularly appears in educational periodicals, and in the form of speeches or conference reports, rarely is the suggestion made that bad or wrong teaching may actively impede learning. Some research studies do report negative correlations but there is almost no tradition of examining negative factors further.

14

THEORY APPLIED TO SETTINGS

> Given the durability of American views of school practice, it is no surprise to find that, with few exceptions, school programs have altered little since the 1890's. Considering the prodigious changes in American society since 1900, it is remarkable, and not merely the result of chance, that only minor rearrangements have been seen.
>
> —Theodore R. Sizer[1]

Surprisingly, remarkably little attention has been given to the design of complete, contemporary school systems. In contrast, our thinking and our public policy about reform and change are predicated on making gradual and usually minor modifications to the antique system that we have inherited, a system now embracing more than 40 million students.

Unless we are willing to examine these structures and elements of the learning environment and make changes consistent with brain-based theory, we will never be able to launch successful efforts at improving the educational experiences and outcomes of students. Settings as used here implies both the structure and the elements that contribute to the environment of the place called school.

BRAIN-ANTAGONISTIC ELEMENTS OF STRUCTURE

There are numerous brain-antagonistic elements built into our current structure. Two of the most powerful are compulsory attendance and the class-grade system.

Compulsory Attendance: Choice Versus Coercion

A key question to ask, and one particularly valuable for staff orientation, is "Why is the student here?" From a brain-compatible learning viewpoint, it makes a great difference whether the student is present under some compulsion—sent to school—or attends by free choice, that is, wants to be there to learn.

Resistance to coercion contributes to student passiveness as well as acts of overt rebellion. Learning—especially the skills and attitudes that form the bedrock of lifelong learning—take the back seat to just getting through the day.[2]

The Class-Grade System

An historical look at the typical school setting throws some light on one of the most stubborn aspects of education's structure, the class-grade system. A century ago, when our class-and-grade system was taking firm shape in a predominantly agricultural country, the school was seen as quite literally providing "book learning." Books and other materials in the home were few. At school the student could be exposed to more of such input as well as hear a little about the world beyond the next farm or town. A traveled teacher might be able to tell firsthand of cities with buildings that towered five and six stories, of ships that crossed the Atlantic with many passengers in only a few weeks, of museums with fossils of creatures that lived millions of years ago. These were wonders to rivet attention.

On the whole, however, children attended school very little and only when their families could forgo their indispensible free labor in the home, garden, fields or in cottage industries or small shops. The basic school hours, 9:00 A.M. to 3:00, still reflect time for children to do their chores before and after school hours plus walking time. The summer vacation, of course, recalls an era when farm work demanded the children full time. Schools now often send their charges home to houses where no adult is present with disregard for the great changes time has brought.[3] At the turn of the century, more women work than do not and many families are headed by only one parent.

Historical Footnote

Lest we underestimate the power of these two structures on other aspects of classroom life, read on. This chapter examines the effect of these structures on ambiance, expectations, and mastery. Chapter 15 further explores the impact of the class-grade classroom.

Also, consider the story of the New American Schools Development Corporation (NASDC) which was formed in the early 1990s to create "break-the-mold designs" for "a new generation" of schools, schools with "completely re-examined assumptions" about "how students learn and what students should know and be able to do." After a well-publicized fund raising effort to amass $50 million and a call for proposals for the bold and new, *not* for "fixing up the design already in place," NASDC faded away, its goals unmet. The clear winner, yet again, is the recalcitrant system and its impervious structures and settings.

BRAIN-ANTAGONISTIC ELEMENTS OF THE ENVIRONMENT

The *settings* of our instructional institutions, whether they be a public school, an undergraduate college, or specialized training center, contain many elements that we have simply come to accept as givens. Many such "givens" are brain antagonistic when viewed with brain research in mind. Four key areas are: *reality, ambiance, expectation,* and *mastery.* Until we all have a workable understanding of why these givens are brain-antagonistic, they will remain rooted in our schools, inherited by yet another generation of educators, parents, and students.

Reality

Of all the criticisms of the public schools, very near the top of the list is their lack of reality. Particularly in curriculum content. As students so frequently lament, "What's this good for?" "When will I ever use this?"

The facet of *reality* brings us back again to the place of the book in education.

Limitations of Textbook-Dependency. The book, of course, ranks among our greatest technological inventions. It has provided the basis for our information age and a good many years are likely to pass before computer retrieval displaces the library shelf. But the book inherently is an *abstract* of reality. A brain-compatible approach introduces a considerable shift from defining an educated person as one "who knows a lot" (possesses much information, or can recite the sacred text, or is familiar with the language of the law) to seeing the educated person as one who *knows what to do* — who can detect the patterns involved and select appropriate *programs that can be implemented.* (While some may still argue that we need a sprinkling of scholars in the old sense, producing them is hardly the duty of our schools and undergraduate colleges or training institutions. We can leave the task to graduate schools.)

In academic instruction, teachers often cling to the book (the text) as though to a life raft. The book does not get translated into doing, or the doing consists mainly of exercises, still remote from acting on the real world. The book is finite and convenient. The instructor can plan to cover the book by going over it with the class at the rate of 10 to 20 pages a week. Examinations can be based on regurgitating right answers on a similar schedule. Incidentally, emphasis on "the" book can hold down use of other books!

As I have noted, reality typically is complex, messy, random, and illogical. It may also be awkward, offensive, controversial, hard to partition off, and subject to many factors producing rapid and sometimes unpredictable change. The well-ordered classroom and rude reality clash head-on, and ordinarily the classroom wins. *The same walls that confine the students as prisoners serve to exclude the inconvenient and often embarrassing real world.*

This conflict between textbook and the real world goes unannounced by bugles and salvos of artillery. The teacher's decision usually occurs all too quietly, all under the steady pressures of tradition and convenience. As a result, pressured teachers may feel the need to "cover the work" faster.

The poverty of instruction that stems from this limiting use of the book becomes compounded manyfold by another invention, the "course." I am far from a pioneer in pointing out that courses are an academic fiction, not to be found in reality. When the setting is built on courses, the door is opened for translating x hours in *y* course into *n* number of point credits, and solemnly maintaining that a certain total of points constitutes an education, or qualification for some credential! Perhaps we should ask another version of the airline question: "Would you like to fly with a pilot who got his certificate points in other courses, without any study of landings?"

The fragmentation introduced by courses appears hard to deny. It becomes still more serious when those giving courses make too little effort to coordinate their efforts, and when the administration or school board accepts traditional and long-outdated notions of what constitute basics.

A brain-compatible approach goes in the opposite direction because the emphasis on patterns tends to unify and to promote natural transfer of learning. Such pattern-concepts (they can be called "grand ideas") as *continuum, feedback circuit, negative/positive, distribution curve, system, energy cycle, life cycle, push/pull or loaded switch, change process* and many more apply in a wide variety of applications. Actual curriculum may almost entirely ignore these true basics.

Recommendation: Ensure a far greater emphasis on reality than on "the book" and on avoiding the fragmentation caused by "courses," and on using unifying "grand ideas."

Changes in Students' Prior Experiences—The Peril in Ignoring Changes in Society.
The students of earlier days, in their hours and months out of school, were drenched in exposure to reality. They helped grow and process food, fed and birthed animals, helped maintain machines and build structures, made many necessaries, wove and sewed clothing, assisted manufacturing and business, knew the community and its people intimately. Their input was varied and often oppressively "real." The school could well afford, on balance, to bring them into a once- or twice-removed, symbolic world. Even so, the basic skills they sometimes acquired were intended for immediate use: arithmetic for ciphering in shops or to keep farm accounts, reading primarily for religious purposes, writing to keep records or occasionally send letters, since travel was very limited for most. Even music, which got much attention, was utilized in church and community events.

But today students are starved for exposure to reality. They have few chores, and these usually are trivial, rather than responsibilities obviously essential to the family's survival as was the case a century ago. They do not see food being grown or necessities being made: milk comes not from cows but from the supermarket. When my friends and I walked to school, we stopped to observe each stage of the building of a new house; today's students most likely whiz by in bus or car. The toys we designed and made have been replaced by those that are bought.

Many children today have no real idea of what their parents do for a living. Terms such as auditor, keypuncher, harness-maker (electronic), long lines installer, change-order checker, renting agent, margin clerk, patent attorney, facsimile operator, interior decorator, actuary, router, manufacturer's representative, systems engineer, dot etcher, flow scheduler, analytical chemist, and the like may have no meaning to youngsters; even titles such as secretary, fitter, cashier, inspector, and executive may relate to little within the child's experience. Many children never see their parents' places of work, or see only the exterior.

They are not likely to learn much of this nature in school, except as they may select specific vocational courses at the secondary level. In most communities academic paths get priority and most of the attention and college entrance stands as the assumed goal. Efforts to stress career education have produced little deep change thus far and where there is no special funding, the program may have faded away. After 12 years of nonrealistic schooling, students usually emerge with few and limited useful skills; superficial and often garbled understanding of the content they have studied; and virtually no substantial knowledge of their communities and how they work, e.g., politics, law, business, taxation, consumer economics, other countries, other languages, recent world history, older and younger people, marriage and the rearing of children, or even the requirements of the fields that interest them. Frequently they have developed no firm ambitions and know so little about occupations that they have no grounds for choice.

Worse, they have had forced on them the notion that the *credential* is what counts, that passing an examination is a license to cease further learning, that the objective of learning is not its application but getting over the next hurdle toward additional credentials.

In at least four areas, the schools, and to a large degree colleges, appear to have allowed their foundation to erode by ignoring the huge changes going on in society:

1. As students have lost the contact with reality most students used to have amply, the schools have failed to bring reality *inside* their walls to offset the loss.

2. As noted above, for centuries schools aimed to *control* what their students learned. Indoctrination and "teaching the book" were the undisputed objectives. New technologies in a different society have wiped out that concept, yet schools commonly act as if control were still possible and desirable and an objective! (For example, conventional schools have detailed curriculums that in practice have little to do with what students learn, inside or outside of school.

3. Similarly, schools have preserved the once valid notion that learning is primarily a youth activity, to be largely terminated as one became an adult. Such a posture may have made sense through perhaps 1940, when change began to occur so rapidly as to make the concept ridiculous. Quite recently, universities have begun to put more emphasis on lifetime learning through continuing education offerings—perhaps more for financial reasons than others. But the schools, where fundamental ideas of education are apt to be laid down, still cling to the old idea.

4. Despite the availability of new understandings of the brain and the potentials of brain-compatible education, most institutions still use instruction that was designed as suitable for an educational factory. Even the first step, recognizing the brain as the organ of learning, has not yet been universally taken, though tens of thousands of educators now pursue this productive path.

Ambiance and the Power of Absence of Threat

As noted in Chapter 11 in the discussion of the role of emotions in learning, the settings for brain-compatible education must be as free from threat as possible, not simply by good intention but by inherent design.

Here again escaping the version of school we have been brought up with is not easy. Though we no longer portray teachers holding an implement for physical punishment, they clearly possess substantial power over students in almost all classrooms, and it is freely used—often perforce on hasty judgment—behind closed doors and with no other adults present to observe, protest, or report. Not only can the power be used as of the moment but it can have long-term, even life-long, effect on the victim when it authorizes an entry on the record or a label on the child. Principals wield similar power, though as a rule theirs must be used more in the open.

Because of schooling history, the power to punish, to hurt, to demean *is built into the system at every turn.* Threat is pervasive, expressed in compulsory attendance, operation by the clock, the incessant giving of tests and examinations, constant use of marks and grades, awarding or withholding of approvals and permissions, and administrative transfer, suspension, and expulsion. Many considerate and good-hearted people work in schools who may soften the threat; but every child knows the adults still possess the power and can use it at any time. The ancient threat of captivity persists over all.

School is not a safe place for youngsters; and when pressures are added by parents hungry for credentials, even the suicide rate can soar. It can be argued that youngsters need trials and not to be coddled if they are to survive later in a hard and uncaring world. But the trials of school are more the result of suffering under a rigid bureaucracy than caused by the complex, interactive, changing problems of the real world. To the degree that such trials cause emotional override and inability to learn, they *lessen* capacity to cope. (I have seen quite a few candidates for high degrees as shaken, as terrified, as deeply into a state of emotional override as primary children.) The fear of examinations does not end early. Yet outside the academic world, and that of the lower end of civil service, examinations have only a minor importance. Those for accounting, law, and some other professions, we may note in passing, have a considerable quality of reality. The problems presented are those likely to be encountered in practice, unlike the quick, academic tests that heavily involve giving remembered right answers and merely checking a multiple-choice question.

Creating a brain-compatible ambiance calls for *deliberately identifying and stripping away sources of threat.* That many students see some faculty members as probably working against them—eager to criticize, mark down, demean, restrict or "fail" them rather than help—remains true today. The adversary role has been widely documented.[4] In visiting many schools, I have been struck by the different attitudes of students depending on their environment. In conventional classroom schools, a visitor is likely to be viewed with suspicion and avoided. In genuinely open settings, however, a visitor is perceived as a friendly helper who can be asked a question or for assistance, even pulled down to the carpet to advise on work in progress.

Equally dispensable are remnants of the factory concept, demanding that all students be present at inflexible hours. One can find administrators who appear to suffer shock at the idea that it is hardly necessary or desirable today to view students as future mill-hands, and that the ability to manage one's own time can hardly be acquired by responding to factory whistles. (Ironically, in literal terms, the whistle has all but disappeared, while the school buzzers or gongs continue in use!) Even more shocking to some (including parents) can be the idea that a certain amount of free, unassigned time, of contemplation, of reverie, even of just resting, can add to productivity. The coffee break, the "take ten" breather, the relaxed lunch period, have all been accepted widely by profit-pressed business and industry, but far less so in education. One might suppose that learning was thought to be a function of the clock, or of how long buttocks remain in contact with a hard chair.

The feeling of *captivity* can be sharply reduced if the value of doing so is seen. Once the factory and classroom molds are broken, practical arrangements present little difficulty, and many models already exist of schools and higher institutions that allow students much freedom of movement and schedule and the opportunity to participate in framing what is to be learned and how.[5] Nor is it difficult to allow students some room to select, rather than have forced on them, the instructors and planning counselors they relate to best. (That arrangement can be equally appreciated on the instructor's side.)

Recommendation: Creating an ambiance that is non-threatening, nonpunitive, and reduces all aspects of captivity to a minimum is the first element to be implemented when creating a brain-compatible learning environment. No other change in curriculum or instruction will result in a shift in student outcomes until emotional override is eliminated on a consistent basis.

Expectations

The schools, and their nonpublic equivalents (more often similar than sharply different) supposedly represent the foundation of *education*. From this base stems a welter of ideas that relate schools and learning, and teaching and learning. Included are beliefs about when children should go to school; what represents basic and normal learning; conditions necessary for learning; desirable organization; the proper roles of students, teachers, administrators, and parents; the functions of the school in the community and its claim to tax monies; and the authority it can, does, and should wield.

Anyone who has closely observed schools over many years from an outsiders vantage point, as I have for several decades, will, I believe, readily agree that "chaos" is not an unfair word to describe this vast, confused, interrelated scene. Schools seem to have great difficulty stating what they are seeking to do, why they are doing it, and what the results are. Examination of why schools are as they are usually finds the reasons, if determinable, far in the past. But so large is the establishment, so huge the amount of money used, so numerous the jobs, that this outdated juggernaut *colors most efforts to comprehend human learning.*

The influence of the school extends upward: much that is done at college level, in vocational schools, and in training programs plainly reflects conventional school practice and the often centuries-old and now plainly defective concepts of human behavior, nature, and learning that schools embody. Against this backdrop, teachers, administrators, and parents wrestle with the fundament query: What should our children at our school know and be able to do? Both the thinking processes and conclusions are, quite understandably, muddled.

The discussion of *expectation* plunges us at once into an unfamiliar area. Schools and colleges provide standards widely taken for granted, as for instance "grade levels" that are used for various purposes year after year without any inquiry into their origins or current suitability.

As I have suggested, the basic idea of brain-compatibility leads to the design of schools that focus on *bringing about student learning* instead of conducting ineffective, ritualistic teaching. From a brain-compatible perspective, expectation has a number of dimensions which remain largely unexplored:

- How fast can individual students learn, given full opportunity? Are we over-influenced by the pitiful outcomes now expected of conventional schools?

- How far up can learning be carried, relative to age and experience? How crippling is the idea of "school" implying group learning, in lockstep? Of age constraining capability?

- How completely can gross failure be eliminated? Seldom do schools reveal how many students fail almost completely. Asking the question may produce instant hostility.

- How well can learning be retained? Conventional schools appear to assume that specific learning need only be retained long enough to deal with the next testing or examination. ("We had that!" declare students. If it is on the record as having been studied, what was retained is considered to be beside the point—and might be frightfully embarrassing to measure.)

On these and related questions, research has been scant and findings few. Books on learning typically do not get into these matters in depth, if at all. Learning has been looked at mostly in relation to classrooms. But although more than two million classrooms go into session each September, reports of solid learning successes seldom appear and the few that do rarely survive critical examination! Where we find individual students who have achieved far above the usual, the conventional classroom may not figure in the achievement, since the student soon goes far beyond its influence.

Barrier to Achieving: Running the Half Race. The core of natural learning is the *desire to better understand how the world* (as experienced by the individual learner) *operates.* From earliest infancy there is a clearly visible, built-in drive to make sense of what seems of value. (As discussed, learning is an innate drive in humans.) But making sense does not mean only an academic understanding. I have previously emphasized that the motor aspect must be involved if one is to act upon the world. One must *do, perform, accomplish.* To stop at academic learning, primarily an act of linguistic retrieval, is to run only half a race . . . *by design!*

The "learning by doing" relationship so closely associated with John Dewey, although embraced by many in education long before and since, should not prevent us from seeing that most natural learning is *for* doing: it enlarges the individual's control over his/her physical and social world.

Learning is the acquisition of programs; programs have goals. A child learns to walk, to talk, to operate light switches and faucets, to ride a wheeled vehicle, to throw and catch a ball, to use tools, *to enlarge the repertoire of what can be done.*

As we inspect settings and ask the question "Why is the student here?" a satisfactory answer from a brain-compatible view must be on the order of "To acquire the programs to do this and that in order to act upon the real world." That is not the kind of answer we often get when we look at conventional schooling. Rather, even the avowed objectives tend to slide semantically away from "do" into vaguer terminology. For example, the student will:

- "Get the fundamentals" of an education
- Learn "basic skills" (probably not sharply named or defined)
- Be prepared for further, higher education
- Be enabled to pass various examinations
- Complete the curriculum

In short, the academic student supposedly will acquire skills and knowledge that form a latent pool, to be useful in some distant, unspecified future, or to pass examinations of some kind: remote objectives, to please or mollify some other party, not the student. The dictionary definition of "academic," in fact, stresses not real, not practical!

Barriers to Achieving: Societal Ambivalence. If learning is indeed a prime objective of schooling, as is so often proclaimed, one might expect that great attention would be paid to learning potentials. But I fear it does not take much study of schooling to see that *by no means can it be assumed that maximum learning is universally desired.* While parents may welcome outstanding performance in certain fields, especially athletics or some form of social approval, it is no secret that many do not jump for joy at having their offspring come home with new and surprising ideas and understandings, expertise that puts parental abilities to shame, or observations that call into question firmly held concepts in religious, patriotic, or economic matters. Interest is likely to focus on credentials. Higher-income parents may see the school as wholly preparatory for college and perhaps advanced degrees. Only a minority can be expected to value learning per se.

Barriers to Achieving: A Topsy-Turvy Sense of Rewards and Failure. If we think of two private teachers, one about to teach 20 beginners to swim and the other to teach 12 to play the piano, we can anticipate their concerns. They do not want failures; they can almost hear voices saying, "I sent my child to ___ and he didn't learn a thing!" In the private setting, any gross failure is a black eye. All children must be made to succeed. Also, the rapid learner is cherished, for each success tends to attract more pupils.

In contrast, in the graded public school, the *sense of failure and reward is reversed.* The lagging pupil can be sloughed off with a label: not motivated, uncooperative, immature, family problems, learning disability, previous failure, language handicaps, disturbed. Whatever the term, it transfers responsibility from instructor and school to the student. The students who do middling well become the blessed, because they more or less fit the syllabus and the standards. At the top end, the bright or gifted students may be nuisances and perhaps threats, apt to become bored, difficult or withdrawn, or heavy consumers of teacher time and effort.

Furthermore, teachers of graded classrooms seldom fail to realize that if they allow students to "run ahead," trouble will ensue from the teachers who receive them in the next grade, the following year. Somehow, the more able students must be prevented from saying "We had that!" when the next term begins. The lockstep grade system puts a cap on what learning students are to achieve.

This lockstep structure also restricts and confines teachers. Within the bureaucratic social system, those whose methods differ and whose students learn sharply better may expect not admiration and emulation but more likely some degree of ostracism. The instructor who produces visibly superior learning becomes a threat to those who don't, and quite possibly a boat-rocker and "disruptive element," in the eyes of an administration concerned with harmony, smooth running, and no problems. Testimony to this pressure for teacher conformity abounds.[6]

In plain and evident truth, accelerated learning can tear apart the conventional school. The economic penalties are apparent, too. If students can complete the present curriculum better in three years less, what will that do to staffing? If reading achievement becomes far better, who will employ the remedial teachers? If the "learning disabled" prove quite able to learn, what will those specialists be needed for? Since students learning with success at their own speed seldom create discipline problems (almost always a sign of impeded learning), why will the schools need all those assistant principals? At present, very few teachers or administrators ever are discharged for incompetence, since historically the failure of students to learn has been easily accommodated by blaming the victim. But suppose the demands for competency continue to rise and student achievement of learning must be demonstrated— what of job security then?

Clearly, some suppression of learning, deliberately and systematically, is essential to preserve the present graded classroom system. But we must wonder at the cost to society and to the individuals held back or diverted by "enrichment."

A setting designed for learning must be so organized that fullest student achievement is welcomed, not feared. That does not imply going through the present curriculum faster, since there exists the widest agreement that present studies are far too narrow, producing graduates with distressingly inadequate skills and a weak grasp of the world they must enter as responsible citizens. Alternative structures already are available, and more can be created, in which brain-compatible learning can be encouraged without constraint,[7] to the great pleasure of most teachers who enjoy seeing learning occur.

Recommendation: Ensure settings in which expectations of student learning are possible and attainable and left open-ended. Also, high attainment should not create difficulties for the faculty.

Mastery

From a brain research and Proster Theory viewpoint, the *mastery* approach appears so simple in concept that one must wonder why it still has the capacity to startle some conventional educators.[8] Presently, we commonly require a fixed period of instruction, such as a semester, at the end of which time each student is given a grade. If passing is 65 percent, credit is given and the 35 percent not-passed portion is forgotten about. For a factory approach, this long seemed a convenient arrangement, even if one built on low standards. The mastery approach turns this upside down: it makes 100 percent attainment of the key elements the goal but leaves the time to achieve it flexible. I have often illustrated the principle by asking, "Would you like to fly with an airline pilot who got 65 percent in landings?"

When mastery is demanded in basic areas of learning, the setting changes from one which emphasizes jumping over hurdles to get credentials, to one in which solid learning takes priority, is expected, demanded, and achieved. The sordid business of cramming for examinations, remembering answers for a brief period, and leaving the gaps in learning still open because a "pass" has been registered, can be ended. Mastery permits observed individual performance, or demonstrated abilities, to take the place of contrived tests. The "right answer," often quick, arbitrary and superficial, gives place to the cycle we have examined in our discussion of Proster Theory: detect the *pattern,* select a stored *program,* implement it successfully.

Mastery (using the term as indicated above and not in some special sense) simultaneously helps create an atmosphere of high standards and achievement within the setting. It also tends to simplify the knotty task of assessment and evaluation currently at the top of many agendas—as though our problem were measuring failure, not forestalling it.

We have noted the difference between *threat,* inflicted upon the individual, and *risk,* selected by the individual in response to the built-in urge for stimulation—to take chances, to dare, to seek excitement and new events, to seek out the novel. When students are always told what to do, the tendency is strong for those who give the orders to set objectives too low for many students. But in settings where students have more room to choose their own, they can often be startling in their originality and level.[9] If a student does overshoot, the results are not necessarily wholly negative—there can be a new appreciation of complexity, a new awareness of the problems involved. On one occasion while in school my son was angered by a librarian's objection to his taking out a book on submarines because she thought it was too difficult for him. (In fact he was able to read a good deal of it and to understand the diagrams.) I have always wondered why she did not see it as simpler to let him take the book and return it, whatever the outcome. What was to be lost? Where the setting offers mastery with a good deal of freedom of choice, students will frequently take on surprising risks and often make good on them. But the setting must allow the time and continuity the projects require. Conversely, students held to short efforts that can be completed within a factory-school time frame are being effectively prevented and discouraged from building experience in undertakings that demand more planning, dedication, and perseverance—all qualities that are highly valued in most settings.

Even at kindergarten level, complaints and labels based on short attention span often turn out to mean that some teacher feels "this child won't stick long with what I want him to do." Yet in the course of schooling, the student may again and again be told, in effect or in so many words, to read a shorter book because the report must be in Monday; to write 250 words because the teacher has no time to read long essays; to forgo an experiment that would take more than a year because "the course will be over before that." Mastery is not only not a goal, but an idea often perceived as a nuisance that interferes with neat bureaucratic scheduling and the dominance of the clock.

Recommendation: Place emphasis on mastery rather than passing, on achieving learning over the demands of the clock, scheduling, and processing.

IMPLEMENTATION IMPLICATIONS

These observations are made to sensibly suggest that not much can be expected from planting flower seeds in concrete. We cannot go far in applying new insights and theory as a new layer on an outdated, obsolete structure, strangled by traditions that fight and impede brain-compatible approaches.

We cannot build on the old foundation; we have to junk it.

But we can begin, at once, to put the new brain-compatible concepts and techniques into use, wherever seeds can find soil. This alone will not free education from the consequences of failure to enter and keep pace with the modern world but it may nonetheless open doors to some urgently needed sweeping reforms.

The discussion of settings obviously involves matters of educational philosophy not to be treated in one chapter of a book on another subject. My intent is only to suggest that a brain-compatible approach, because of the nature of the brain, should guide us in designing settings and in becoming more critical of, and thus more willing to leave behind, the now decrepit settings we still struggle to use.

NOTES

1 *Places for Learning, Places for Joy* (Cambridge: Harvard University Press, 1973), p. 28.

2 Editors Note's: For a extensive, and challenging, compilation of socio-logical data regarding the effects of schooling, particularly the coercion of punishments and rewards, see Alfie Kohn's *Punished by Rewards: The Trouble with Gold Stars, Incentive Plans, A's, Praise, and other Bribes* (Boston: Houghton-Mifflin Company, 1993) and *Beyond Discipline: From Compliance to Community* (Alexandria, Virginia: ASCD, 1996).

3 From 1950 to 1977 the percentage of married women in the labor force rose from not quite 25 percent to 47 percent; in 1995, more than 60 percent were employed. About 48 percent of women 16 or over had or were seeking jobs; in 1995, 52 per-cent. Of the female labor force, higher percentages of divorced women work than married women. (*United Business Service*, September 4, 1979, p. 353 and *Facts on Working Woman*, September, 1996, pp. 1-2.) The trend appears to continue for women with school-age children to seek employment. Nearly six out of every ten women, age 16 and over, were working or looking for work in 1995. Women account for 46 percent of the total United States labor force (1995).

4 Much evidence suggests teachers and other people working in schools are deceived, or deceive themselves, on how their stu-dents regard their efforts. For example, *The Fleischmann Report*, a massive study of New York State elementary and secondary schools, found that "Students generally felt that teachers did not help them to do their best, did not understand their prob-lems, did not help them improve their skills and were not concerned with their future. More than simply not enjoying school, many students indicated that their school experience was actually painful. . . . Teachers appeared largely unaware of the negative feelings of their students." (New York: The Viking Press, 1973), pp. 46-47. Other studies also show wide differ-ences between teacher and student views of what is happening.

5 Editor's Note: Both the constructivist and bodybrain-compatible learning movements emphasize the importance of students learning to sit in the

driver's seat during their learning. Both recognize that student passivity in the classroom is antithetical to learning to become a lifelong learner.

6   A considerable body of literature that might be called teacher "confessions" has appeared over the years, among the most insightful being those of James Herndon, *The Way It 'Spozed to Be* and particularly, in relation to staff relationships, *How to Survive in Your Native Land* (New York: Simon and Schuster, 1971). For a penetrating discussion from an expert outsider's viewpoint, see Seymour B. Sarason, *The Culture of the School and the Problem of Change* (Boston: Allyn and Bacon, 1971). On teachers' anxiety about colleagues' opinions, see James P. Comer, *School Power* (New York: Free Press, 1980), especially p. 115. This book gives a case history of efforts to improve schools and how and why "teachers close the doors and try to survive." There can be little doubt that the pressures on teachers usually are intense, complex, often amorphous, and contradictory. Teachers bear the brunt of the system's crazy unsuitability. In my opinion they do too little to protest it, having given scant thought to alternatives.

7   The furious interest in experimental approaches and structures that began in the 1960s and continued into the 1970s scarcely affected the great majority of classrooms, it has become clear, but did provide a considerable body of thinking and experience that has not yet been digested and summarized. There seems no question that many viable alternative plans exist, often in bits and pieces not organized into a system—in large part, I suggest, because of the lack of a comprehensive theory of learning until now. The literature is vast and highly variable in quality. Some starting points might include: Harriet Talmage, ed. *Systems of Individualized Education* (Berkeley: McCutchan, 1975); Allan A. Glatthorn, "Creating Learning Environments" in *The Teaching of English, 76th Yearbook of the National Society for the Study of Education* (Chicago: University of Chicago Press, 1977); Mario D. Fantini, editor. *Alternative Education* (Garden City, New York: Anchor Books, 1976); and Harvey B. Scribner and Leonard B. Stevens, *Make Your School Work* (New York: Simon and Schuster, 1975). Also see the April 1981 issue of *Phi Delta Kappan*. These give a sense of the great range of alternatives. My study of school organization and its effects, *The Classroom Disaster* (New York: Teachers College Press, Columbia University, 1969)

remains one of the few discussions of the kind and contains a description of a plan subsequently elaborated into a blueprint for a complete system known as IROSS. Few such full-system blueprints seem to exist.

8   The term mastery is associated by some with the work of Benjamin S. Bloom, who has pursued this approach. In using it here I am not necessarily referring to those specific applications but to a principle I advanced in *The Classroom Disaster* (see Note 7). Others have expressed similar ideas, notably John Carroll, at least as far back as 1963.

9   On the other hand, it should be noted that under present conditions students given choice at secondary levels may seek the easiest courses so they can pile up good grades for college entrance. This was a more serious problem when the struggle to get into college was more intense, but it may still influence many students who have been pressured into chasing credentials.

15

THEORY APPLIED TO SITUATIONS: THE CLASSROOM, EDUCATION'S CURSE

For more than 50 years now, studies have been documenting the effectiveness of nontraditional school programs in the United States. This research should cause us to question 95 percent of current educational practice.

—Wayne Jennings and Joe Nathan[1]

To observe *situation* as I am using that term here, we bring the camcorder inside and zoom to close-ups of the student's day-to-day immediate surroundings and routines. Most of the time while attending school, and for hours at a stretch, the student will be in a classroom.

Here again the past dominates and that monstrous invention, the classroom,[2] colors all thinking in schools and far up the educational ladder. As once people referred to "horseless carriages" because they could not imagine carriages outside of the context of horses, we speak of *non* classroom schemes. Or we have used such locutions as "open classroom" which, at best, is a contradiction in terms. As yet we do not even have convenient words to describe arrangements free from the blight of classrooms!

THE CONVENTIONAL CLASSROOM

We can define the graded, conventional classroom as an arrangement for learning—or perhaps more accurately, for teaching—that calls for one teacher and a group of students, normally 15 or more, to maintain a fixed relationship for a period of months. In the graded version, as opposed to the rare nongraded, the students are considered to be at a more or less uniform level of attainment. This may be on the basis of chronological age—an utterly fictitious criteria since age tells little about what a specific group of students know or can do or what experience they have had individually and thus bring to the situation.[3] As a result, the teaching is geared to a level which denies the actual variations; the inmates of a classroom most often are there by assignment or as the consequence of forced, limited choice. In the terms of this definition, it matters little whether the classroom be elementary, secondary, or post-secondary.

The Classroom's Impact on Teachers

The classroom today *puts the teacher into an assignment where success is virtually impossible.* There is simply no way to deal with the huge variations the students exhibit, other than to teach and let the chips fall where they may. If there were really a desire and aim to individualize, the first step would be to abandon the standard classroom. *It was designed and established in the mid-1880s for precisely the opposite purpose: to process the students with minimum regard to their individual backgrounds, previous achievement, and needs.* The classroom preserves the old approach of "school as factory."

In my experience, which includes meeting with teachers and other educators literally by the thousands, in hundreds of places over a period of decades, a baffling aspect of schools is the apparent inability or refusal of practitioners at all levels to see or acknowledge the tremendous, horrendous effect the classroom organizational device has on *them.* On occasion, some may complain bitterly of their current frustration but overall they find it hard to conceive of *not* being in a classroom or of schools that function other than as a collection of classrooms. Even those who write or lecture as expert observers and analysts appear to assume the classroom is inevitable and inescapable.

Why, one might ask, this inability or refusal to see and examine the negative effects of the classroom? It may be tempting here to guess at teachers' motivations. Do they at heart love the classroom because it puts them in full power to control? Because it is a hiding place, where they can work behind closed doors and so out of view of possible critics? Or because, for at least some, so they can be "stars" performing to a captive audience? Or because many fear having to deal with other adults as is required of most people who hold jobs? We can find evidence for many such speculations but with little profit. What is of prime concern here is that it seems cryingly obvious that the classroom severely limits teachers' options (both real and imagined) and constrains their efforts to teach. In fact, we might well say that it coerces them to pay less attention to student learning and more to "classroom management" and to strongly aggressive instructional approaches that prove highly brain-antagonistic. When it comes to the classroom, there are no winners.

Barrier to Flexible Grouping. As one clear example, the conventional classroom makes difficult, if not practically impossible, any *flexibility of student grouping.* To work with one or four or five students, the teacher must find some way to keep the others busy. To divide the class into three reading groups, as is often done, requires that two be neglected while one is given attention. It cannot prove too surprising that the instructor who feels obliged to manage or "drive" the entire class finds frequent relief in going to whole-class activities. In contrast, in the true open or informal classroom and in Montessori programs, a skilled teacher has no problem concentrating attention on one or a few students for many minutes at a time. The other students continue their activities.

I am no all-out advocate of the open classroom (why have the classroom at all?) but ample observation shows clearly that it creates a great difference in the teacher's practical ability to have close contact and interchange with individual students on matters involving learning. In conventional classrooms, teachers seldom spend as much as 30 seconds in such discussions, and usually less than 10, and may dominate all talking to such a degree that weeks may pass before a student makes, in class sessions, a self-initiated remark of any consequence![4]

The Gap. A number of studies agree that conventional classroom teachers behave in ways that they vigorously deny when presented with observations. Such is the pressure of the classroom's demands that *a huge gap develops between the intentions of even good, experienced teachers and what they actually do.*[5] Further, the pressure pushes most such teachers into behaving in quite uniform patterns.[6]

"Driving" the Classroom. The essential concept in the classroom teacher's role appears to be that of "driving" the class. We can suspect that some mix of several elements contributes to the overall posture and behavior of teachers. Some of these are old, such as surviving bits of the religiously-derived notion that children are born evil and must be firmly disciplined for their own good (originally, to be "saved"); or the idea, from the old, deadly dull days of rote schooling, that students must be forced into learning which would occur no other way. Other concerns are current and practical such as the worry of many teachers that their charges might rebel or get seriously out of control (a nightmare of newer teachers) or that noise or exuberance might disturb the teachers of adjoining classrooms. There may be a niggling worry that a school board member, parent, or other potential critic might pop in and misconstrue or disapprove of what is going on. Prominent is a feeling that the assigned year's work must be "covered" at all costs so the teacher can't be blamed however well students learn or don't. And, always there is anxiety about the unknown—what might happen if the teacher does not drive all the time.

Student Passivity. This kind of aggressive teaching, of course, puts the students into passive roles. The classroom is a place where one is *told* what to do, criticized or punished for not fully complying, and not allowed time or opportunity to do anything else. (Many teachers do reward students by permitting them to play games or read what is available but this is regarded as a temporary cessation of instruction.)

Exams As a Coercive Tool. Examinations, of course, bring more of the same driving of students. In addition, examinations can be observed in blatant use to intimidate or "motivate" students: "You better pay attention, Leroy and Tim, you're going to have a test on this Friday." Teachers displeased with a student's attitude or behavior may mark a quiz harshly, thus getting even, with a show of objectivity. As many have observed, rather seldom are test results used diagnostically and followed up with re-teaching. For administrators, standardized or official evaluations may serve to show the public that the school cares about learning results or is serious about outcomes—with again perhaps little or no real effort to seek to rectify failures.

Power is hard for anyone to resist. In classrooms, with no other adult observing (genuine supervision of teachers long ago virtually ceased in most schools),[7] teachers may easily come to use their power oppressively, even while convinced that they are concerned, kindly, and helpful. Classrooms provide little corrective feedback and students who take home complaints may find parents receive them with disbelief, scant sympathy, or even approval: "Good, you need to be made to toe the line!"

Impact of the Classroom on Students

Students learn early that in classrooms one suffers. That is *school*. The object then becomes survival, by whatever strategies will work. Since students regard the school as representing adult authority, their contempt and alienation may extend to learning in general and all "authority."

When we evaluate this situation in brain-compatible referents, we are forced to regard it as about as brain-antagonistic as could be contrived.[8]

Teachers become the victims of this antagonistic situation along with students even though, unlike their captive students, they have the option of withdrawing, which they do in large numbers.[9]

Impact on Beginning Teachers

Beginning teachers in schools are often appalled, as many personal accounts show, at the realities of their working situation. Their high ideals, aims, and spirits may rapidly evaporate. But the beginning teachers, often in their early twenties and with limited experience as employees, have little expertise and less status to apply to changing the institution. Bucking the social system of the school may well bring resentments, criticism, and early loss of job. Like students, teachers are under much pressure to comply—or face the agonizing choice of making a fresh start in some other field, casting aside several years of what was supposed to have been training for just this kind of work. In the open market, they may be aware, a bachelor's degree in education is not an impressive credential. And many may eagerly *want* to work with youngsters.

The Invisible Line: Teacher Dissatisfaction and the Classroom Structure

It can hardly be surprising that periodic surveys find many classroom teachers dissatisfied with their jobs.[10] The frustrations of instructors, who want to produce learning results and to treat students as individuals yet are nevertheless thrust into situations where doing either is extremely difficult, are all too apparent to anyone who has much contact with teachers. Curiously, in my experience, few relate their frustrations to the graded classroom. Most of them never think about the structure and its effect — the classroom is "invisible"[11] because *it is taken for granted as the standard setting for instruction.*

THE CLASSROOM AND RESEARCH

In spite of tons of so-called research on classroom operation, there exists virtually no knowledge base that could support successful classroom teaching of the conventional kind. Teachers are assigned jobs that no one knows how to do in terms of creating demonstrable learning outcomes.

What we do know about prevailing teaching in classrooms is that the learning results, such as those shown by NAEP surveys[12] are appallingly low, with more than 90 per cent failure of high school graduates to attain what would seem to be reasonable, modest goals. It is hard to think of any widely used organizational device that works worse than the standard school classroom.

What's more, the learning that does result is heavily of the recall, right-answer kind, valuable not for real-world applications but for answering examinations or achievement tests — *precisely the kind of learning that moves away from the excellence and understandings we urgently require.*

A person unfamiliar with educational research might assume that if anything whatever was known it would be what goes on, minute by minute, in classrooms. Those more sophisticated will know that such observations have been avoided rather than vigorously explored. A variety of "outside" studies, however, have thrown some light on the question although none as yet, to my knowledge, attack it directly in an adequate way. Overall, findings suggest that *sizeable chunks of school time do not get used for instruc-*

tion[13] but go to "management" and distractions. Further, large variations in time use from classroom to classroom have commonly been noted. As we stand outside the closed door of a "classroom," that term in itself gives us virtually no specific notion of what is going on inside.

In schools where classrooms are closed-door "boxes," as most are, administrators also can only guess what actually transpires. Though the public tends to assume that principals frequently visit classrooms, today much visiting simply does not occur or visits are merely perfunctory. While exceptional principals can and sometimes do work wonders by leadership, principals' authority has been stripped away over the years. To discharge a teacher for inept teaching, for example, has long been impractical in typical settings and, in fact, rarely occurs.

My own observations suggest that when classroom instruction is measured on a stopwatch basis, excluding the time that goes to disciplinary remarks or action, class management, giving out and collecting, housekeeping, tests and examinations, clerical matters, internal and outside interruptions, and so on, the net time shrinks typically to under 90 minutes a day, and often far less.[14] *If this teaching is looked at in brain terms of input and program building, the amount of useful instruction falls incredibly low, perhaps scraping zero.* Time given to individual attention, so cherished by the public, by my calculations comes out to be about six hours *per year per student.*

In the higher grades, it may be that the proportion of teacher-instructed time tends to rise in academic subjects; but here we find a marked increase in lecturing. Still, a 1970 study using video tapes showed teachers behaving with striking overall similarity of pattern, in grades 1, 4, and 11.[15]The teachers had varying experience and their subjects were mathematics or social studies. However, these factors did not seem to much affect behavior. The classroom exerts an overriding influence on what teachers feel they can do, and do.

This same study, supported by recordings that could be looked at again and again to verify findings, brought out another characteristic of the classroom situation:

> Changes occurred frequently and rapidly. For instance, in the most active classroom, a change of one sort or another occurred on an average *once every five seconds.* In the least active classroom,

there was change every eighteen seconds. This means that there were 371 activity episodes in the average lesson.[16]

If this butterfly changing translated as variety of random input, it might be welcomed. But of course most of it presents very little that could be considered input for pattern extraction purposes and the frenetic pace produces a blur. Most of what the teachers presented was *information* to be remembered, the centuries-old rote approach, diluted and disguised by currently conventional techniques. Very little time was spent on having students *do* anything.

These findings, I am painfully well aware, tend to infuriate teachers and many administrators who believe that they are all wrong for *their* classrooms or schools. One can understand and empathize with well-intentioned people trapped in graded classroom schools who abhor facing the quite obvious facts and prefer fantasized versions of their activities that let them maintain some semblance of morale and mental health.

When we put workers in any field into situations that make success exceedingly hard to attain, we treat them cruelly and they will respond by quitting, working in a "get by," disinterested way, or grossly distorting their estimate of their performance. When, in addition, we give teachers shamefully poor training, weak support on the job, and public blame for results, we end up with the pitiful outcomes we wrestle with today in the great majority of schools. *And we fail to use the enormous total of energy, good-will, enthusiasm, intelligence and creativity that teachers will willingly provide if given opportunity,* as I have had ample chance to witness.

So myopic are many researchers, so eager to find some ray of hope for the conventional practices, that expensive research fails to reach the obvious conclusion: *if classrooms fail so blatantly, we should find other arrangements that don't.*

Sober thought also tells us that any suggestion that some two million teachers be retrained to change what they do in classrooms must be called wishful. We have no means of reaching teachers isolated in classrooms, no inservice apparatus that might be effective, and no reason to believe teachers will alter their accustomed ways in unchanged settings, where all the biases support use of old programs.[17] *Only in new settings can we hope to bring about new teacher behaviors and only if instruction rests on solid, brain-based theory.* Freeing teachers from the classroom structure and providing needed retraining of teachers is a chick and egg affair. And as a farmer might counsel us, it is wise to have both at the same time.

LEAVING THE CLASSROOM BEHIND

Here is a critical question: Can a strong, expert teacher apply brain-compatible approaches and principles with effect, even in a conventional classroom? Observation tells me that the answer may be yes, depending on how persistent the teacher is and how secure he or she is in using brain-compatible techniques. But the deadly constraints and awkwardness of the classroom will not go away. The teacher will be swimming against a strong current. Furthermore, although short-term progress has been readily demonstrated, long-term implementation is ephemeral.

Starting Points

In brief and in general, how can the classroom and its procedures be replaced? The answer is not hard, at least in terms of organizational objectives:

1. Students should not be held captive in one room with one teacher but should be free to circulate in a much larger area, working with a number of helpers: fellow students, volunteers, visitors, aides, apprentice teachers, teachers, instructional specialists. All of these can be providers of feedback on a one-to-one basis as well as providers of input on an individual, small-group, or large-group basis. The idea that input should come from a single teacher proves disastrously restrictive.

2. Groupings should be formed *as required for the work in hand* and continued only so long as that grouping is suitable. In college, a student may at various times work alone (as in a library), with one or two others (as in a laboratory), with a small group (as in a discussion, carrying out a project, planning an event, conducting a survey or study, or rehearsing a play), in a class-size group (as for learning a language by rote or listening to a presentation), or in a large group (as in a lecture hall, assembly, theatre, or concert hall). Similar flexibility is quite possible in schools, from kindergarten on.

3. The use of language by students should be facilitated by providing continual room for asking questions, genuine student-originated discussion, working jointly, making announcements and broadcasting, writing real reports (not dictated exercises) and private or public communications. Student contact with people *outside* the school should be frequent and varied.

4. Much of the learning and application of so-called basic skills should be in relation to *real* events (not contrived) and a large proportion should involve the outside world. A good deal can stem from following local, state, regional, national, and international news, and real projects (having some observable outcome) of great variety, especially those selected by individual students.

5. Students' work should not be interrupted by changing periods but rather should take precedence over the clock. Students should not be required, especially after the primary-grade age levels, to be in a particular room at a particular time or, at times, even to be in school if their work can better be done elsewhere. Schools should, as feasible, reject the role of custodians.

6. Students coming to school hungry because of family conditions or emergency should be fed. Those needing rest or sleep should be permitted to do so. Just as adults regularly take breaks and relax, children should be allowed, at individual option, to do nothing for reasonable periods. (Since they become bored quickly doing nothing, this is not likely to be a problem, except as this behavior indicates another serious problem.)

7. Students should be exposed to, but should largely self-select, perhaps *ten times as much input* as ordinarily characterizes the conventional graded classroom. Much of the increase occurs automatically when the school walls are not permitted to shut out the real world. Even more input derives from escaping the classroom routine with its long waits and many no-input intervals and from bringing the real world into the school, via visitors, speakers, radio, television, film, performers, craftspeople, and so on. Having the students go outside the school—not in awkward class-size

bodies that defeat the purpose in most cases and generate much strain for teachers— but in groups of appropriate size, far easier to transport and supervise.

8. Most teachers should be relieved of the power and obligation to give marks and grades and make evaluative entries in permanent records. That power by its existence makes every person who has it an active or potential judge and punisher which, for students, puts a premium on conciliating teachers and "apple polishing," to use the politest term. In addition to the severe threat aspects, *the power to grade prevents frank relationships between faculty and students and encourages teachers to place the blame for learning failure wholly on the student.*

9. The progress of each individual student should be closely and continuously monitored, *with corrective action taken as indicated.* This is not done in the conventional graded school. Instead, teachers customarily take no responsibility for deficits in learning of children they receive and simply pass them on at the end of a year. Principals today, especially in larger schools, rarely know how well individual students are achieving except as acute problems or occasional remarkable successes occur. Counselors, with many pressures, seldom even attempt routine monitoring. Any quality control aim must be based on friendly, helpful, consistent monitoring, not simply recording and punishing.

10. Schools should be places where *courtesy and respect for others* is both demonstrated and learned. One of the most striking features of typical classrooms, to the outside observer, is the rudeness of address, the lack of civilities, the tone of voice conveying lack of respect for students, or mistrust, and the frequent "hollering" that students often find the most objectionable classroom teacher attribute. Students should have the option of avoiding such behavior just as they may have to some extent outside the school. Courteous teachers have courteous students and situations far more suited to learning accomplishment.

Cautions

Experience tells me that when some of the concepts enumerated above are advocated, many readers or listeners at once form an image of wild confusion, with children running around in great excitement, jumping pointlessly from activity to activity, while anything that can be called discipline vanishes. In truth, some examples of the free-school movement, involving schools set up by well-meaning but naive parents and romantic teachers have collapsed after a brief period for these reasons, among others. Let me suggest, if it be necessary, that nothing of the kind need occur.

Instant Change Is a Myth. First, we should realize that children who have been for years captives in traditional classrooms can hardly be expected to acquire wholly new programs just by virtue of being transferred en masse to less restrictive environments. New patterns must be understood and *new programs built.*[18]

The Inborn Need for Structure: A Home Base and Limits. Second, what is being suggested is not that there should be no structure but rather a different and more suitable structure. Students, like other people, like structure—they want to know the rules of the game and they need and want their "home base." In early enthusiasm for open schools, that word was at times taken literally, students were dumped into great expanses without walls. The human species has spent too much time crowded into caves and tents and huts to feel comfortable for long in such areas. We like the security of some walls, some dividers, some markers of space such as rugs, furniture, arches, and the like; outdoors we use fences, hedges, or boundaries such as brooks or roads. Individual children, like adults, prefer a chair, locker, cupboard, space, or something that is *theirs.* At home, each member of a household normally has a fixed place at table, a certain place to sleep, and closets and containers for personal effects. "Mine" is a powerful word for humans; to suddenly ignore it in schools invites serious troubles.

The situations proposed above do not leave students (after suitable orientation) wondering how to behave—they can see very clearly what is expected and what will not be tolerated. If we allow students to learn from many teachers and other adults, that does not prevent assigning students, with a good deal of choice and flexibility allowed, to "guiding" teachers who must accept a substantial responsibility for their students' achievement. But fundamentally, students must develop their own ability to manage themselves. When they are kept in four-walled rooms, required to have a hall pass to go anywhere else, and incessantly told what to do and not to do, they are being systematically *prevented* from developing judgment and taking responsibility. Only in fluid settings and situations can these be realistically asked for and expected.

Without necessarily realizing it, aggressive teachers and ritualistic taskmasters may come to think routinely in *confrontation* terms: teachers try to drive classes, to force behaviors; students seek to escape, evade, avoid. When opening up structure and the time frame as suggested, many such adults may see the student (the enemy) as winning. But once the student is treated with respect, given some room to self-direct and learn in an individual way at an individual pace, the confrontation disappears.

One of the most arresting aspects of a genuinely brain-compatible plan is that it virtually ends the discipline problem! My observation, confirmed by a number of associates, is that *any need for corrective or punitive discipline signals that learning is being actively prevented.* (In individual cases, of course, personal clashes may occur, as they do in office or plant or hospital; and some problems may arise outside and be brought into school — family break-up or fights, financial emergencies, sudden illness or death, or fear of street attack, for example.)

When months and years rather than days or weeks are allowed for mastery and fulfilling achievement, the wholly artificial and arbitrary pressures and threat stemming from the teacher's drive to cover the term's work roll away like heavy clouds. An ironic aspect of the conventional classroom is that the uninvolved observer can plainly see teachers working hard to make problems for themselves — clinging to unfruitful and at times disastrous programs as though to an oak in a hurricane. Continuing to act *without regard to outcomes* is, of course, the essence of ritual.

The effort to force students to learn in strongly brain-antagonistic situations must and does bring about intense frustration for teachers. Some adjust, accepting failure as the norm and glorying in rare transient bits of success; others shrug and do their job in the easiest way, eyeing retirement; some break down mentally or physically; some grow mean, bitter, and shrill. Only a few look for real alternatives. But their number is growing as it becomes "polite," even politically correct, to talk openly about the constraints discussed above.

But alternative situations such as I have broadly described are practical and viable, beyond question. In the better English open schools, and Montessori schools, millions of students have prospered. Thousands of schools in the United States have demonstrated a great variety of formats. Some have not endured as when key leaders have left or ritualists aided by budget squeezes have reversed progress; but others have. Few, of course, have had the benefit of the sharp, scientifically based theory of human learning now available. But to doubt that nonclassroom schools (and their images cast on education and training at higher levels) can function, can be real, can work is to argue with an impressive body of consistent experience that is now rapidly expanding.

In contrast, conventional, rigid, confrontational schools continue to produce abysmally low learning results, coupled with dismaying behavior problems and sagging staff morale.

In my direct personal experience with school change, I have again and again observed the surprise of teachers who move to brain-compatible, non-classroom approaches. They have trouble believing that students can behave so differently after a short transition during which old biases are altered, and that "school" does not have to mean an endless war between students and teachers. Over and over school people have spoken or written to me in terms of having found a "new world" or a "new life" that they did not know could exist.

For a half century and more, we should again note, an American system of schools flourished and produced citizens with basic skills with astonishing success considering the tiny resources allotted: the one-room country school. It had no classroom organization, no periods, no real grades. Students tutored students; groups formed and dissolved as needs indicated; the teacher had to view students as individuals and work with them on that basis. Reality was as close as the stove that had to be kept glowing, the winter path that no custodian was there to shovel. The books, though very few, were real books, not basals. If no standardized testing went on, the teacher hardly needed it—she could observe each student at work. If input was small because of resources and not every student made great gains, it can be said that few if any were prevented from learning. *The yellow school bus ended it all . . . in favor of schools with a thousand times the resources, that do prevent learning.*

The classroom did not come from Mount Sinai. It came from militaristic, regimented Prussia, imported by Horace Mann.[19] Never has it worked to produce adequate student learning. Today, I submit, evidence is overwhelming that we cannot tolerate the continued dominance of "classroom" concepts and operations if we are to obtain the schools we desperately need for national survival.

NOTES

1 "Startling/Disturbing Research on School Program Effectiveness," *Phi Delta Kappan*, March, 1977, p. 568.

2 Editor's Note: Of all the conditions of schooling that Leslie Hart railed against, the classroom itself—as a structure, situation, and mindset—merited his full wrath, an anger that leaps from the page with no sugar-coating. While his words may wound or anger, his message is an important one. Applying the patterns-programs concepts of how the brain learns, the heart of Proster Theory, Hart presents a creditable case for why the classroom is, in his words, a disaster for both students and teachers alike.

Upon first reading Hart's view of classrooms, I considered it a bit overdrawn. Now, 15 years later, after involvement in many statewide and local improvement initiatives, I must confess that I wish I had trusted in his wisdom much earlier! Please read this chapter with an open mind and the 20/20 vision of hindsight.

3 It is shocking to realize that a clear and definitive exposition of student differences was made by two prestigious educators, John I. Goodlad and Robert H. Anderson, as long ago as 1959, and published in a widely noted book, *The Nongraded Elementary School* (New York: Harcourt, Brace and Company). They pointed out then that: "Grade-mindedness has left so deep a mark on the teaching profession that its by-products are everywhere and it often blinds teachers to the real facts of professional life." (p. 188). Two decades later it is hard to maintain that there has been substantial change. The welfare of children has been pushed aside, particularly by administrators and school boards, for the convenience of keeping a senseless status quo.

4 See Thomas L. Good and Jere E. Brophy, *Looking in Classrooms* (New York: Harper & Row, 1973), pp. 25, 27.

5 See John I. Goodlad, M. Frances Klein and associates, *Looking Behind the Classroom Door* (Belmont, California: Charles A. Jones, 1974).

6 See Raymond S. Adams and Bruce J. Biddle, *Realities of Teaching* (New York: Holt, Rinehart and Winston, 1970).

7   See *Supervision of Teaching, 1982 Yearbook* of the Association for Supervision and Curriculum Development, Alexandria, VA. "In many school systems, formal feedback on teaching performance may come no more than once a year and then in a quite perfunctory way. One of the tragedies of American education is that teachers work in isolation. Their immediate superiors often have only a rather generalized perception of their teaching performance. . . . There is little contact among colleagues, classroom doors are seldom opened to each other, and teachers who are members of the same staff in the same school, even in the same grade or discipline, maintain a collusive and almost deliberate ignorance of the work of their peers." Robert J. Alfonso and Lee Goldsberry, p. 91.

8   Wayne Jennings, long-term principal of the famous and successful alternative open school in St. Paul, Minn., has observed with reference to conventional school structures: "It may be that current practice is the worst possible arrangement for the education of the young." See his article, with Joe Nathan, "Startling/Disturbing Research on School Program Effectiveness," *Phi Delta Kappan,* March 1977, p. 571. The article provides a devastating review of major studies and their findings, which have been persistently ignored.

9   Dropout rates in the teaching profession have always been high; more leave than stay. Among many factors in the decision to leave the profession is fear of violence. (See the annual surveys conducted by Phi Delta Kappan and NEA.

10 Issued in July 1977, the study found morale at its lowest in years, despite higher salaries and improved working conditions. Only 38 percent felt sure they would choose a teaching career if they had the choice over again. More recent reports confirm the despair, including those from 1982 teacher unions' conventions. The trend continues.

11 See Leslie A. Hart, "A Classroom Is a Classroom Is a Classroom — and Invisible," *Toronto Education Quarterly,* Autumn 1971.

12 See the report of the National Assessment of Educational Progress, September, 1979.

13 *Beginning Teacher Evaluation Study, Report V-1* (San Francisco: The Far West Laboratory for Educational Research and Development, June 1978). See particularly Chapter 4. The massive study contains reports of many classroom observations. CEMREL, Inc., is located in Chicago. See publication "Teacher Resource Allocation: Consequences for Pupils," March 1978.

14 See Leslie A. Hart, "The Case Against Organizing Schools into Classrooms," *The American School Board Journal*, June, 1974, p. 34.

15 See note 5, above.

16 See Leslie A. Hart, "The Case Against Organizing Schools into Classrooms," *The American School Board Journal*, June, 1974, p. 29.

17 Editor's Note: This is Hart's most important observation on why classrooms are so powerful in fending off significant change. According to Proster Theory, if biases don't change, behavior doesn't change. The effects or biases of being in the situation called "classroom"—and the interlocking biases produced by it—make change in behavior by teacher or student all but impossible on a long-term basis. Thus Hart's conclusion: the classroom must go.

18 Editor's Note: The Kovalik ITI model has an unusually effective yet simple approach to teaching students attitudes and behaviors that enhance academic learning and, for teachers, make the day more pleasant.

19 Educational historian Michael B. Katz states: "The structure of American urban education has not changed since late in the nineteenth century; by 1880, the basic features of public education in most major cities were the same as they are today." See *Class, Bureaucracy, and School* (New York: Praeger, 1971), p. 105.

16

APPLYING THEORY TO ACTIVITIES

Teaching is a skill so complex that no single factor can fully explain or describe the qualities of an effective teacher. In fact, it may not be possible to distinguish between "good" and "bad" or "effective" and "ineffective" teaching. Some education researchers . . . admit that they "do not know how to define, prepare for, or measure teacher competence," despite the urgent need for skilled teachers and for understanding teacher effectiveness.

— Allan C. Ornstein and Daniel U. Levine[1]

As we now *consider* how theory applies to activities—both those of students and of teachers—we must ask the key question: What should be done, and not done, by teachers to produce effective learning by students? Answers to the question what should NOT be done are every bit as important as what should be added anew, continued with modifications, or continued as is.

We must remind ourselves (as frequently as possible!) of this dual process: on one hand, to stop and discard practices and uses of time and effort that prove harmful, inhibitory, or wasteful, and, on the other, to introduce or expand those that help. In other words, we must *cease* what is brain-antagonistic and *expand* what is brain-compatible.

LOOKING FOR ANSWERS

Here we are at the crux of schooling, the key interface between students, supposedly there to learn, and teachers, charged with bringing about learning. In one direction extends the upbringing and experiences of the students, their families and resources and their environments. In the opposite stretch the far reaches of the educational establishment, its thousands of school districts, millions of employees, huge plant, and budget that far exceeds the total budgets of most nations on earth.

The interface site will usually be the conventional, one-teacher, "box" classroom. Here at the very heart of teaching-learning, what do we find to guide and support this staggeringly huge, critically important effort and activity?

The answer shocks: substantially, *nothing.*

Incredible as it must seem, this vast educational enterprise lacks a knowledge base—a foundational body of experience, understandings, and practice.

A Comparative Look

People generally are used to the idea that the great majority of workers in any specific field have well-defined jobs by which they make a living and serve society. We also expect a certain level of competence of those whose services are thus offered—although plainly that level is affected by individual training and experience. We assume that the waiter will not spill the soup down our neck, that our tax adviser will not land us in jail, that the carpenters' roof will not blow away in the first storm. Whether it be the bus driver, the nurse, the drug store pharmacist, or the travel agent, we credit them (in the absence of warning signals) with having and using a knowledge base that warrants reasonable trust in their day-to-day expertise.

We also assume that such persons can learn to do their jobs well by using the accumulated experience of their mentors. In short, a knowledge base for each role exists. The nurse, for instance, must follow certain procedures; the carpenter must conform with good practice and local building codes. The knowledge base not only exists intellectually but has given rise to implementing tools, machines, instruments, furnishings, and working arrangements which normally are made available. Think of the auto service station, the barber shop, the stockbroker's office, the corner delicatessen. Each provides suitable setting and equipment that experience has shown to be desirable.

In contrast, the teacher typically is given an empty room, perhaps boasting an antique chalkboard and several sets of textbooks as the sum of equipment. Too often the working space has *negative* aspects: too noisy or crowded, ill-painted, ugly, chilly or too hot, poorly lighted, badly furnished. No matter—"Teach this class, in this room, with these textbooks," he or she is told. But nothing like a substantial, practical knowledge base is provided!

While an intermittent assortment of trainers, supervisors, and consultants may proffer advice, evidence is scant that following it will bring student learning. *Teachers are hired to do a job that, to shocking degree, no one seems to know how to do.* The teacher has little choice but to try, to hunt for something that will work, and to follow common sense and local custom however dreadful the outcomes may be.

By pointing out this lack of knowledge base, we do not mean to demean teachers, especially those who valiantly apply resourcefulness and "people abilities" to address the problems inherent in their task. But learning is a *brain/bodymind* function and all too often teachers have been "trained" by college people who profess no expertise in this area, may have little interest in it, have never applied a brain-compatible approach in actual teaching in school, and have themselves only paper credentials: courses completed rather than student learning brought about. Even worse, they may have notions about "thinking skills" that seriously mislead, being based on erroneous ideas about the biology of learning.

WHERE TO BEGIN: STUDYING THE GAP

If you find this picture disturbing, you're not alone. In fact, the story has yet an even more distressing turn. According to John I. Goodlad, a knowledge base of sorts does exist *but is not being utilized within the education establishment.* In his book, *Teachers for Our Nation's Schools,* Goodlad refers to "a massive body of research relevant to learning and teaching" but not yet put into a unified, accessible form likely to empower teachers. In addition, classroom teachers' supervisors are not necessarily focused on producing learning.

Rather, there is a broad assumption that if the school operates from day to day, the students will by some rather obscure process, become "educated." Furthermore, if the school is traditional, teachers can lose their jobs for many reasons: poor attendance, not doing paperwork properly, alcohol or substance abuse, or political activity — but rarely for simply not bringing about student learning. Since the teachers started their work with students at a wide range of ability and achievement levels, even measuring the teachers' competence to produce learning can be difficult.

There is now the broadest admission that school teachers get, typically, miserably inadequate and incoherent preparation for their important work. The nearly 3,000 institutions that grant would-be teachers certificates have increasingly been under most severe criticism for their poor quality. Reforms are much talked about but little achieved. We should note that even those trainees who obtain the best experiences in their college work will still likely be taught and urged to use the conventional, old, "no knowledge base" methods that bring dismal school learning outcomes so reliably. Neophyte classroom teachers understandably fall back on using the methods made familiar to them during the dozen years or so that *they* were in classrooms as elementary and secondary students! They also try to observe what their current fellow teachers do — far from easy when they have little chance to escape even briefly from their own classroom's confines. We get a hint here of one aspect of the difficulty of getting new concepts and techniques to teachers and of why inducing schools to change can be so daunting a task. The old ways that have long failed are nevertheless passed on like a torch that spews cinders.

CLARIFYING THE OLD BASIC BELIEFS

The great majority of teachers at all levels of education and training tend to operate on one or more of the following basic beliefs, derived from their search for a way to survive in the catch-as-catch-can world of the conventional school:

- The teacher has been hired to *teach* and therefore should *aggressively* instruct the students, incessantly.

- The teacher should take and maintain tight *control* of the classroom, telling the students what to do, when and how, and when to stop — usually in great detail. To keep control, and obtain compliance, the teacher stands ready to *punish* students to whatever degree may be necessary.

- The teacher should seek to *cover* the material assigned for study during the year, semester, or other period. "Cover" means that in some way attention is given to syllabus, curriculum, texts, or mandated topics. It does not mean that acceptable learning has occurred.

- The teacher, by virtue of that title, should act as *judge* of conduct and *evaluator* of achievement in relation to discerned capabilities and should systematically *report* such judgmental findings to the administration, parents, and possibly others. Most reporting will use "marks" and scores.

That teachers in conventional schools tend to arrive at these bases for behavior seems apparent from simple observation as well as incessant references in the current literature and reports. We should be aware, however, that *there is virtually no connection between these four guiding concepts and producing student learning.* To oversimplify a bit, the classroom shapes the behavior of those in it, making teacher's main concern "managing" the room and so retaining employment. Most classroom teachers, we can feel confident, would be delighted to see their students learn. But in practice, that would come about almost by accident or, as is so often the case, through some personal, individual, probably intuitive behaviors of the teacher that probably would involve violating to some degree the four bases described!

When we realize that the classroom is the standard operating format, with far over a million in constant use from coast to coast, in schools considered our best or worst, we begin to see more clearly why learning results can be as bad as they (now undeniably) are. However incredible the statement may appear to be, the key guidelines teachers usually apply have virtually no validity for producing student learning!

An Analogy to Chuckle Over. A friend who lived a long time in Iran told me that when the Shah was pushing modernization at breakneck speed, various foreign companies were hired to build railroads. In some instances, engineers failed to agree in advance on the gauge of the tracks (the distance between the rails). So where lines of different gauges met, there could be no connection, though a map might show the desired meeting. In education, we have an analogous condition. Such knowledge base as exists does not reliably connect to the classroom!

TURNING TO A NEW KNOWLEDGE BASE

While teachers are commonly committed to their work, energetic, resourceful, and somehow able to persevere despite appalling odds, rarely in reality do we find a teacher answering the question, "How do I accomplish this body of desired learning?" by turning to a basic understanding of how learning can be brought about. Robert Gagne has written that, "the essential task of the teacher is to arrange the conditions of the learner's environment so that the processes of learning will be activated, supported, enhanced, and maintained."[2]

The same thought has been expressed by many others. But in practice classroom teachers rarely seem to feel either powerful or competent enough to carry out such a mission. As anyone like myself who has labored in the harsh landscapes of educational reform can testify, many classroom teachers seem almost swamped by "what do I do Monday" worries and may become impatient with those (including myself) who attempt to interest them in theoretical or longer-term considerations. One can empathize with their distress and anxiety even while seeing that large problems are not going to be relieved by having some plans for keeping their charges occupied on Monday.

Much of this bind can be avoided, we now can be confident, by deliberately taking a broader, theoretical, brain-compatible view.

Making the Shift

To at least some significant degree, any teacher can shift from brain-antagonistic practices to brain-compatible ones, even within the rigid classroom framework; however, such a shift, I believe, can have effect only if the theoretical base is well grasped and the teacher knows in depth what is being done, and why,[3] rather than using the primitive "let's try this" trial-and-error approach. After all, it does help to have some clear idea of what one is trying to do, and why.

For clarity, let us briefly review here the brain concepts put forward in the earlier chapters of this book. The human brain was not "designed" for the classroom, nor for school. It developed over periods of millions of years in the species from which modern humans evolved. It is a brain for *surviving* in a tremendously *complicated* world.

Brain Fundamental #1: Pattern-Seeking

The first duty of the brain is to detect *patterns*, extracting them from the confusion of the "real world." For example, one looks at a tree and observes thousands of "leaves." The leaves are not identical but have a common pattern. Or, one can detect "rain clouds" in the sky, "grass" on the ground, feel "heat." The human brain is so subtle that it can detect melodies and rhythms, or even such insubstantial ideas as "celebration" or "suspicion."

The brain, then, continually detects patterns and so answers the questions, "What am I dealing with? What is this? What does this imply for my immediate safety and welfare?"

The human brain *does not need to be taught* to do this pattern detection, any more than the heart has to be taught to pump blood. Efforts to teach it how to do its job[4] will likely have *negative* effect—it may interfere with and disrupt the natural process. Commonly, people who see themselves as educators, and genuinely want to help students to learn, find this fact difficult to accept. As we have noted, teachers typically have been trained to be aggressive, active, and in control. It can be hard for them to realize that an effort to help may in fact hurt. Students who are constantly told to stop talking don't get the experience they need in using language; those who are continually told what to do are denied experience in making their own decisions and are literally taught to be passive and "unmotivated."

Brain Fundamental #2: Program-Building

Having answered the question "What am I dealing with?" the brain moves to asking "What should I do about it?" It seeks a *program* that can be implemented—the most appropriate program it can select from the stock of programs it has built and stored in the brain or that can be speedily re-combined for improvising. For example, "That animal looks as if it may be about to attack me" (*pattern recognized*). "I need a *program* to deal with it; shall I run? hide? call for help? find a weapon?"

This is the ancient *pattern-program* cycle that has kept humans surviving for thousands of generations. It lies deep in the brain. It will not suffer being pushed aside. *It is the rock-bottom foundation of learning:* the brain wants to learn more and more patterns, to be better able to detect and recognize them and extract them from confusion and it wants to build and store more and more programs so that there will be a choice of action, ready for any need. The need may be routine or minor — today we don't often have to deal with a charging lion although we may have to leap for the curb to avoid a speeding car. Children normally are tremendously "motivated" to learn, if they feel such learning will give them a better understanding of the world (by grasping patterns) and how it works (gaining more control over it by building programs). But the brain developed its *pattern-program* way of working many centuries before classrooms existed. *Our human brain is not going to change to suit schools.* Schools must change to suit the brain.

Not All Learning Is Conscious

While we can fairly readily observe how the brain operates in the pattern-program modes, the detailed mechanisms are presently beyond our ken and have to be described as in "subconscious" realms. When early in the century Freud's fevered speculations popularized the notion of an "unconscious mind" as a sort of sub-cellar in the brain that hid some horrifying secrets, this term took on disturbing connotations. Today it is easier to see that the bodymind performs a great variety of "automatic" chores for us. I do not have to "think" about how to walk across the room. My brain willingly directs all the balancing and muscle movements required. If I have learned to drive a car, I do not have to give attention to pressing this pedal or that. The car magically does what I wish it to. *As we learn any program, the mechanics of it transfer to this "non-attentional" aspect of the brain.* Not only is this "brain service" (for lack of a better name) exceedingly expert and reliable, it is also fast — far more so than pedestrian, laborious linear "thinking" which the schools often try hard to bring about.[5]

Among many modern psychologists, debate has raged as to how "smart" this brain service is. Arranging experiments that clearly show this can be technically difficult. In June 1992, however, the journal *The American Psychologist* reported on a group of studies that reflected growing interest and progress in this area. Of particular value was one by Dr. Pawel Lewicki in which sophisticated subjects were required to try to anticipate which quadrant of a computer screen would be next selected by the computer's undisclosed program. Their scores improved with experience, showing that they were somehow learning, but none could explain how the program worked—even when they were offered pay to do so! Clearly their "subconscious" apparatus was doing the learning of the intricate rules of the program—a crisp demonstration of the brain's ability to "extract patterns from confusion," even when the patterns are complex and subtle.

This function of the brain surely is among our most common, universal experiences. Yet as we get into the literature and rhetoric of schooling, we find scarcely a mention of this extremely effective kind of learning that teachers see accomplished and exhibited every day. I would suggest that the bulk of durable learning that occurs in conventional classrooms actually occurs not as the result of the ostensible "teaching" going on but rather through such individual student unconscious/subconscious pattern seeking. As teachers observe with some puzzlement, all of a sudden the student somehow "knows."

Unfortunately, this natural, effortless, rock-solid learning may be ignored and even suppressed in favor of conventional, non-brain "teach 'em, drill 'em, punish 'em!" approaches that fail miserably. However, we cannot expect many teachers, themselves fighting for survival, to challenge the conventional wisdom head-on unless they have new, brain-compatible understandings of how learning comes about.

A note on speed of learning may be needed here. The "unconscious" learning may often be accomplished much faster than that by conventional instruction but close study shows a great many exposures or "trials" may be needed. For example, a novice driver finds making a neat right or left turn into a cross street not at all easy at first. Steering and speed must be precisely adjusted. But in a single driving session, the learner may try 40 such turns. In 10 days, that means 400 trials, and in a month over 1,000. In the same way, throwing a ball, skipping a rope, or operating a cash register call for a great many rapid trials, as does typewriting, dancing, playing an instrument, or even using speech. But the activity must produce some result, which provides some sort of feedback on correctness. To fill in answers on a worksheet produces little if any inherent feedback and does not provide the same levels of trial-with-feedback opportunities as in the examples above. Low-trial classroom activities in which a student may experience perhaps only one or a few trials an hour versus those that may provide many dozens result in vastly different learning.

APPLYING THE BRAIN FUNDAMENTALS

Pattern and program are hardly the whole scope of how the brain works to learn but together they form the core. If we look at the activities of the classroom in brain-compatible terms, we can make surprisingly valid estimates of what will and will not serve to bring about learning. Let us look at the main activities of the standard, conventional classroom.

Theory Versus Lecturing

For centuries before printing, books were few and very expensive. The teacher in any institution either had the book or, more likely, knew it by rote. The students did not have it and had to learn its contents. Lecturing made very practical sense. It makes no sense today but the tradition continues and a large segment of classroom time goes to lecturing. Standing in front of a captive audience and talking is relatively easy, particularly if the speaker is not too likely to be challenged on fact or concept by a critical listener. A teacher can say, "Today I told them about dolphins . . ." or "I explained right-angle triangles . . ." and feel this was a productive effort. In fact, an earnest and thoughtful teacher, accepting the classroom as the model, may even wonder "How else could you do it? How else could I transfer the knowledge as fast or as easily?"

"Handing Over." Such a teacher, of course, is thinking in terms of "handing over" information—facts, "content," right answers to questions. Schools seem still obsessed with "information," today so available (and transient) that most of it has short-term value as something to be taught and remembered.

Here we must again remember the nature of the brain. To ferret out and recognize patterns, the brain must be subtle, sensitive, and capable of very complex processing—not in words, not "logically," and not by moving along a single path in linear fashion. For example, see the pattern "city" in Chapter 8, pages 134-5 and 141-2. When the brain is *told* a fact or bit of information, it will usually not accept this shortcut. It prefers to process this input in its ancient, time-tested way.[6]

We can draw a powerful analogy here with *digestion.* The human way is to take food into the mouth, masticate it, mix it with saliva, then transport it to the stomach where it is dealt with by powerful hydrochloric acid and agitated before being passed into the small intestine and ultimately the large, where further processing completes the complex procedure. One can imagine a meal of largely pre-processed ingredients—but it would still have to go the same digestive route.

In parallel fashion, the brain will not swallow knowledge pills, so to speak. No shortcuts! Whatever we tell students the brain receives as more *input to be processed* in the usual fashion. Earnest teachers and mentors and parents universally labor over exactly what to tell students; we might call that the Great Instructional Error. It is hard indeed for adults to realize that the exact words they employ in attempts to transfer hard-won knowledge into the heads of youngsters seldom matter—such a precise transfer is not going to occur other than by pure rote memory. *The brain will not "listen" and record as on a CD disk.* It receives the words of wisdom only as so much more raw input, to be added to other input and what is already "in the head," to be digested and organized the way that particular brain wants it. Frustrating, if one expects something else, but liberating if we realize that this is the way the brain works and that each brain processes input in its own individual way. Approached on its own (brain-compatible) terms, the brain can learn with amazing efficiency.

Lecturing, as critics have long observed, has only a feeble effectiveness with younger and secondary students; yet some students appear to teachers to have learned a good deal, so why didn't all? The hidden factor here is that previous experience (and in a related way, *age)* plays a role simply because how much one can understand from a lecture depends in large measure on how much *previous* learning one can bring to the lecture. If I know a good deal about Bach, boating, or Barbados, hearing a lecture on one of these subjects might provide input to fill a gap in pattern understanding or to add a verbal program I can later execute in a discussion. But should I know nothing about Caribbean islands, I must depend on rote memory of *words* to be able to regurgitate anything on

Barbados the next day. Listening passively to a lecture is a poor way to develop even rote memory.

The speaker may attempt a logical presentation: location, size, topography, agriculture, economy, history, without in the slightest adding to my grasp. (There can be, of course, innumerable "logical" presentations.) A key point to note is that the lecturer controls only what is uttered and *has no control whatever as to how the input is processed or utilized in the individual brains of the audience.* As we have seen, brains don't work logically. Rather, each brain will weave together bits and pieces or old and new input to construct or reconstruct a pertinent pattern.

Lecturing has long been thought of as pouring knowledge into an empty vessel or some such metaphor. We can see, however, that the importance of *previous* learning and existing patterns (to which new input can be added), produces a surprising anomaly: the emptier the vessel, the less the lecture will fill it; the fuller it is, the more chance of something more entering! This explains the familiar classroom phenomenon: certain students appear to profit by a lecture, giving the teacher some encouraging bits of feedback. The teacher then proceeds to lecture all the more. The vicious cycle aggravates the failure of those who need instruction most.

Learning as Program Building. When we define the second stage of learning as the acquisition of useful *programs,* we illuminate to the fullest the hopelessness of lecturing. No program can be built by listening but only by *acting* in some fashion. Parents, too, often seem oblivious to this fact, and endlessly *tell* their offspring to shut doors, turn off lights, wipe feet, hang up clothes, wash hands, brush teeth, not interrupt, and so on, with only the slightest success. But whether we use the terms lecturing, telling, explaining, or orienting, the activity must fail to bring about any substantial learning of new or changed programs unless students *do* something—act in some fashion. There is another, serious negative: while teachers talk, students by and large cannot. Yet, *it is the students who need to talk.* To talk is to use and enlarge communication programs, to develop the essential skills of presenting and receiving ideas, to exchange views and reach mutual aims and agreements.

Theory Versus Telling Combined with Demonstration

At first glance, this approach seems a sounder way to instruct. But the same pitfalls exist. Those who readily follow the demonstration step-by-step are probably those who need it least; others may watch and listen with no idea what is going on, especially when, as is often the case, "something new" is being introduced. But the brain does not learn anything completely new to it except by rote and under duress; rather it persists in *attaching any new learning to previous learning,* enlarging and refining *pattern* recognition and expanding the store of *programs.*

First of all, there is the basic problem we have examined in defining the first stage of learning as the extraction of patterns *from confusion.* The more clearly a teacher explains or the "neater" the demonstration, the less the student is able to extract the pattern for himself, or herself, as is essential to grasp it and the more the desired learning does *not* occur. If this seems to give common sense a drubbing, we must remember that the brain does not work by "common sense" but only in its ancient, nonlogical manner.

To accept that this is the way the brain works, and that the conventional teacher-talk of the classroom has negative results is assuredly not easy, even when the teacher constantly sees how poorly most students are learning. Yet there are thousands of "open" classrooms of various styles that demonstrate that teachers can reduce talking to the whole group to a few minutes a day, clearing the way for other activities that are brain-compatible and productive.

Second, one does not generate programs by merely *watching* a demonstration, however expert it may be. One develops programs through practice. Thus, the demonstrating or "showing" technique can be made more effective if the students participate in some fashion, have some emotional involvement, or have hands-on inputs as individuals which can also arouse interest. For example, doing a "magic" trick may bring intense interest in learning the program necessary to perform it, hands-on. But the teacher who shows at the board how to solve a new math problem can expect only yawns.

Theory Versus Seatwork

Seatwork constitutes a large part of instructional time in most conventional classrooms. It is hardly a professional secret that seatwork helps keep students quiet and at least looking busy while giving the teacher considerable respite. Much seatwork involves the use of workbooks or prepared sheets which means that once again students are being told, in detail, what to do, in what sequence. And here again the student who has learned the work is able to move through it rapidly, learning little if anything more and suffering boredom, while one who has yet to grasp the task struggles painfully, often actually practicing doing the work wrong and thus building programs that will produce further error and bafflement!

One essential found lacking in seatwork is feedback—nothing *happens* when a wrong figure or fill-in or choice is entered. There is no equivalent of shooting the basketball at the hoop and seeing it miss. Likewise, although a computer can provide an immediate right/wrong response, which may be helpful to a degree, such feedback is an arbitrary answer from unseen authority, not one deriving from reality and thus may not help the student see why the answer is right or wrong or help him/her grasp the pattern involved.

The principle is simple: a learner can improve by practice or exercises only when the learner has some way of knowing what has been executed well and gets such feedback at once, not next week or even the next day. *We build programs by doing things right, even if clumsily,* very gradually working toward mastery. But much seatwork consists of many right/wrong alternatives in small units with no gradations. If we were to allow a student in gym to shoot for baskets, closing the eyes as the ball left the hands, we would have the equivalent. Unable to follow the flight of the ball and gradually refine it, the student would find it extremely difficult to improve. It would not help much to be told later, "You got 13 in out of 60 attempts."

The bulk of seatwork done in classrooms with commercial or teacher-generated materials simply wastes time and often has negative effect, especially when students are unable to see how they are acquiring any programs useful to them. While seatwork is being done, some teachers may wander around the room, peeking at the work and offering some help or correction to individuals. Such attention potentially can be of value; but when a stopwatch is held on the contacts they usually prove to be only seconds in duration and the total for the class a scant few minutes per day. Teachers may have the impression (perhaps partly wishful) that they are spending substantial time on individualization. But building programs is a slow process. While a quick bit of feedback helps, a huge quantity of practice with immediate feedback is needed for effective learning, not occasional dribbles.

Theory Versus Recitation

Recitation, like lecturing, dates from teacher-has-the-book times and like lecturing tends to aggravate the problems of the less successful learners. To call on a student who cannot give the desired (and largely directed) response is to embarrass both student and teacher. To move the lesson ahead, the teacher needs the answer, and so goes to the student most likely to supply it, possibly allowing more time for a reply than is afforded the poorer achiever.[7] The assumption is constantly made that if one or a few students can answer, the whole group grasps the point—the most obvious of fictions. But in any case recitation normally provides no appreciable contribution to learning. Patterns are difficult to sort out from slow, painful questioning that often brings wrong, garbled, poorly expressed or inexact answers. The student responding cannot give an answer unless it *already* has been learned! Recitation tends in large measure to be a highly inefficient, boring form of examination, with the input level extremely low. Furthermore, being called on to give such a public performance is also a form of threat for most students and so brings on emotional override and a significant shutting off of cerebral cortex functioning.

Theory Versus Discussion

Discussion has some popularity with less rigid teachers in conventional classrooms because on the surface it appears to give students a participatory role and does permit more utterances by students than other activities. But observation suggests that groupings of 20 to 30 are far too large for genuine discussion and that again the stopwatch will show the teacher still talks more than all others together while many students do not talk at all or give only minimal replies under pressure. For the verbally clever student, discussion provides a golden chance to manipulate the teacher by playing up to known teacher views. Like other people, teachers tend to regard those who agree with them or accept their values as admirable. Those students who deliberately "earn Brownie points" this way may indeed be learning programs: for dissembling and "faking out" adults in authority. But, otherwise, discussion ordinarily provides very low input and the purely verbal exercises seldom reach the level of true communication — students talk because the teacher calls for talking. To be sure, some discussions do take off and may reveal student interests and views that otherwise might not come to light. That can help the teacher; but often the discussion gets into shaky ground and is choked off. Individual students talk hardly enough to matter.[8]

Theory Versus Testing

Testing — whether "standardized" achievement, IQ, aptitude, diagnostic, or other, along with quizzes, weekly tests, teacher-generated or institutional formal examinations and the like — seems to come into increasing use as learning failures come more to public view, a sort of reflex response to the public's criticism of its schools. Absurdly, administrators and boards seem to feel that doing more testing will of itself prove the school effort is more rigorous! But giving tests simply takes time (and money) *away* from instruction and learning; and the more tests are emphasized, the more the teaching focuses on learning of right answers to test questions, with deadly results for genuine learning.

As I have suggested, so-called "diagnostic" tests at best disclose areas of weakness in answering other tests. They may fail utterly to show *why* there is weakness and, even when they do, rarely are they followed up sufficiently to result in successful remediation. Most likely, more work will be assigned in the general area of what are seen as the weak areas with a repeat of the same teaching that failed in the first place. Altogether, the outcome is just the reverse of what is wanted!

The notion that students learn from giving wrong answers and being so informed (usually a good deal later) persists.[9] It would seem evident that one cannot build useful programs via wrong answers. Even if one learned what not to do, that is hardly a substitute for learning what to do and how to do it. Examinations, whether of the pencil-and-paper, verbal, or chalkboard variety, produce virtually no learning, except perhaps for building programs for answering examinations.

Heavy use of so-called "standardized" tests has introduced a new category of teacher effort: preparing students to take such tests in the hope of "raising scores" a couple of utterly meaningless points. Commonly, such drilling goes on for months, with minimum success in outcomes and maximum waste of time and effort. Since this type of machine-scorable test does not even require the student to "know" the answer, but only to *recognize* which multiple choice may be it (the right answer is provided) the whole procedure may be called ludicrous but is nonetheless destructive.

Theory Versus Rote Learning

In breaking away from old-style parrot learning, educators have tended to downplay rote. The irony is that most classroom progress is still measured by ability to give right answers and the answers depend heavily on rote acquisition. Teachers drill their classes over and over to answer expected examination questions. The more pressures are put on teachers to have students attain minimum competence or to teach the basics, the more rote methods come to be used, often with little realization that this is what is happening. Consequently the rote teaching is done weakly.[10]

The rote method, or what used to be called "learning by heart," can be both highly effective and useful if done well. As the Proster Theory makes clear the program-building aspect of rote, it works effectively under the following conditions: we learn by rote not by listening or silent effort but by acting—usually declaiming with vigor the poem or table or formula we wish to retain, or playing over and over the piano piece to be performed, or running through the intricate steps of a football play. Rather than "by heart," we learn by muscle or, more accurately, by bodymind. If rhythm can be added, learning is speeded; melody in addition will help further. The alphabet, for example, can be picked up rapidly and permanently to the tune of "Twinkle, Twinkle, Little Star." A marching band represents complex rote learning, blending maneuvers and the playing of music on instruments. A huge amount of practice may be required—a reminder that we build programs slowly and only with far more repetition than we tend to realize.

Although rote learning also makes "parrot" learning possible—learning in which comprehension is not necessary—comprehension significantly increases the rote learning process. A grasp of the pattern of the football play or of the band's formation certainly will speed learning. So will insight into the relations of numbers and the patterns they form aid mastery of multiplication tables. Likewise when driving in a strange city: while I have learned at times to drive to destinations by a rote sequence of turns, I am always unhappy until I can see a map and get some idea of what I have been doing.

Even when comprehension is not possible, such as in the arbitrary sequencing of our alphabet, understanding of the use of what is being learned can greatly assist the rote learning process. For example, knowing the alphabet can help one find a friend's phone number in the phone book.

The combination of pattern recognition, words, rhythm or music, and vigorous muscular activity means that much cross-modal power of the bodymind will be used. The learning that results often is amazingly sure and durable; with a little brushing up, one may easily recite a long poem learned decades before. Most people have to say aloud or in suppressed speech "6 times 8 is 48" to recover that "fact"—demonstrating that we do not really recall a fact but rather *implement a program* that produces those words.[11]

IN SUMMARY

This review of activities of the conventional classroom will, perhaps, profoundly discourage and upset some who conduct aggressive teaching in conventional ways. (As we have noted, teachers tend to be unrealistic about what they are actually doing, and to think that criticism for clinging to antique methods applies to other teachers, not them.) To suggest that lecturing, telling, explaining, recitation, seatwork, discussion, and testing are in sum almost totally ineffective and probably a negative factor in producing learning can be a shock throughout the establishment.

The most common response, I have found, is the protest, "But that does not agree with the obvious facts! Our students do learn." Certainly students learn to a degree across the years of schooling but that is not quite the issue. What I am submitting is that they do not learn appreciably from the aggressive classroom instruction

I have been describing. The great bulk of evidence shows a profound inability of instruction by these techniques to produce learning. If they did, we should have millions of reports of such success; we have almost none.

It would seem simple enough for teachers to routinely test before a lesson or unit is given and test after it. But it is easy to see why that is seldom done. If the teacher finds on the pretest that a third or half of the students know the material, what is to be done with them while the others are taught? If the post-test should show little learning resulted, who wants that information? Nobody stands to gain love and applause by proving that the rituals are only rituals.

Students learn to a degree outside this main body of instruction, by reading texts and other books, by getting help from parents and friends, and from the huge input they get from all media and experience out of school. It has long been apparent that how well students do in school, on the record, relates closely to family income and their out-of-school resources,[12] and that conversely those students who lack such alternative support tend to do very badly in school.

Such studies as those of the National Assessment of Educational Progress and more recently competency testing by states or localities increasingly reveal how shallow and limited actual student learning has been. But this is hardly surprising: the literature critical of the aggressive teaching methods we have reviewed fills libraries to overflowing. It is not radical to suggest that lecturing, for example, is ineffective. What I have tried to do is show that, in brain terms, it *must* be ineffective; no other result can be expected.

As I observed in Chapter 1, teachers have long been thwarted and puzzled by the failure of teaching to "get across" to students. But producing learning results has not been mandatory or even necessary to draw salary, get increases, or win promotions. Times may now be changing, as public and educational customers at all levels become more and more unwilling to accept and pay for empty rituals. Well-proved, practical brain-compatible techniques now offer attractive and rewarding alternatives. Teachers at last can free themselves of century-old brain-antagonistic ideas and practices, many forced on them by a defunct system which they and the public have inherited, with little or no change, from the mid-1800s.

NOTES

1   "Teacher Behavior Research: Overview and Outlook," *Phi Delta Kappan*, April 1981, p. 592.

2   *The Psychology of Teaching Methods, 75th Yearbook* of the National Society for the Study of Education (Chicago: University of Chicago Press, 1976), p. 42.

3   Editor's Note: It is my belief that the number one cause of failure of reform efforts at the secondary level over the past decades is that structures, such as scheduling, were changed before teachers learned new instructional strategies and curriculum approaches. Pouring old wine into a new bottle doesn't change the wine; if anything, it merely heightens awareness of the contrast, thus increasing dissatisfaction.

4   Editor's Note: This brings into question the validity of many "critical thinking" programs with their "models" for thinking critically in various situations. Perhaps the best preparation for critical thinking is abundant opportunity to think—to solve worthwhile and, to the learner, interesting problems, on a daily basis. Sporadic lessons during which one is told how to think critically are not consistent with how the brain naturally, and thus most powerfully, works.

5   Editor's Note: This notion of brain function raises some interesting questions for the teaching of reading. The strongest readers in terms of comprehension and accurate spelling are those whose decoding skills are automatic and non-attentional. Forcing such students through prolonged phonics instruction is likely to be detrimental, slowing them down and taking up processing capacity with unnecessary, distracting details. Research into this question is underway.

6   Editor's Note: This requirement of the brain reinforces the constructivists' view of education: in order to learn each student must construct his/her own meaning.

7   Various studies suggest that when the "wait time" of the teacher is increased from about one second to two or three, student responses greatly increase. For example, see Mary Budd Rowe, "Give Students Time to Respond," *School Science and Mathematics*, March 1978, or in *Education Digest*, May 1978.

8   Perhaps because teachers may want students to talk, they tend to overestimate greatly the amount of time that they do—

usually only a few seconds. I have often suggested to teachers that they tape some class sessions (the presence of the tape recorder is soon forgotten) to replay for themselves later. As yet, I have never known a teacher to take this simple step. It may be that teachers feel they have enough problems, without doing research of this nature to discover some more. I have, however, witnessed some impressive discussions that were student-led, with the teacher resolutely sitting apart and silent. Students had prepared for these sessions, which usually were held elsewhere than the regular classroom (in one instance, in the principal's office!). The biases of the classroom may inhibit talking freely. Groupings of not over 15, and preferably not over 12, work best for discussions.

9   Editor's Note: The average teacher spends a high portion of his/her non-student contact time grading papers and tests. The hours per week rise significantly in departmentalized middle and high schools. Such non-immediate feedback is largely wasted time in terms of helping students build useful mental programs for using what is being learned and in storing knowledge and skills in long-term memory. Such time used in planning and preparing would be much more effective in producing learning.

10 For a further discussion of rote use and emotional override under threat, see Leslie A. Hart, "The Three-Brain Concept and the Classroom," *Phi Delta Kappan*, March 1981, p. 504, and "Brain Language and New Concepts of Learning," *Educational Leadership*, March 1981, p. 443.

11 This was strikingly brought home to me when I met a woman who had spent her early school years in France. She then moved to the United States, where she acquired excellent English and for 35 years rarely spoke French, except when doing arithmetic, which she could not do unless she whispered her numbers tables in French!

12 The factor has shown up consistently in a long series of studies over recent years, from *Education and Income* by Patricia Cayo Sexton (New York: Viking Press, 1961, 1964). *The Fleischmann Report* (New York: Viking Press, 1973) noted: "The most striking fact that emerged from our studies of school performance in New York State is the high correlation shown between

school success and socio-economic origin of pupils. This is true at all levels of the performance scale." (p. 25)

17

WHAT WORKS: SOME DIRECTIONS WE CAN GO

> There lies ahead of us the enormous task of translating what we know of language acquisition, language development, and the nature of learning into structures by which teaching and learning in school may be organized. Too often today the call for "structure" takes the form of demanding the preservation of, or a return to, lockstep procedures that grew up in ignorance of the nature of learning and reflect a mistaken view of knowledge, and hence of curriculum. In this task teachers must take a lead, both as to theory and as to practice, if the structures devised are to be workable and grounded in experience. The further participation of linguists, psychologists, and sociologists will be essential.
>
> —James Britton[1]

When this book first appeared in 1983, the educational storm threatened but had yet to break. Highly critical reports, not a few of them real shockers, had begun to make some headlines but these were only the first winds of the hurricane. In the next few years it would bring numbing reports of failures and shortcomings literally by the hundreds. The storm had begun but most educational practitioners were busy indoors with the windows closed and shades pulled down. What could be ignored, was. The prime response was denial: Schools were not that bad, learning not that sparse, discontent not that pervasive—no? The criticism was confusing, and somehow remote. Surely these biting criticisms could not be intended for us!

Indeed, not a few practitioners in the schools continued intent on the day-to-day demands of their jobs and pooh-poohed the whole idea that great changes were needed and wanted. Problems that entered the schools with students, such as those from inner city areas, often were seen as those of society; fix society — that was the cure. Typically, the more experienced school people were (up to and including board members) the less open they were to suggestion that massive change was needed. During this period, I was meeting with teachers by the thousands; they were interested in hearing about the brain but had hardly begun to think about departing from long familiar ideas and practices.

As criticism and complaint intensified, pundits, politicians, and assorted certified wise men offered superficial "common sense" solutions. The rhetoric thickened, year by year. Yet somehow the core concept, that *schools no longer worked adequately well,* seeped in to reach something like a majority of the practitioners, at all levels. Looking back, that astonishing shift seems to have come about rapidly although it is yet far from complete. Within half a dozen years, a genuine search for solutions began—even while some of the simplistic, common sense "solutions" persisted and are still on the scene as "choice," "technology," "critical thinking," and the like, all of which avoid serious study of *learning.*

At this point we have happier tidings. The same decade has also brought considerable actual experience with brain-compatible schools, and substantial success in outcomes. Little such in-school brain-compatible experience existed in 1983.

But as was noted in the previous chapter, education's knowledge base is far from consolidated; even the findings from implementation of brain-compatible approaches have yet to be well gathered and organized, at this writing. But we can declare with confidence that the brain-compatible approach, and the body of experience with it, convincingly support the conclusion that we now *know what to do* amply well enough to greatly improve our schools.

THE WORK AHEAD

We can progress on two levels in quite different ways. The first seeks to change schools by making many specific shifts, from old, traditional ways of schooling to brain-compatible ways, eventually arriving at a quite different school; this is the topic of this chapter. The second way puts more emphasis on theory, on deep and broad concepts of *what schools are for* and on *how learning comes about*—a bolder and more sweeping view that when implemented can take education further; this is addressed in Chapter 18.

SHIFTING FROM OLD TO NEW

We have looked at activities in the graded classroom in terms of what the teacher does because in those settings the teacher is aggressive, in charge (or in trouble), and drives the group and its doings, making or imposing most of the decisions. As we turn in contrast to brain-compatible settings, we need to look rather at what *students* do—students who are now permitted, encouraged, and helped to act as the aggressive learners they are by nature.

The role of teacher now changes to that of facilitator—the role Gagne described (see page 258) as "to arrange the conditions of the learner's environment so that the processes of learning will be activated, supported, enhanced, and maintained." We must note that "learner" here must mean *individual*. The aggressive teacher runs a group but aggressive learners largely direct themselves and 25 or 30 students may go in as many different directions. It may seem at first as though the teacher must abandon everything associated with the ancient role of teaching but that, we shall see on further consideration, is an overstatement.

The Biggest Challenge

As I (and many others) have remarked, the harder part of change is not adding the new but dropping the old. This applies strongly in moving from old conventional to new brain-compatible instruction. Some people, we can suspect, are attracted to teaching because they enjoy using power—"pushing people around" as the vernacular bluntly puts it. But observation of neophyte teachers suggests that as they must deal with the problems of controlling students, they see power as a necessary means. Authority implies the right to give orders and compliance is seen as necessary to keep school running. The beating of students, with "hickory stick" or other instrument of torture, has a prominent place in the traditions of education. There are still many schools in which the staffs resist outlawing corporal punishment.

But the great majority of neophyte teachers, most observers agree, burn with eagerness to help children and produce learning. New secondary teachers hope they will inspire and help launch careers. It is only as they become disenchanted with a bureaucratic, brain-antagonistic system that most teachers, I believe, come to see power as needed for class control and their own protection against administrative, parental, or political criticism or complaint. From contacts with thousands of school people, I feel sure a great many would happily choose a nonconfrontational approach if they saw that as a feasible option.

Obviously practitioners cannot be expected to give up what is seen as a job benefit and protection at a mere suggestion. Many teachers have never actually seen a good "open" program or Montessori school in operation, where for hours on end there is no need to make a single disciplinary remark. Some do not believe this other world of instruction exists.

Needed Support

To make the transition from conventional aggressive, driving teaching to fully brain-compatible approaches, teachers and the administrators who will support them need specific kinds of assistance: the gift of time, quick help when needed, and protection.

Time. People cannot sensibly be expected to change long-used behaviors overnight. A comfortable amount of time must be allowed by which the expected changes are to be implemented. And, very importantly, time to be thoughtful and plan with colleagues must be provided on a regular, ongoing basis.

Quick Help When Needed. As with students, immediate feedback is essential. Someone who can answer small or larger questions by telephone or otherwise must be readily available; ideally a consultant on call for the purpose.

Protection. During the "tender"phase of the change-over, there must be persons who are prepared to deflect or fend off unfriendly criticism. Teachers also need protection from conflicting demands emanating from the district office.

Permission to Drop the Old

The specific activities—what students do—feasible in a brain-compatible setting and situation have few limits and need hardly be set down in a definitive list. If the *principles* are well grasped, activities can be chosen and assembled in ways suited to local needs and resources with confidence and success. This effort can be undertaken, however, only when "the old has been dropped" and staff no longer thinks of "school" as a building where youngsters are rounded up, confined, and then processed in a uniform way to have certain knowledge (the curriculum) and certain "skills," especially reading and mathematics, pushed into them. This processing conventionally goes on for a dozen or so years at least, with little heed paid to the individual's differences, aims, preferences, and abilities. This whole approach, we now are reminded almost daily, is enormously unsuccessful but continues in wide use because the people in control don't know how to break away from it and perhaps lack eagerness to try. Also they do not have a clear image of what they could change to: the brain-compatible school based on Proster Theory.

(I apologize for singing so many verses of this sad song but we cannot get to brain-compatible operation, which has proved highly successful, without seeing the need to "drop the old" and then *doing* just that.)

THE TARGET: FOUR IMPORTANT BRAIN-COMPATIBLE AIMS

We can consider four of the most important brain-compatible aims and some means for implementing them:

- Input
- Talking and communicating
- Feedback
- Risk

Input

We have seen that input serves as the raw material from which patterns are extracted from confusion—the first of the two basic stages of learning. Setting, situations, and activities must all provide a huge amount of input. As a rule of thumb, I have suggested ten times as much as is typical of our present low-input schools. There are several major factors that can help raise input; none are difficult.

Increasing the Hours of Input. Increasing the number of hours during which high input is provided (possibly lengthening the school day and week, if not necessarily the teacher's work-week), the school year,[2] and increasing the net use of each hour. Once aware of the crucial need for input, teachers can readily choose high-input activities that, experience has demonstrated, do exist and escape from low-input formats which also tend to be boring. (But more "teaching time" will not help if it is not used for brain-compatible purposes; indeed it may hurt.)

Providing Exposure to Many People. Schools must ensure students are exposed to and interact with *many people rather than very few,* for example, a *team* of teachers, other staff, apprentices, volunteers, visitors, older students, peers and other helpers. Techniques for accomplishing this are known and not difficult. One key concept is that of the "MILU" or Multi-Teacher Interactive Learning Unit (pronounced "milieu"; for a description of MILU, see page 285).

Providing a Variety of Input Sources. Schools must provide a great variety of *machines, devices, equipment, and materials* (usually possible at minor cost if the resources of the community are called upon)[3] and ample opportunity for students to use them, for example, drafting tools and materials, machine for making blueprints; microscopes, portable bunsen burners; hand tools for woodworking, auto repair, plumbing, dental work; measuring devices of all kinds (liquid, solids, metric); cameras, videocameras, splicing/editing equipment, recorders, players; desktop publishing and office machines; educational brochures from businesses such as a vet's office, realtor, or park (local, state, or national); marketing materials from nonprofit and profit organizations such as zoos, airports, cattlemen's associations, plumbers, hotels . . . and much more, as available from parents, local businesses and manufacturers, or other sources, as gifts, loans, or via funding. And don't forget live animals, guests for the day, animal of the curriculum's weekly topic, and/or classroom mascots.

Varied Presentations. Schools must offer hundreds of **presentations** to students in such forms as visitors' talks and first person narrated films and slides; exhibits and demonstrations (real, not performances); and multimedia events. These can be organized, arranged, and perhaps presented by staff, students, parents, volunteers, local businesses and professional people, local or other governmental employees and officials, etc., in any combination. Sometimes called "sparks," these presentations can deal with any topic so long as it is real and can be provided to large groupings, usually in an hour or less. Properly done, sparks provide students with a wide range of input they would not otherwise get and allow them to meet non-school people for a glimpse of the real world, with opportunity to ask questions and follow up on their interests. As many as 100 such sessions can readily be offered in a school year.

Field Trips. Arrange many **field trips** of varying duration, most often with a small number of students making the trip at any one time and then reporting to other students using various media and so building communication skills to real purposes.

Tying in Current Events. Tie in closely with **current news**, news events, television programs and specials, local public issues and emergencies, openings, dedications, ceremonies, inaugurations, and the like.[4]

A school, in short, can be transformed through emphasis on high input. A dreary egg-crate of classrooms, largely isolated from one another and almost empty of anything real one might learn from can become a vibrant center where there is constant fresh encounter with the richness and variety of the real world. Large and small *new* experiences and adventures thus replace grinding monotony.

When the potentials of input in instruction are grasped, each bit of input material can be thought of as a magical door that opens on the world. If we are looking at something as "simple" as a common pencil, for example, we can ask when such products came into wide use; who invented or developed them; what the "lead" actually is, how it is put inside the wood, what the wood is, where it comes from, why yellow is a preferred color, and even about the source of the brand names. Is lead pencil use increasing or falling off and why? In these explorations we get into a variety of school subjects: from geography to economics. More important, each input window opens on the *real* world, not an academic abstraction. The difference is like that between hearing a lecture on expert driving and taking a car out into a variety of city traffic. While there is a place for academics, the school, at any level, should not become a place where the students are separated from (even "protected" from) reality. The effort to select relatively tiny bits of reality and call this "curriculum" to be taught to all students while the vast, infinitely complex rest of the world is ignored, has become absurd on the face of it.

Talking and Communicating

Students must **talk and communicate** to learn well. Few disagree that a good command of language, an ability to convey ideas and information in speech and writing, and to receive and understand communication is an essential body of "skill" to function well in almost any role in society. Yet conventional schools expend a huge amount of energy and time *suppressing* talk, and communication becomes corrupted into exercises to be marked for grades. Desirable brain-compatible activities, then, include talking about what one is doing (especially important for youngest students); talking within small teams working on common tasks or projects; asking questions for guidance, information, or clarification; public talking such as in making announcements or addressing an audience; and communication by speech directly and via writing or some instrumental means. Communication means that an actual exchange occurs and "something happens." (Exercises are not communication.) If writing (memo, report, proposal, request, complaint) is used by both students and faculty as a means of effecting some action, its usefulness becomes apparent.

Feedback

As used in a brain-compatible frame, feedback takes on a very different definition. **Feedback**[5] is necessary for learners to find out whether their pattern recognition and extraction is correct or improving and whether programs have been appropriately selected and executed. As we have noted, the right/wrong responses of teachers, often delayed, provide poor quality feedback. What is wanted, and should influence selection of offered activities, is *feedback from reality* rather than from an authority and feedback that is graduated rather than being classified either right or wrong.

Avoiding Black and White, Right and Wrong. Programs are acquired by progressively refining the initial crude and clumsy execution so that it becomes smoother and more exact after many trials. If the slow or halting or inaccurate early performance is called "wrong," the feedback gives a false message. *We build programs by having a correct general idea of what we are trying to do and then gradually reducing error by getting and heeding feedback.* To tell the learner who is on the right track that an effort made is wrong because performance is poor is to confuse and inhibit, as we see in early reading when the student is permitted no error and gets corrected on every wrong word. Inevitably the learner becomes a word-by-word reader, trying to use a dreadfully wrong overall program. In general, brain-compatible instruction requires that students not be permitted to pursue wrong programs at the outset nor to practice making errors. Practice and drill should be assigned and encouraged only after the student is clearly on the correct track and has begun refining a desired program.[6]

Using Real Rather Than the Contrived. Feedback stems better from using real rather than contrived learning devices and materials. A child using a typewriter, for example, sees at once whether the intended keys have been struck and if the spacing is as planned; one connecting an electric circuit finds out quickly whether it works. *In many instances, practical, useful learning can be achieved only through reality:* nursing students may start building programs by using a dummy but sooner or later they must experience real patients, responsive or resistant.

The Power of Involving Students in Design Work. A key word may be suggested here: *design.* In the familiar aggressive-teacher situation, students deal almost always with what other people, usually unseen, have designed and they have much the same experience outside school. My experience with students suggests that most have utterly no idea of how books are written, news is transmitted, products are developed, or large works are constructed—all these seem to come out of thin air, mysteriously and presumably reflect the efforts and powers of people never encountered.[7] This ignorance may well contribute to both a feeling of being powerless and to alienation from established society. Preschool age and primary-grade children quite normally like to design structures built with blocks, sand, or snow; sculpture and engineering models built with construction toys or materials, and the like. Conventional schools tend to crush design activities, providing neither time nor materials, and forcing other people's design on the students. In some instances, "design" is limited to graphics on paper as though three dimensions did not exist.

Yet design, in the broadest sense, provides some of the most productive kinds of feedback. Students designing a special-purpose space, a cage for an animal, or scenery for a play quickly discover whether the design works, whether parts fit, whether it provides what is needed. At the same time, shortcomings in their sense of pattern must come to light, as grasp is increased of how complex even apparently simple projects turn out to be. Design tasks, whether they involve words, drawings, plans, construction, decoration, invention, arrangements, mechanisms, or aesthetics, give a student or small team opportunity to "play God," to experience the process of choosing among alternatives and making the compromises engineers call trade-offs. Inherently design entails problem solving, and builds those frontal-lobe super-programs by which previous knowledge can be transferred to fresh applications.

Risk

Risk, as we have noted, is what the individual voluntarily assumes to meet the built-in human need for challenge, excitement, variety, adventure. Threat, in contrast, is imposed and usually involves a sense of powerlessness. We have examined the emotional override of the great human cerebrum under threat that effectively inhibits cerebral learning. Obviously brain-compatible learning demands activities that offer students the degree of risk they choose (within reason), and the opportunity to carry them out in no-threat or very low-threat circumstances.

Eliminating the Sense of Captivity. Captivity is the first aspect of threat that must be attacked. Emphasis on sitting in compulsory places for compulsory periods, a flagrant denial of the movement so characteristic of youth, must be eliminated if the learning situation is not to generate friction and confrontation interminably. Even when a student must be kept in the antagonistic classroom situation, it is both feasible and easy to set up an area to which he or she may withdraw from the prevailing activity — in adult terms, take a break. But that seems an extreme minimum. If the school is seen as a safe place, adequately supervised, there seems no reason why students should not move freely about it as their needs dictate. That this approach is practicable has long been demonstrated. In contrast, rigid schools fight a constant battle, often lost, to control students' whereabouts and behavior.

I have put forward, without claiming originality, the concept of MILU, a group of rooms and spaces around which a unit of about 75 to 125 students may circulate during most of their earlier half of schooling. Formed of three or four teachers and their students, the MILU (Multiteacher Interactive Learning Unit which may be called "milieu") offers students a wide range of resources and facilities.[8] Such an arrangement demands no great architectural changes in existing school buildings, yet permits an enormous variety of activities to be readily accommodated. Older students may circulate still more freely, in some cases doing much of their work outside the school.

This larger than classroom unit is inherently more flexible and able to use the various talents and enthusiasms of the assigned teachers far more effectively as well as end the "lonely teacher" problem. Teachers who are moving to brain-compatible approaches, experience shows, readily learn to work as a team and become mutually supportive.

Reducing Testing and Grading. Threat also can be sharply reduced by ceasing the practice, centuries old, of continually *marking* student activity—the systematic recording of all failures in a Doomsday Book—and by reducing all testing and written examinations to a barest minimum. As activities multiply in number and variety to provide true individual choice, the group examination becomes less and less usable. Individual student progress can be far better followed and guided by reporting *observations of accomplishments* as they occur. The shift is made from what the student knows (often meaning "remembers for the moment") to what the student actually does in appropriate circumstances.[9] The student writes a clear message; solves a real arithmetical problem; translates a foreign newspaper story; takes and processes some good photographs; seeks out and compiles some needed information; designs a rack for chemical equipment; chairs a meeting; reviews an unassigned book; keeps accounts for the store; plans and arranges a visit by the mayor; paints a portrait; or plays a part in the orchestra.

Whatever the achievement, it is recorded only if it attains an acceptable level of mastery—it is pointless to record failures except to lay blame on the student. I have suggested that, using computer record-keeping resources, each student's progress can be rigorously followed, with lack of progress made a signal for investigation and possibly corrective action.[10]

In this way, *school then becomes a place where ordinarily students succeed,* not one where failure is endemic and, to a considerable degree, expected. (Students enrolling in commercial or industrial schools to learn typing, accounting, welding, or lifesaving, for examples, expect to succeed to at least practically acceptable levels and in legitimate schools usually do. Some drop out, mostly on finding they do not like the work or lack physical aptitude, but few fail in such large percentages as they do in conventional schools The high-input approach provides both much chance to find *areas in which one can succeed* through **interest** and aptitude and *room to enlarge success areas.* We may note, too, that the student who is enjoying clear success in any learning area of importance is likely to have a self-image and confidence that encourages wider achievement—and such a student is little likely to present behavior problems. In contrast, the student in a conventional school who, because of competitive marking and grading attains no clear success over years on end but has many spotlighted failures, easily may come to have a low self-image and to look upon the whole formal learning process with strong distaste. Quite correctly, the school is viewed as a punishing enemy.

Using theory, we can analyze what helps, what hurts, what doesn't matter, for both group or individual. In effect, we can deliberately "factor in" success. Staff can then become able to predict to a useful degree what activities will help and which should be dropped.

TAKING A BRAIN-COMPATIBLE VIEW OF CURRICULUM

Curriculum today is still arrived at by a process ludicrously defective because it embodies two flagrantly untrue propositions:

- What is taught will be learned and

- What is to be learned can fit into a neatly packaged, exactly timed course.

With these two misconceptions, curriculum-making becomes a process of decisions as to what courses shall be taught at particular times. The courses are further broken down to syllabus or topics to be covered; these in turn to units, sequences, and lessons to be aggressively taught. Teachers constrained to execute these ill-conceived efforts break them down further, eagerly seeking "things to do," all of which must square with the limitations of *course* and the oppressive demands of classroom management. What the individual teachers select will vary greatly, reflecting many differences in personality, experience, training, and personal beliefs, prejudices, convenience, aptitudes, and intuition.[11] The end of this chain, students' activities (what the students actually do) becomes almost lost to sight (we have very few studies reporting what students do), haphazard, heavily ritualized, and out of control. Where the learning must take place there is only confusion.

Curriculum as Structure for Doing

Brain-compatible "curriculum" must start from the other end, from the realization that *the entire structure exists only to provide student activities* which give students ample opportunities to practice pattern-seeking (making meaning) and to develop mental programs for using (and storing) what is being learned. What learning is desired? Not passing courses, not accumulation of Carnegie points, not certified attendance for a certain number of days, not obtaining paper credentials—these are hardly learning. But we can state what learning is desired in a broad way that is acceptable to virtually all citizens: *The child should become familiar with and able to operate successfully in the complex world in which he or she now operates to a limited degree and will soon operate to an adult degree.*

This is, historically, a new concept. Even a century ago many and perhaps most people felt that youngsters should be exposed only to carefully selected slivers of the real world and that their learning should be tightly controlled and limited. If such a plan was feasible then, obviously it is not today.

If we observe the infant and preschool-age child, we see plainly the vigorous natural-learning attack on the world, which at first is limited largely to crib and mother's arms, but rapidly expands. Today's five-year-old has had experience in many ways beyond that of the fifty-year-old of past centuries—exposure to mass media, to a variety of locales, to perhaps several thousands of miles of travel in family cars alone. Input has climbed enormously and with it opportunity to grasp real-world patterns and to build programs useful in that world. It seems clearly desirable that this process should continue in school and not run into curriculum in the antique, restrictive sense. The brain-compatible school must be one in which *the process of world-discovery accelerates and broadens.* In contrast, courses narrow and focus attention and interest. To move from broad input to narrow is natural and makes sense in terms of results; to try to start with a few narrow approaches and then broaden slightly with a few more optional courses is plainly inadequate, in concept and in outcomes.

Searching for Transferability

One compelling reason to avoid the narrowness of courses is that the most important, insightful, and transferable pattern under-standings transcend courses. Such concepts or "grand ideas" — such as energy cycles, systems, negative/ positive, innovation/obsoles-cence, new generation, probability, causation, critical mass, and feedback — apply in almost any field. To illustrate, the negative/ positive concept has critical usefulness in mathematics, photogra-phy, molding, chemistry, accounting, politics, electronics, and in education. Only as these multiuse patterns are detected, recognized, and employed to select programs do learners establish the base for easy, rapid acquisition of narrower learning through courses. Narrow study through courses before broad application of concepts during the learning process is putting the cart before the horse.

THE POWER OF INTEGRATION

Here we see why the *integrative concept — rather than fragmented subjects —* that is currently gaining ground is welcomed and appre-ciated for its effectiveness by teachers who have learned this technique. Rather than sequentially plodding along a narrowly-defined "course," students explore a "theme," examining it from many aspects in an interesting, welcoming way. Such a theme allows students to follow a concept wherever the real world takes it/demonstrates it. This is the natural way of learning for the brain. Interests thus aroused can be followed up, instead of being choked off because the teacher is trying to hold to the course topic and perhaps a neat lesson plan. Instruction becomes more a web, less a thread — far more robust, more interesting and engaging, and much more brain-compatible because the brain takes in input without the slightest regard for what is "logical" or tidy or what is within a particular subject area . . . or convenient to a bureaucratic program. Themes may vary widely in the time they take, from less than one day to even a year, giving teachers new flexibility.

One approach to integration, now widely known as Integrated Thematic Instruction (ITI),[12] is designed as a brain-compatible approach to both curriculum and instruction. Developed by teacher-trainer Susan Kovalik of Kent, Washington, a notable pioneer and leader in brain-compatible applications, it is a model designed and updated annually to respond to emerging brain research. It should be noted that ITI and its brain base in practice facilitate changing from outmoded and failing class-and-grade schools to newer and far better models which are now demonstrating their ability to produce superior outcomes.

OTHER FACTORS TO CONSIDER

Some other factors besides the "big four" deserve at least mention:

- Freedom to explore and manipulate

- Addressing learning to immediate and later uses

- Freedom to function in natural, rather than logical, ways

- Rote ("right answer") learning that is vigorous, multimodal, and individualized

Freedom to Explore and Manipulate. Young children especially must **manipulate** what they deal with. Manipulation remains helpful, if less essential, at later ages. Manipulation demands not only "hands-on" but also freedom to explore in unhurried style what is being examined. It should not be simply doing what teachers direct step-by-step.

Addressing Learning to Immediate and Later Uses.

Learning must always be dominantly **addressed** to immediate and later uses, not to testing or examinations, and not to a future use beyond the ken of the learner. ("You will need algebra to get into college" or "Develop critical thinking you will use later on." Students who are told such advice find it frustrating and infuriating.)

Freedom to Function in Natural, Rather Than Logical Ways. The freedom of the human brain to function in *natural* (as opposed to logical) ways should not be infringed and its output as a result should be accepted and honored.[13]

Rote Learning Should be Vigorous, Multimodal, and Individualized. **Rote** ("right answer") learning should be used judiciously. When used, it should be achieved by vigorous, fast-paced, preferably multimodal means, and only as individually helpful to achieve mastery.

IN SUMMARY

What will be learned by students can be directly affected if activities have these characteristics:

1. The brain-compatible principles permit broad recognition of individual differences and accommodate a wide range of learning styles. Student conflict with the institution can be greatly reduced without the school giving up control of main, consequential objectives. Providing students with many choices in interests and short-term strategies for learning and exploration should be a deliberate aspect of the program, rather than a coping strategy for releasing frustration with the inflexible demands of the system. Students acquire ability to take responsibilities through experience in taking responsibilities.

2. Appropriate settings and situations and selection of activities largely by student initiatives can increase input up to tenfold, while student exposure to a rich variety of people and the real world is greatly enhanced.

3. Spoken and written language for actual communication purposes (in contrast to exercises) can be stepped up enormously.

4. Feedback from reality, rather than from authority, can be greatly enhanced by making available activities with this built-in characteristic.

5. Including design tasks can greatly increase reality feedback, foster a sense of control of the student's world, add to problem-solving experience in a real context, and strengthen

skills in transfer of patterns and programs to fresh applications (a capability often referred to as creativity).

6. As threat is reduced and the setting becomes safe for the student, emphasis can increase on mastery rather than partial learning, and on actual accomplishment, with the opportunity to stress quality and excellence rather than pen-and-paper test answers.

7. Student activity and accomplishment can be readily and meaningfully followed to monitor and assure progress, with success expected and obtained.

8. Curriculum can shift from meaning "what teachers do" to broadly-planned provisions for "what students will do."

9. Grand ideas or concepts that transcend courses can readily be incorporated in student activities, especially as integrated plans of instruction are importantly put into use.

10. Particularly for younger children, manipulation activities can be provided for and encouraged.

11. Natural thinking (intuitive, heuristic, frontal lobe directed) can be encouraged and accepted.

12. Rote learning methods can be vigorously used where appropriate for a purpose.

13. What the student does can be largely oriented to the real, outside world rather than to school artificialities, recognizing that the student already inhabits this real world and will take on increasing responsibilities within it.

While this even in summary is a long list, it is not, I submit, a "laundry list." The elements in it intertwine and interrelate and become mutually supportive. They stem from a common source: a brain-compatible approach.

NOTES

1 James Britton, *The Teaching of English, 76th Yearbook of National Society for the Study of Education* (Chicago: University of Chicago Press, 1977), p. 37.

2 Most Japanese schools provide 240 or more days per school year against our 180, and students are engaged in learning perhaps 85 percent of the time compared with 25 percent or less in our schools. See "Japan: The Learning Society," *Educational Leadership,* March 1982, p. 412.

3 Two points should be noted here briefly. First, almost everywhere but in education managers think in terms of equipment/labor trade-offs, introducing equipment when it will more than offset labor costs. Schools and other similar institutions tend to remain a century or more behind and as a result fearfully expensive, to the point that much desirable is not done because of labor costs. Second, school people seem to believe that everything needed must be bought from special school suppliers. But actually much useful material and equipment can be obtained at no cost, or by modest expenditures, as good open-style teachers often demonstrate. Expensive equipment in schools is frequently found, unused or needing maintenance, in closets and storerooms.

4 A quick survey of my neighborhood children after a recent significant space shuttle flight revealed that three had followed at least the landing in school but most had not watched or discussed it at all. One might find it hard to think of an event that afforded more high-interest "handles" for science, mathematics, geography, and language arts.

5 As observed previously, I am using the term loosely. Also required here is "feed forward," as those familiar with this concept will realize. One feeds forward intention, aim, or plan, and gets feedback that tells how well it is working. This permits revised, better feed forward. Steering a car down a winding road provides a good example.

6 Rising interest in computers puts emphasis on the "debugging" process. After a new program is written, it must be tested for bugs, or faults, which normally show up. Their elimination, at times a difficult and tedious task, is viewed as an essential step

that may increase understandings and skills. In times past, when students did more writing in school, many teachers insisted on the debugging of essays in somewhat the same way. Today, this valuable process in learning more likely gets scant attention—the effort is marked right or wrong, errors are circled in red but not followed up, or an overall grade or mark is given.

7 Having no idea of how industrial nations produce manufactured goods, the cultists assume it is the result of magic. They may erect sticks that look like a radio antenna in the hope that this will bring the radio receiver. The problem is only to find the right magic, an idea that prevailed in Europe for centuries during the heyday of alchemy and associated metaphysics. To today's students, auto parts may be seen as coming from the auto parts store, with the magical aid of money.

8 See Chapter 16, Leslie A. Hart, *The Classroom Disaster* (New York: Teachers College Press, Columbia University, 1969.)

9 Editor's Note: Four very relevant and useable indicators of mastery and competence come from Renata and Geoffrey Caine:

- The ability to use the language of the discipline or subject in complex situations and in social interaction

- The ability to perform appropriately in unanticipated situations

- The ability to solve real problems using the skills and concepts

- The ability to show, explain, or teach the idea or skill to another person who has a real need to know

See *Making Connections: Teaching and the Human Brain* (Menlo Park, California: Innovative Learning Publications, 1994).

Another set of indicators to guide a teacher's judgement of mastery and competency are two questions from the Kovalik ITI model: "What do students understand?" And, "What do you want them to do with what they understand?"

10 See Chapter 20, *The Classroom Disaster*. This idea has since been developed further: to create a separate office and function, that of the evaluator, who follows in detail the progress of each student throughout the years of attendance and is the prime reporter to both parents and administration.

11 One consequence of classroom organization is that teachers duplicate rather than pool efforts, a huge and constant waste of effort and salaries.

12 Editor's Note: For more information about the ITI model, see Appendix C.

13 See Chapter 16, Leslie A. Hart, *How The Brain Works* (New York: Basic Books, 1975) for discussion of natural thinking.

18

PROSPECTS OF CHANGE: CAN SCHOOLS SURVIVE?

> There are two very significant signs of our being at the end of one era, even if we cannot yet discern the character of the next. First, principles previously unquestioned or questioned only by "radicals" begin to come in for more serious, popular questioning . . . second, the less tenable long-established principles come to be, the more intense the ceremonial rain dances by those who fear the personal consequences of new ones.
>
> — John I. Goodlad[1]

Even the reader who has questioned or taken exception to one or another assertion that I have made in this book will, I think, agree with the overall thrust: that current educational effort tends to be choked with antique structures and cobwebbed ideas and rituals. Nor can it be seriously argued, in the light of literally hundreds of recent studies of learning achievement and general public dissatisfaction, that schools and other educational institutions function with acceptable success. While some educators feel the storm of public criticism may include excesses and inaccurate charges, it would not be easy to find one of prominence who does not feel that major changes are needed. And there are many high political officers and others who speak of the present situation in terms such as "crisis" and "disaster." "School reform" has become something of an industry.

A dozen or so years ago, any suggestion that schools as we know them could not survive much longer brought sharp and angry reactions. Today that notion, if far from universally accepted, hardly raises eyebrows.

Can schools really change? Do the new concepts of learning now available offer practical hope? Do we know how to move from the old to the new? These seem pertinent questions to address in this concluding chapter.

Our educational system, based on and dominated by the public schools, involves an intimidating bulk of payroll, plant, and peripheral interests. Employees are numbered in millions, students in the tens of millions, and expenditures run into hundreds of billions of dollars each year. Countless suppliers of all kinds have a huge stake, and influence. The greatest portion of this whole rests firmly in the hands of bureaucracies, usually multi-level, in conflict with one another, and inherently resistant to change. Unions, associations, and interest groups fiercely defend against moves they see as threatening, often in knee-jerk fashion. Public influence is sapped by the prevalence of myths, a lack of information, diverse interests and attitudes toward children and education, massive demographic and economic shifts (including massive legal and illegal immigration), racial conflict, and the difficulties of penetrating the bureaucratic citadels.

To even contemplate trying to move such a mass in a particular direction can be dismaying. Yet I remain among those who after many years of engagement with the harsh actualities of "school reform" feel that we may well be on the eve of rapid change. But it may not be polite, orderly, expected change. It may prove to be more a period of collapse of many old props, even as radical new concepts take hold—a messy time of confusion and shocks hard on those involved—but offering opportunities for rapid gains. As Goodlad suggests in the quotation that opened this chapter, the threat of an era ending may provoke more intense rain dances of resistance. In fact, the current thrust for reform, nominally supported at the highest political and bureaucratic levels, seems aimed more at *preserving* the bureaucratic, assembly-line concept of "school" than trying to bring on the more "human" view that springs from brain-compatible approaches.

SHIFTS TO BE MADE

Here we reach the crux of the change problem. How practical is it to ask people long committed to traditional approaches to play by new rules so to speak? Consider a few of the shifts to be made: giving up the belief that curriculum must be made up of a certain body of knowledge, escaping from the concept of school as a collection of classrooms, and ending the focus on "teaching lessons" rather than on learning as the measurement of the job to be done.

Giving Up "Canon"

The concept that there is a certain body of core learning that every student must strive to master above all else has long been accepted as academic bedrock. But today it has become hard to win agreement on what the canon should include and, even harder, to suppose that in a fast-changing world there is or could be a canon that remains valid for long. The whole idea of "canon" suggests a longing for simpler, less frenetic times. As we take a brain-compatible approach we have to favor seeing the brain as an active process, not as a storage file. Going a step further, we come to see that any practical "core" would consist of *programs,* a collection of things one knows how to *do* (perform or execute) rather than in the academic sense of write or talk about or pass an exam. Such a collection would have to be flexible, responsive to the current real world. That is not the idea of canon.

Escaping From the Concept of Classroom

The common concept of "school" as a *collection of classrooms* will no longer be tolerable as education moves to brain-compatible approaches. The classroom as an organizational device came into use understandably enough as the result of circumstances (see Chapter 15) and the rise of bureaucracy in education, at a time when attention and concern for individual students would have seemed to run afoul of the proverb "beggars can't be choosers." Schools were devised to be cheap and easily operated by ordering youngsters what to do, not "catering" to them. (There are still many who share this view and are forever annoyed or angered by the fact that young students cannot be stamped out like coins but differ as humans relentlessly do.)

To watch a highly skilled teacher "manage" a classroom by bridging differences or pretending they are not there, or can be pushed aside, is to see how absurd and restrictive the classroom device can be. When individual differences become too painful, of course, the offending students are thrown into a barrel labeled "learning disabled" or "special education" and such. The compensatory and "remedial" programs then necessary typically prove far more expensive for the school to provide, and strikingly unsuccessful. Remedial measures notoriously fail to remediate, and may readily make matters worse when the basic effort can be described as "try once again what has failed many times, only this time try harder and longer." Even with a lower student-teacher ratio, failure is predictable.

Fierce struggles ensue over whether a child should or should not be "in a classroom," meaning a room in which the teacher-student ratio is about the usual. This witless debate persists but seldom leads to serious consideration of the inherent defects of the old classroom concept and effort to teach. The argument is over whether the student would be less troublesome in room 103 or room 108. The classroom scheme ensnares school efforts as a spider's web does a luscious bug, wrapping strand after strand. All the arrangements contribute—even the physical building, which provides not flexible space but all too solid walls. Since virtually everything provided has been created *for classrooms*, including texts and teaching aids, schedules and rules, and even terminology, teachers and principals who want to change often must struggle endlessly with a sticky past. The teacher who says: "I don't want to run a classroom" may win the rejoinder: "You'd rather be unemployed?"

A teacher joining the staff of an existing school feels pressure to "fit in" and conform at least for a year or two. The same applies to a supervisor or principal. The culture of schools does not encourage rapid change. So long as the main expertise of teachers lies in "running a classroom," I suspect most teachers won't have rapid impact on encrusted schools. The classroom type of school, we have all too thoroughly demonstrated, seldom produces acceptable results.

Only as teachers and supervisors can shift to nonclassroom situations can the door be opened to the benefits of brain-compatible approaches. Encouragingly, an increasing number of practitioners have come to realize that alternatives to the classroom exist.

Ending the Focus on "Teaching Lessons"

When my wife and I first set up a household, times were uncertain and money scarce. Our supply of china was minimal. Opportunistically, we bought what we could and gradually the kitchen shelves filled, as gravy bowl and eggcups joined the fish platter.

For generations schools have viewed knowledge as a *collection,* by which bare mental shelves might be filled in much the same way — but the knowledge the school delivered was perishable and could (as it usually did) disappear. All the educators could do was keep elaborate records of what was delivered. That was the school's job: retaining the collection was the student's responsibility. Delivery was by means of what were called "lessons." Each lesson was like a plate or cup within our metaphor. It should have helped fill a shelf. The record showed it had been delivered — the school knew in detail what "had been taught." It also knew, from too ample experience, that what a student actually "retained" for a while could vanish like butterflies in a breeze.

Convincing teachers that giving lessons is not a brain-compatible activity is by no means impossible but it does take time for people in any occupation to set aside old ways and adopt new. The bright aspect is that the much greater success of brain-compatible instruction becomes evident quite quickly, without need for clumsy tests to provide "scores."[2]

WINDOWS OF OPPORTUNITY

Despite painfully slow visible progress, I feel that there are a variety of changes afoot that may open the way for the emergence of truly significant change in our public schools. The most notable windows of opportunity are fluctuating enrollment, public discontent with runaway costs, public demand for learning, availability of coherent theory, and other societal influences such as the civil and women's rights movements and competition.

Fluctuating Enrollment

Changes in enrollment could provide considerable opportunity for change. Increases bring additional funding; decreases require (or should) dialogue about priorities. However, in institutions such as the schools, growth tends to hide and ease problems, while shrinkage not only intensifies them but adds all the pain and strain of cutting back. In the past, for example, the new floods of immigration have often brought problems that outweighed relief generated by the additional funding. Rather than use fluctuating enrollment as a positive opportunity for change, schools retrenched, often in the crudest, blindest way, as boards of education tried to cope with changing conditions. Likewise, under the dubious banner of "back to basics" (as though basics were sound and successful, not the site of the worst failures), confused and quarreling local leaders tended to retain all the hoariest, costliest, and least productive forms of effort. Much as strains accumulate before an earthquake, the stage was set for deep-seated, fundamental change while little showed on the surface. Enrollments, however, continue to fluctuate, each time giving us an open window of opportunity to rethink what we do and why we do it.

Public Discontent with Runaway Costs

General inflation, especially during the 1980s, plus an accelerated rise in costs in education have hit taxpayers hard. The combination of rising expense for fewer students chilled those who had already been showing an increasing tendency to resist higher tax loads. Even in communities where only a few years before citizens had boasted of how lavishly they spent on schools, budgets already trimmed were defeated. In a few dramatic instances, schools shut down for periods as funds ran out. In a great many more, individual schools closed, perhaps permanently. Shortage of money is now chronic for most school systems. Committees commonly form to agitate for lower taxes on property owners.

The coincidence of inflation and rising costs had significant potential, not always noted, for facilitating change. So long as members of school staffs usually felt impregnably secure in their employment, they and their unions could look at proposals for change as less than compelling. But teachers and others who see closings, dismissals, and forced retirements all around them acquire new worries to add to those about reduced prestige, personal safety, and depressing conditions of work. Much as one may deplore these hardships, they clearly make continued resistance to change harder for boards, administrators, staffs, and unions to maintain.

Public Demand for Learning

Whether by happenstance again or because of the influences mentioned above, for the first time in recent American educational history *the amount and quality of learning achieved by students* has become an urgent issue. Though it sounds absurd to state baldly that interest in learning is new, historically that seems to be precisely accurate! The schools have worried about control, order, socialization, moral considerations, manners, and compliance; but grossly inadequate *learning* has been blamed on the individual student (or the student's background) even when failure to learn was massive and pervasive in the student body, even when middle-class as well as poor and "minority" children were victims. While some schools boasted of scholarships won and college admissions obtained, on the whole schools have long evaded or avoided publicizing "the bottom line" — student learning outcomes. When some years ago a few big city systems began to publish reading scores, the move was regarded as radical in the extreme.[3] Talking about learning, it seemed, made many educators uneasy, as if under attack and insulted. For generations it has been assumed that youngsters went to school and thereby became "educated" as they spent time in the halls of education. Was proof really required?

But public demand to know outcomes has risen steadily over recent years, fueled from a variety of sources. Employers found candidates unqualified and unready, colleges complained of freshmen grossly ill-prepared, the armed forces had to reject large numbers of potential recruits as hopelessly lacking in elementary skills even though many were high school graduates, at least on paper. A long series of studies and reports, led by those of the National Assessment[4] kept winning publicity as they brought dismal confirmation of poor learning, grade inflation (lowered standards), alarming gaps in knowledge, and stunted skills. Falling college entrance test scores (their importance absurdly exaggerated and over-publicized), glaring shortcomings in the study of science, mathematics, and foreign languages, all induced public worries. Concern arose about "our ability to compete" as a nation, accentuated as imports took larger shares of markets we had long regarded as ours, such as automobiles. As the disturbing findings came in, they inspired more studies, and more wondering about whether educators knew their business. Many pundits and politicians rushed to proffer them a dizzying range of usually simple-minded "solutions."

Disappearing Myth #1: Protective Cloak. If in general the schools appeared to pay little heed other than by hasty window-dressing, some important (and much trivial) movement nevertheless occurred. The old myths and attitudes that had long protected the schools from pointed criticism on *learning achieved* began to crumble and educators found themselves confronted with legislation in most states that now *ordered* the schools to produce a minimal amount of learning. Such laws may be considered essentially foolish—one cannot legislate learning. But the message was clearer: much higher student achievement was now demanded of the schools. The fashionable term "accountability" became essential; yet, if it meant anything it was "You *make* 'em learn, y'hear?"

If I may venture an observation, not a few boards of education and administrators still seem to regard this demand as one more patchwork quilt to emerge from state capitols, another pin prick to be endured. But others, especially at higher levels, appear to concede that this extraordinary change in the rules of the game has a broad public base and has come to stay. It seems clear that pressures on schools to produce real, substantial, useful learning will increase; it is not at all clear that school people know how to bring that about. My own informal sampling, down to the building principal level, suggests a much expanded willingness to consider alternatives and—cautiously—undertake leadership. A new question is repeatedly asked: *what can we do that will work?*

At the highest levels, concern has intensified over those many students who not so long ago were written off as failures and thrown on the junk heap to fend for themselves. Today it is apparent that if our national junk heap gets larger, it will sink us as a nation. We simply cannot afford to have a multitude of student failures. We need a work force and society of men and women, of all backgrounds and sources, who have an education that will help them to contribute to the nation's and their own success. Schools must bring this about if *they* are to survive. Such ideas as vouchers, "choice," home schooling, and new kinds of private, for-profit suppliers or managers already nibble at the core concept of *public* schools.

Disappearing Myth #2: "One Best System." The notion that we should have "the one best system," to use David Tyack's term[5] has already begun to fray badly. The more schools we have that offer brain compatibility in a variety of ways, the more the opportunity grows for brain-compatible schools to demonstrate outcomes far superior to those of the defunct class-and-grade system. We do not need many such successes, I believe, to have potent effect, if the successes are substantially unquestionable. If even a scattering of schools in a variety of typical communities can show virtually zero failure in the basic skills (including children from low-income and non-English-speaking homes, and the millions imaginatively called learning disabled[6] or otherwise improperly labeled) and can achieve much better results in quality and range of other learning, then the mere existence of such schools can be used as a wedge to crack resistance elsewhere.

Until recently, exemplary schools have been hard to find, and usually content to claim only modest superiority, to avoid flack. But the "critical mass" of such schools may even now have become enough to inspire a giant shift from class-and-grade to brain-compatible schools.

Parents and public clamor for better schools; employers tend to scream in frustration; colleges are painfully aware that their students all too commonly are grossly ill-prepared. The suspicion that crime and drug abuse has a closer connection with failing schools than we like to think is not far below the surface. In cold fact, most parents do not want to get involved in schools—they want to send their youngsters to schools where they will be safe and reasonably successful and happy, without putting onerous demands on the home and causing feelings of guilt. They have, understandably enough, a limited concept of the role of the brain; but experience show they will accept brain-compatible schools in most cases on the evidence of how their children respond.

By the mid 1990s, successful brain-compatible schools at all levels had become easy to find and the brain-based movement was flourishing at a pace that would have seemed incredible even two years earlier.

Availability of Coherent Theory

In Proster Theory, and other such brain-based theories of human learning as may come forward, we have at last the crucial element that can accelerate successful change: coherent theory to guide planning and implementing.

Not having ever experienced great advances, people in education generally have neither expected them nor looked for them, in large part because they had *no programs, no procedures, for obtaining major improvements and advances* within the parameters of ordinary, sanctioned behavior. Only individuals who felt very secure, or were daring by nature, ordinarily ventured into new ground. But today new pressures seem to be changing that generality, pushing people into action because the status quo has become intolerable and threatening. In such a push-pull environment, the availability of radically new theory beckons them to consider breakthrough possibilities never before seriously studied.

Experience with brain-compatible approaches suggests strongly that the theory not only leads to learning successes but also gives a lot of highly practical assistance to effecting the changes that can convert an old, conventional school or system to a new, brain-based one.

Much is now known about how to do this and how to interest staff in what becomes an appealing, exciting and rewarding adventure. While it may take up to two years for teachers and others to fully grasp and accept Proster Theory, results of beginning to apply it may become strikingly evident within a few weeks. As they see firsthand that the theory "works" (and that working from theory works) their enthusiasm for real change is likely to flourish. The contrast between this process and the usual telling of staff what to do is of course extreme.

Other Influences

Three trends that may operate to push or encourage major changes should be at least mentioned, although their effects must be speculative.

Civil Rights Movement. The *civil rights* movement which has produced large gains for "minorities" in many ways (reminding us how fast large-scale changes in society can occur, once they get going) seems currently to have encountered more resistance. A flood of immigrants and refugees has complicated schooling problems, putting new strains on the classroom system and its efforts to deal with youngsters as if alike.

For a long time African-Americans parents believed, as an article of faith, that if their children went to schools with whites, learning would follow. Unfortunately, they enormously exaggerated the ability of schools to bring about learning achievement for students. This fact now is coming more to light, to meld with other acute (and justified) dissatisfactions such as the tight link between family income and all levels of educational credential achievement.[7] In my experience, African-Americans, Latinos, Native Americans, Asian-Americans, and other immigrants have been slow to see how classroom schools harm their children the most, and the most cruelly, because their differences in background and experience are neither fully understood nor accepted. While many teachers struggle to be fair and supportive, they must work within a structure and tradition that does not encourage responsiveness. The standard classroom was intended for white, middle-class children (insofar as it can be said to be "intended" for anyone). It may well collapse as more parents of "other" children demand a fairer deal, long overdue.

Women's Rights Movement. Women's rights, too, have made rapid progress. As women commonly spend less time in the home, gain more exposure to the world of work, and speak with firmer voices, women's demands for more effective and desirable schools may well become stronger and less patient. In general, the schools appear to have ignored these changes, and even continue, often, to complain about lack of parental involvement, as though major social changes could be dealt with as naughty behavior. Some day, too, feminists may be willing to confront the low regard for women built into the classroom system.[8]

Competition. Competition is the third influence, and perhaps the most inscrutable. The near monopoly the public schools have long enjoyed has obviously been crumbling. Non-public schools appear to be gaining, albeit slowly. Should the trend accelerate even a little, perhaps aided by vouchers and "choice" plans of some kind, the impact on public schools, already shrinking, could be shattering, and could spur even sleepy schools to change. In the immediate offing looms a new component: the host of electronic developments, including video cassettes and low-cost home computers which can make any of 100,000 pictures or pages instantly available on a television screen, or present motion which can be reversed and repeated — tools made all the more powerful by internet access. The potentials are staggering and the cost already relatively modest. Each such device — more are on the way — makes the conventional school look more primitive and feeble. For the conventional class-and-grade school, alternative schools, public or private (even purely for-profit schools) also offer direct competition that may only have begun. The greater flexibility of such schools and their willingness to consider new approaches could quite possibly lead to their explosive growth, even if some pioneers fail.

But the notion that "competition" and "choice" will have magical effect seems one more instance of trying to find success without having brain-based theory as foundation for producing learning. The desire to find some gimmick or bit of magic that will solve the "school problem" without having to recognize that the old class-and-grade system never worked adequately continues to blind us. Theoretical gimmicks hold no hope but do appeal to the common sense, logical, would-be fixers who do not yet understand the role of the bodymind in learning and that the new system must be brain-compatible and focused on *producing learning.*

Currently we have vast amounts of energy going into testing, and even a proposal for national "standards," as though having contrived standards would automatically result in having adequately prepared staff focused on producing learning and working in schools designed for that purpose. We must wonder at the rhetoric of those who pursue this foolish path (which of course produces income for those who follow it as hired researchers and policy-makers).

COMING FULL CIRCLE

We have come full circle. When Horace Mann took up his new office a century and a half ago, he looked at the schools of his day and found them wanting. Sensibly, he wasted no time on tinkering but set out actively to seek a replacement system. In Prussia he found a model to adapt. The American class-and-grade system that resulted was a smashing success in meeting the political and funding needs of a common-school system; it was equally a disaster for producing reliable learning, a consideration given scant attention at the time. It has been a curse to us ever since. *Today our clear need is to look actively for a replacement system that will bring about learning.* If momentarily there seems to be more moaning than looking, it hardly appears impossible that looking may be the next step—a very large step away from lifting the drawbridge and defending the status quo castle. For our educators to say out loud, "What we are doing does not work and must be replaced," is a giant step forward.

Throughout the sixties and into the seventies, a spirit of looking found much sustenance, in part, oddly enough, due to the success of the Russian space experts in launching Sputnik and so proving they were far ahead in that dramatic technology. Both private and public funds flowed into experiments and new formats and arrangements. At almost any conference—and there was then money for many conferences—innovation was a prime topic. The criticisms of the dominant system that compose a portion of this book were then aired in detail and with vehemence, verbally and in a succession of books that found wide readership. The Johnson administration attacked the problem of student failure on a huge scale, lavishing funds on "compensatory" programs to unheard-of extent. For a time it seemed probable that sweeping change would indeed come, fueled by the emotions of civil rights drives, lubricated with easy money, and guided by many of the most creative, enterprising people within education.

Yet not much happened. *The old system survived, unchanged.*

A study of that period is beyond the scope of this book. Much more literature on it would be welcome to explain why a period of ferment brought only fragments of permanent change at best.

Avoiding Fragmentation

Some of the largest programs, especially in compensatory education, were based on logical plans innocent of substantial learning theory. As one collapsed, another was put in its place. Project Head Start, for example, was intended to prepare certain children to fit the schools they would attend, not to prepare the schools to fit the children. Hailed in revolutionary terms, it was actually a massive effort to bolster the failing status quo.[9]

The Whole Is Greater Than the Sum of the Parts. Because the cheerful, hopeful, well-intended blunderings into unmapped regions were largely unrelated to each other, they failed to add up. *Cumulative effect requires theory; there was no theory.* Good intuitions of the sort sensitive educators have had for centuries were mixed in with novelties, hot fads, of the moment, buzzwords, old and tired conventional curriculums and materials, new "teacher-proof" programs from academic ivory towers, and ancient traditions and folklore. "Open" approaches for classrooms, corridors, or schools, some more or less inspired by British experience, ranged from expert to inept, from well considered to crackpot, with "open" nonetheless taken as a meaningful descriptor by researchers who solemnly wrote up comparisons with graded classrooms. The same foolish use of vague labels was made with team teaching, ungraded classrooms, flexible plans, and other formats.

Lessons from the Ashes. To imply that this era of change produced nothing of value would be incorrect. Obviously, a great deal was learned about what not to do and the difficulties of bringing about change in complex, loosely-coupled school organization came to light to provide sobering lessons to naive enthusiasts. But amid the failures and wash-outs there was much that worked.

Perhaps most important were the thousands of demonstrations that *arrangements other than the conventional graded classrooms were viable.* They could be set up, usually in existing buildings; they could be staffed with teachers and others with conventional backgrounds, after training; they could continue for years to serve not only the hand-picked but also the broad flow of students. Once established, costs fell within normal range or even lower. For a number of years I have checked informally on the effects on disciplinary and attendance problems; they almost always decrease strikingly in nonclassroom settings, particularly in substantially brain-compatible environments. Equally, teachers who have a year of experience in such situations strongly prefer not to return to conventional classrooms.[10]

Despite retrenchment and the often mindless "back to basics" cry, thousands of exceptions to the conventional classroom continue to function, even if they total only a small percent of the whole.[11] Unfortunately, to my knowledge no adequate studies of any large sample of these departures from the conventional have been made and reported.

Survivors of the era of change have tended to maintain low profiles, rather than beat drums for their successes. As the brain-compatible approach has spread and taken hold, a considerable number of examples of this radically different effort exist but they, too, scatter over a range from early beginnings to well developed. Again, many practitioners feel it expedient to keep profiles low and claims of achievement more modest than may be warranted. (Conventional teachers who have moved into brain-based activities often seem hesitant to "flaunt" their outcomes, at least in public, for fear of arousing opposition.)[12]

We have, in short, a rich body of ore to turn to, once there arises the desire to prospect. And whereas the graded classroom is over-aged, exhausted, and feeble as a device, these newer forms usually stand at the threshold of their development. Seldom are they integrated into a system or vigorously supported with resources.

UNDERSTANDING FORCES THAT RESIST CHANGE

The forces that resist change are numerous. Some are central, others strong contributors. Some seem evident[13] while others represent complex, crisscross forces, a welter of factors treacherous to analyze.

Contributing Factors

Contributing factors which have proved particularly powerful include:

- **Many of the experiments were not carried into practice.** They were protocols on paper, resisted in the classroom by teachers who often resented them and continued doing what they had always done, though sometimes using new labels and terms in mock compliance.

- The great majority of efforts were **fragmentary rather than systemic,** concerned with students at a limited age range or level. Others dealt only with certain topics, subjects, or groups.

- **Implementation** was often grossly inadequate, with little attention given to the needs and views of teachers and others at the working level. The "new math," for example, was thrust on ill-prepared teachers. "Open" techniques were jumped into hastily, with little provision for training and support. Also, administrators and staffs, it may be suspected, failed to support, even sabotaged, the programs they disliked or feared.

- The problem of **evaluation** was frequently left for later; or methods designed for the old system were applied to new efforts, leading to endless wrangles about outcomes.[14]

- **"Change agents"** who supposedly could introduce the new techniques and arrangements came into hot demand but moved frequently to take advantage of better job offers, leaving vacuums behind.

- School staffs, little involved in and mistrustful of change pushed on them, bided their time and when possible **reverted** to old, comfortable ways. Even where new approaches took some root, boards of education and administrators who felt their own expertise and control diminished made no effort to build on the success and allowed it to slough off as the enthusiasts for it moved or retired.[15]

- **Money** was flooded in. Educators had long used lack of funds as an all-purpose excuse for not solving problems and shortcomings. Generous funding wiped out the excuse but at the same time the money itself created new bureaucracies. Those bureaucracies attracted people eager to share the bonanza while it lasted but who often were little interested in building programs that could endure on regular funding. When the foundations, disenchanted by scant results, turned off their money, projects tended to slide into oblivion even when they had merit and promise.

- **Teacher prep** by the institutions that presumably exist primarily to train teachers for the schools — more than 1,500 of them — should have provided a safe haven and vigorous support for innovators and pioneering theoreticians but fell down almost completely on that opportunity. The sad state of those programs has been described and evaluated in a number of studies, notably that headed by John L. Goodlad and reported in the shocking book, *Teachers for Our Nation's Schools*. With rare exception, these institutions for the preparation of teachers not only failed to offer leadership but persisted in passing along to the new generations of certified candidates for school jobs all the failure-encrusted concepts and practices of the conventional class-and-grade school, while maintaining a ten-foot-pole stand-away from actual schools and the best achieving teachers. Teacher education, Goodlad comments, is simply "one of our nation's neglected enterprises."

- Although the various forms of brain-compatible schools do not appear to demand substantially rebuilt or new buildings and plants, the problem of **retraining staff** at first looks formidable. Experience over a decade, however, suggests that "converting" typical "class-and-grade" schools to brain-compatible ones can be accomplished smoothly and rapidly when there is desire to do so and procedures and techniques that have shown success are known and utilized. Retraining can be difficult indeed when the people involved do not want to change, see little point to learning new ways, and have little desire to master new programs. It can be quite another matter when the goals are most attractive, seem well-conceived and attainable, and very quickly produce visible results as the new approaches are implemented with strong, on-site support. The shift to brain-compatible instruction should be mostly on-the-job and real, rather than by lecture and meeting as in feeble, futile in-service programs that have a high content of pious talk.

Crucial Factors

The overwhelming reason why this era of change produced so little in proportion to the rhetoric and effort now stands clear—the more so if this book has served its aim. The efforts went in all directions because **there existed no unifying theory.** One enthusiasm, one experiment, was as good as another. Foundations and government funded almost anything that might work, even where admittedly the proposals had conflicting rationales.

In addition, it appears pertinent to point out that Proster Theory itself suggests strongly how effective retraining can be planned: by *identifying the new programs sought* and *changing the biases* so that old ones will not be called up from the proster.[16] *Teachers left in classroom settings will likely revert to old ways.*

More About Teacher Preparation and Retraining

The exhaustive survey Goodlad reports found little effort by teacher preparation programs to develop teachers as professionals who comprehend the uses of theory and to provide serious exposure to the newest and best ways to translate theory into practice.

Even scattered incidence of more successful and productive schools could not, without useful theory and theoretically prepared leaders to apply it, be of general help. As cognitive psychologist Donald Snygg pointed out astutely over a quarter-century ago:

> Knowledge of what has happened in one situation cannot, without a theory of why it happened, enable us to predict what will happen in any other situation if it is different in the slightest degree. . . . Without a scientific theory of learning, teachers and administrators have to meet new problems with inappropriate routines that were devised long ago to meet other problems or to base their decisions on folk beliefs about learning which, although thoroughly disproved in the laboratories, still pass for common sense.[17]

Educational philosopher Harry S. Broudy is among those who have stressed the same thought, noting the fundamental impact of "the lack of any body of accepted theory or expertise in terms of which one can tell in advance something about the viability of a project or experiment." But Broudy has gone further to observe:

> Between the theoreticians and operatives there must be an interposition of practitioners enlightened by theory from mere rule following. The almost farcical attempts to evade the task of providing this professional layer are the prime cause of most of the ills from which the schools of America suffer.[18]

It would be pleasant to report that the institutions that train teachers, administrators, and specialists now offer leadership and courses to meet the needs Broudy identified but such programs remain exceptional. However, when teacher's colleges and departments of education also feel the shaking-up effects of lower enrollments and the demand for learning achievement, they may well respond in due course.[19] That interest in the brain approach has steadily risen seems hardly disputable and a sprinkling of largely self-directed graduate students and holders of doctorates have taken brain-oriented paths. As long ago as 1979, a yearbook of the Association for Supervision and Curriculum Development, a long-established, conservative organization, offered these blunt views:

> As practiced, schooling is a poor facilitator of learning. Its persis-

tent view of learning as product interferes with significant learnings connected to such complex processes as inquiry and appreciation. What often passes for education is noise that interrupts the natural flow of learning. Schooling too often fragments learning into subject areas, substitutes control for the natural desire to learn, co-opts naturally active children for hours in assembly line classroom structures, and ignores both individual and cultural differences. . . . The formal educational system often destroys opportunities for learning from elders, from each other, and from the new generation. . . . Much is known about the learning process but little has been applied to education. . . . The American education system is not making use of brain research findings, findings which shatter the S-R learning myth.[20]

If useful theory can be valuable to those directly engaged in instruction, it would seem just as valuable to those who undertake to train teachers and administrators. To be sure, colleges cannot offer programs on brain-compatible approaches until they have people to teach them. This is a hen-and-egg problem that can lessen in a few years. The institutions that take the lead may find it less onerous than those who trail.

SUCCESSFUL PATTERNS OF BRAIN-COMPATIBLE SCHOOLS

Many designs for brain-compatible schools are possible. Positive factors can be emphasized and negative factors eliminated by an infinite variety of combinations of elements. The engineering can take many forms. Certain patterns, however, are likely to be common to all successes, including aspects of organization, instruction, curriculum, interaction, student progress, atmosphere, and retraining.

Organizational

The old Horace Mann "classroom" will largely vanish, to give way to flexible, temporary groupings of a size suitable to the activity in hand. Most teachers will work mostly as members of teams—students will no longer have "my teacher" who has multiple powers as instructor, evaluator, judge and boss. Almost all instructional staff will have guidance functions relating to assigned students and these will not automatically cease at the end of the year or semester. Students will not be in grades or seg-regated by age and will not be tracked. Schools will generally be smaller than they have been and often divided to avoid deperson-alization and "factory" effects. Required years of attendance will be made flexible and subject to individual determinations, not automatic "for everybody."

Instructional

In place of aggressive teaching, students will usually come to instructors (of all kinds) for assistance with perceived needs, and for continuing individual guidance. Students will be able to fol-low individual interests for short or long periods—even years. With classroom gone, old classroom ideas and procedures will vanish, including "management," control, lock-step "covering" of material, recitation, seatwork, uniform homework, constant grad-ing of student work, quizzes, exams and most testing, and the use of report-card grades. The old "lesson" concepts of learning to order, teacher as dispenser of knowledge pills, and logical-sequence courses will all give way to brain-based understandings of how learning occurs.

Curriculum

"Curriculum" will no longer mean "courses all students are to study" but rather the broad sweep of what may be investigated by one, a few, or many students according to interests. Students will be guided, however, to attain within certain, few areas com-petence in "basics" such as use of language, fundamental math concepts, civics, science, health, and the like. in a free, flexibly scheduled, cumulative way, without predetermined sequence, and with attainment measured mainly by ability to *apply* and *per-form*. Much work will be integrated around themes. Students will be far more engaged with realities, much less with writing at a desk or dealing with abstracted, academic work. Acquiring factu-al knowledge will be de-emphasized, but skill and experience in locating or retrieving information will get constant practical attention and application.

Interaction

Students will talk with, work with, and learn from a wide vari-ety of individuals, only some of whom will be on staff. Frequently, people from the community will come in to discuss their functions and expertise with students, as will visitors and parents. On-going collaboration with fellow students of various ages and grades is also important.

Student Progress

Progress of each student will be known in detail and reviewed frequently, with failure not acceptable to the school. So-called "standardized" fill-in tests will be used little if at all.

Atmosphere

The school will become a *learning center* for all in it, including staff rather than a punitive institution where confrontation is normal and teaching staff merely repeat their activities from year to year.

Staff Retraining

As the Proster Theory makes clear, a shift to brain-compatibility will not happen unless current biases are changed and new mental programs are developed for implementing curriculum and instruction. Retraining of current staff—all staff, not just teachers—is therefore a critical prerequisite. We must have people who (1) have theory and (2) know how to use it. While common sense suggests that one school can imitate another that appears to be a successful model, in fact that proves difficult, and rarely happens—unless the grasp of theory provides the bridge. Also, of course, schools lack the means, time, and desire to study a model, even if aware of its existence. Petty pride may negate the option—it is not uncommon for principals to reject an advance simply because it was "not invented here" or "by me" or because of reluctance to squander their "honeymoon" period on cleaning up problems left behind by the departing leader(s).

Brain-based theory, even in its early stages, gives us what has never been available before: the ability to *design* settings and methods likely to work much better to produce student learning. The broad objective of brain compatibility can be *factored*, i.e., the theory strongly suggests what elements will impede learning, facilitate it, or be neutral. True experiments become feasible, not aimed at trying to determine the influence of one variable in a complex situation (an effort that has wasted millions of research dollars) but at designing and conducting actual instruction for a period and reading the outcomes against what theory predicted. If a model is available, it can be studied in the light of applied theory, rather than by superficial imitation.

Pilot Implementation

Experience in converting schools to brain-compatible operation has shown the usefulness of a technique well-known in most large operations — the use of "pilot" innovations. The retail chain with 3,000 stores does not have to try to innovate in all of them at once. It is far easier to select four or six and see how the changes work in these. Once the pilots succeed, what has been learned can be applied rapidly elsewhere. In addition, a cadre of people with some experience has been created. What at first may seem a slower and roundabout approach actually proves to be easier, less risky, and faster. For obscure reasons, educators (and politicians) appear to get bogged down in large scale attempts that may waste years before failure becomes clear.

It should be noted, however, that the changes being tested in the pilot examples should not be watered down or timidly made. The idea is to make the changes "whole hog" but on a scale that permits easy staffing, low initial investment, and clear focus on implementation issues both large and small.[21]

In medical research, awareness is keen of the great differences between *in vitro* or test tube studies, and those in *vivo* or in actual living bodies, where outcomes can be unexpected and highly variable with individuals. In the end, only in vivo success has broad, practical human value. In education, the in vivo efforts, without good theoretical design, have been of necessity blind, "try it and see" investigations, and as Snygg pointed out, of little use for prediction if even a single element is changed.

Working from *theory to factors*, from factors to *design of complex situations*, permits experiments that can rapidly refine both basic theory and the "engineering" necessary to apply it. At the same time, the outcomes of trials can be analyzed in theory and factor terms, producing far more understanding of why they developed as they did. This technique, used virtually everywhere except in education, also yields steadily *cumulative* results — each pilot effort brings more knowledge of what to do and how.

Expected Outcomes of Brain Compatibility

Those who have never really seen the achievement of learning by all students as the objective of schools will be slow to scrap old ways of instructing. And those who have never seen a tight connection between brain and learning will have trouble adopting and developing brain-compatible approaches and techniques. Practitioners who have worked for years believing that only coercion will get students to learn (even while they see the miserable results coercion produces) will resist moving to the new concepts. Conversion requires first finding the staff who want change and who see the potential of getting away from a structure that has failed miserably. As even a few leaders demonstrate that brain-based ways clearly work, those more timid (or longer oppressed) may quickly follow.

Fortunately, when brain-compatible settings and techniques are introduced, visible improvement in student learning occurs very quickly, though it may take far more time to convert the school as a whole, and teachers must be allowed time to revise their own long-held concepts. The even faster changes in how students behave in themselves give staff an early reward that often proves more than a little astonishing to participants.

Unfortunately, the brain-compatible movement still has much organizing and consolidating to do, though progress is notable. And the vast, chaotic, little-disciplined educational establishment, especially at the college level, has yet to wake up appropriately and offer the needed brain-compatible training. To many academics (certainly not all) the non-logical realities of the brain, which threaten the rhetorical towers of "the discipline" are seen as an anathema to be ridiculed and defended against.

Years ago, when television was all black-and-white and color waited on the threshold, I was peripherally involved, and recall the seemingly insolvable dilemma: color sets could not be made at reasonable cost except in great volume; people would not buy receivers unless there were a lot of color programs to make it worthwhile; broadcasters could not afford expensive color programs unless there preexisted a large audience able to view them in color. Somehow the problems, involving many parties and hundreds of millions of dollars, were resolved. In contrast, the difficulties of setting up a modest number of pilot brain-compatible schools seem relatively simple, and the time seems ripe.

Pictures of Brain Compatibility in Action. We live in days when changes come with a rush. Let us speculate on outcomes that seem possible:[22]

- Student failure or serious lagging, even where endemic, might well be virtually eliminated so far as core learning is concerned.

- Most students would go far beyond present grade levels, achieving much more solid and in-depth learning.

- The discipline problem would largely vanish, as it already has in many nonclassroom schools.

- Teachers would find their burdens sharply reduced as confrontations gave way to enhanced individual learning, with teachers taking on much more professional (and gratifying) obligations and roles.

- Administration could become far more focused on education rather than often minor, time-consuming duties.

- The cost of schools could be substantially reduced by a variety of savings, especially by reducing non-productive efforts.

- Public and community would be directly and continuously involved, and supportive.

- Youth crime and drug abuses, at least the portion attributable to school failure, boredom, and age grouping, might be reduced.

- Student and staff morale could show great improvement, as the tone of schools changed to successful, cooperative effort rather than conflict and decline.

- Students from poorer or certain "minority" homes would escape many current disadvantages.

- Students would emerge from secondary school far better prepared for further education or work, with substantial grasp and experience of the real world.

In Conclusion

Beyond argument, learning is a bodybrain function. This new knowledge of how humans learn can have profound impact on students and their learning. To welcome it and to explore the potential of bodybrain-compatible approaches is our personal responsibility as educators and an obligation we owe to our grandchildren.

NOTES

1   "Can Our Schools Get Better?" *Phi Delta Kappan*, January 1979, p. 345.

2   Editor's Note: See *The ITI Classroom Rubric* and *The ITI Schoolwide Rubric*, two excellent guides for examining progress toward implementing a brain-compatible environment. Stage 3 from both documents appears in Appendix B.

3   Innumerable individual teachers and others, of course, have taken personal interest in their students' learning achievement, and to some this has been a source of deep concern. On institutional levels, however, it is difficult to find evidence of similar distress. Bottom-line reports remain a rarity, and at best tend to be rigid, statistically overwhelming, and obscure as well as very limited in scope. Instances of deliberate manipulation or falsification of scores are not unknown. Dismissal or demotion of employees primarily because of poor learning outcomes seldom occurs. The success of individual practitioners and administrators is not known, nor is direct reward often feasible.

4   The National Assessment of Educational Progress was set up by joint action of several parties in 1969, over widespread opposition of educators. It periodically samples student attainment by special examinations and issues public reports. For more information, contact NAEP, Rosedale Blvd., Princeton, NJ; 609/734-1327.

5   David B. Tyack, *The One Best System* (Cambridge: Harvard University Press, 1974). This much noted revisionist history documents a number of observations made in this chapter. Tyack writes: "In most cities failure in school was a way of life for vast numbers of children" (p. 200).

6 This dubious condition, which has at best only a rambling def-inition, has become one of the many vested interests, as well as a convenient blame-the-victim way of dealing with poor learning outcomes.

7 The correlation with family income has long been common knowledge. Recent studies also show similar linkage for SAT college entrance scores.

8 Leslie A. Hart, "Classrooms Are Killing Learning," *Principal,* May 1981, especially p. 9. In the parent involvement area, Salt Lake City public schools have been in the lead in showing what can be done, even as more parents work.

9 The value of Head Start continues to be debated. Possibly, however, some improvement in achievement may be attribut-able to the better feeding and other incidental factors of the program rather than to the instructional aspects. In general, Head Start enabled needy children to get more attention in many forms, no small benefit.

10 For a striking example, see James H. Lytle, "An Untimely (but Significant) Experiment in Teacher Motivation," *Phi Delta Kappan,* June 1980, p. 700. The article shows the sacrifices teachers were eager to make to continue in the famous Philadelphia Parkway Program.

11 The growth of alternative schools within larger systems, intended to give parents some choice, has been impressive. From a handful in 1970, these schools now number in the thousands. See Vernon H. Smith, "Alternative Education Is Here to Stay," *Phi Delta Kappan,* April 1981, and other articles in this issue. A still greater number of nonclassroom programs exist within conventional schools, some as alternatives parents or students may select.

12 Editor's Note: The Bay Area Middle School Program (BAMS) funded by the David and Lucille Packard Foundation and administered by the Center for the Future of Public Education from 1990-95 witnessed classic cases of the system's unrelenting destruction of excellence. Two of its three model schools were abruptly dismantled by forcing out the principal, both of whom were strong and effective leaders.

13 In 1972 the Ford Foundation issued a frank and valuable summary, "A Foundation Goes to School." The foundation was a leader in encouraging and supporting reform and experimental efforts but later severely cut educational efforts, presumably because of the unrewarding outcomes.

14 For a number of years I have sought evaluations of results when I have visited or heard about innovative in-school programs, only to find they seldom are made. One difficulty is that standard forms of testing may be unsuitable. Another difficulty in finding information, I believe, is that those in charge of the new programs avoid "making waves" and seek a low profile.

15 Seymour B. Sarason, in *The Culture of the School and the Problem of Change* (Boston: Allyn and Bacon, 1971), has brilliantly explored these difficulties, illuminating the emotional factors involved, but often not given sufficient attention. Some of his readable reports on encounters provide good examples of the effect of threat, as that term is used in Proster Theory. See also the valuable study by Philip J. Runkel et al, *Transforming the School's Capacity for Problem Solving,* (Eugene, Oregon: Center for Educational Policy and Management, College of Education, University of Oregon, 1979).

16 See Leslie A. Hart, "Necessary Ingredients for Retraining Teachers," *Bulletin, National Association of Secondary School Principals,* December 1973, p. 9.

17 Association for Supervision and Curriculum Development 1966 Yearbook, *Learning and Mental Health in the School* (Washington: National Education Association, 1966), p. 77.

18 *The Real World of the Public Schools* (New York: Harcourt Brace Jovanovich, 1972), p. 67.

19 As a considerable straw in the wind, see the October, 1980 issue of *Phi Delta Kappan,* a special one concentrating on reform in teacher education.

20 Norman V. Overly, ed. *Lifetime Learning,* p. 107. ASCD headquarters are in Alexandria, Virginia.

21 Editor's Note: In addition to the many changes internal to the school, a very large factor in predicting success is the district's willingness to allow those involved in the school pilot to "dance to a different drummer," i.e., to allow the school leeway in following the bureaucratic rules and procedures when those rules and procedures contradict elements of brain compatibility.

22 Editor's Note: If these snapshots of the outcomes of brain-compatibility surprise the reader or seem a bit fictitious, please see the following excerpts from the rubrics for assessing implementation of brain-compatible education using the Kovalik ITI model. The "expectations" listed are descriptors of what actually occurs when the implementation of bodybrain-compatible curriculum and instruction are as described. (Of the five stages, only the third stage of each is included in Appendices A and B.)

APPENDICES

APPENDIX A—ITI CLASSROOM STAGES OF IMPLEMENTATION

Assessing Implementation of Brain-Compatible Learning

By Karen D. Olsen and Susan Kovalik

Stage 3

Stage 3 assumes that a brain-compatible learning environment has been established and is consistently nurtured and maintained throughout the day (Stage 1) and that the tools for developing brain-compatible curriculum are consistently and effectively used during the time targeted for ITI curriculum (Stage 2). Stage 3 represents a refinement of implementing a brain-compatible environment and curriculum for students. Targeted time for ITI curriculum increases to approximately 25 percent of the year in Stage 3.

If either Stage 1 or 2 is not fully in place at this time, do not attempt to apply this rubric stage regardless of the amount of teacher-developed curriculum being implemented. It is the quality, not the quantity, of ITI curriculum that is key. The power of the ITI model lies with its brain-compatible underpinnings.

Curriculum

- A yearlong theme, prominently displayed on the wall for both students and teacher, serves as the framework for content development. On average, more than 25 percent of instruction during the school year is based upon bodybrain-compatible curriculum developed for this theme.

- Curriculum content, as expressed in the key points, enhances pattern-seeking, making it easy for students to perceive and under-

Instructional Strategies

- Immersion and hands-on-of-the-real-thing are the primary input used to supplement and extend *being there* experiences.

- All instructional time during the theme and for a growing portion of time during the remainder of the day is based upon the progression of "*being there* > concept > language > application to the real world" rather than the traditional approach of

Expectations

- Students demonstrate LIFESKILLS throughout the day (in and out of the classroom); students are self-directed.

- Students as well as the teacher use the 3Cs of Assessment as a means of assessing learning.

Indicators

- Celebrations of learning and social/political action are key assessment tools for each component; they are designed to allow students to demonstrate

- stand the most important ideas and concepts in the curriculum. Inquiries are designed to help students make connections to the real world, to practice using the concepts and skills of the key points, and to develop mental programs for long-term memory. Inquiries that provide experiences in citizenship, such as social/political action activities and collaborative grouping practices, occur weekly.

- Most of the time, the curriculum includes almost all of the elements that appear as a natural part or extension of the *being there* focus, e.g., science, math technology, history/social studies, and fine arts, as well as arithmetic, reading, writing, and oral expression, including second language acquisition.

- The content of the theme is consistently used as a high interest area for applying the skills/knowledge currently being taught in at least one basic skill area (e.g., math, reading, writing).

- Curriculum for collaborative assignments is specifically designed for group work.

"language > concept application."

- Collaboration is used daily whenever it will enhance pattern seeking and program building.

- Time is allocated in accordance with the nature of the tasks and student and teacher need for adequate time; such time allocations are made in recognition of the need to develop mental programs for using knowledge and skills in real-world contexts.

- Peers and cross-age tutors substantially increase teaching and practice time for students in areas of individual need.

- Students exercise more shared leadership while doing collaborative activities and actively seek connections to and applications in the real world.

- Student absentee rates drop to less than 3 percent; visits to the school nurse due to emotional, upset-based problems drop significantly. Library circulation rates increase by 50 percent.

- Parents report student levels of interest in school and learning as being higher than ever before. Parents' support levels are higher than ever before; volunteerism has doubled.

mastery and application of the key points in the curriculum.

- Selections, for the portfolio folder, of work completed as part of the theme are made primarily by the student.

APPENDIX B—ITI SCHOOLWIDE STAGES OF IMPLEMENTATION*

Planning and Assessing Schoolwide Implementation of Brain-Compatible Education

By Karen Olsen and Susan Kovalik

Stage 3 *School As a Mirror of Real Life*

Stage 3 of the schoolwide ITI implementation rubric assumes that Stage 1 has been fully implemented, and maintained, and significant progress has been made implementing Stage 2. If not, it is inappropriate to apply this stage of the rubric. Elements of a later stage depend upon success in creating a solid foundation during the prior stages.

Learning and Working Environment

Training and Implementing

All staff and involved parents and community understand the new brain research definition of learning as a two-step process: detecting/understanding patterns and acquiring mental programs for using what is understood. Staff have also learned to apply Levels of Use to their work.

Expectations

Staff can and do apply the stages of pattern-seeking and program development to their own learning of the skills and knowledge needed to create a brain-compatible environment. As learners, staff members know what to ask for and when in their learning process, e.g., clarification of a pattern or the relations among patterns, examples of how the skill or knowledge relates to the learner's work, or the need for more practice in applying what is understood in order to complete the mental wiring of mastery for long-term memory. Staff can also apply Levels of Use to their learning processes; content for staff development at the school site is organized by those levels.

Indicators

Staff understand and frequently discuss how the new definition of learning reduces the strain of transitions and applying new work skills—how to do on-going jobs differently (in a manner consistent with the mission of providing a brain-compatible learning and working environment) and acquiring new skills to do newly created jobs. Staff development, in formal and informal settings, is conducted in ways consistent with the new definition of learning; it is appropriate to individual and group needs and is followed by frequent, one-on-one and team coaching.

Training and Implementing	Expectations	Indicators
An understanding of patterns and programs, particularly as they apply to learning new behaviors and trying to modify old ones in real-life settings at home and on the job, is a recurring agenda item for formal and informal discussion.	Knowledge of how to build programs is being applied to the change process at the school. Staff recognize and are learning positive coping strategies to deal with the personal stress caused by the transitions being made.	Staff understand, and can recognize in their own behaviors, the difficulty of extinguishing old programs and how old learnings often interfere with learning new patterns (e.g., creating resistance to new knowledge and its implications for implementation and slipping back into old behaviors, thus forcing new learning to disappear).
Early in this implementation stage, know-ledge of pattern and program is used to adopt/adapt/develop brain-compatible curriculum for the school's first chosen content area of focus.	The curriculum analysis process provides an opportunity to apply, and deepen understanding of, the brain research concepts of patterns and programs and to determine age-appropriateness.	All teachers are using the new curriculum as a basis for creating curriculum in their classrooms on at least a weekly basis and find it a useful (and brain-compatible) beginning point for developing key points and inquiries.
Staff are changing their traditional work assignments in order to create a more viable sense of community for their students. They are experimenting with ways to create a greater sense of school and classroom family by moving to looping and multi-age configurations.	Looping and multi-age assignments are viewed as a way to accelerate academic achievement as well as personal/social growth and citizenship skills, particularly leadership skills for lower and middle achieving students and collaborative skills for all.	All teachers expect to make changes in their working structure within three years. The needed staff development has been analyzed, budgeted for, and scheduled. Student data and teacher input from current looped and multi-aged classrooms are carefully analyzed; recommendations are used to improve implementation.

The role of public education—the creation of responsible citizens and the patterns and programs students must learn to become responsible citizens—has been thoroughly discussed by staff and involved parents and community members in large and small groups.

Training and Implementing

Preparing students for responsible citizenship is progressing along two paths:

• ensuring that classroom studies reach out to locations in the community (for "being there" experiences and for application of social/ political action opportunities) and

• establishing a schoolwide micro-community which mirrors the governance, economic, and social patterns of the community.

Establishing a schoolwide micro-community:

In establishing a schoolwide micro-community, the patterns of local governance structures, such as city council/county board of supervisors, law enforcement (police/sheriff and court system), governmental administration, and regulatory bodies have been accurately replicated in terms of number of mem-

Expectations

Ensuring that classroom studies reach out:

To ensure that classroom studies will reach out to the community in meaningful ways, curriculum planning (at schoolwide and classroom levels) focuses on concepts rather than on factoids. Linear, sequential curriculum has given way to efforts to make clear the attributes of the patterns inherent in the concepts being studied and to provide practice in applying those concepts to real-life situations. Site visitation is a key curriculum development and instructional strategy used by every teacher within at least one curricular area.

Establishing a schoolwide micro-community:

The knowledge and skills needed to operate, and to competently interact with, these entities are integrated into the curriculum of the classroom and school; such skills include the basic skills of listening, speaking, writing, and reading plus the social and

Indicators

Classroom studies reach out:

Students are clear about how what they are learning applies to the real world as a result of their social/political action projects. The school is known for its ability to engage students in their learning. The school's formal assessment tools and procedures include measures that assess development of mental programs for long-term retention of what is being learned.

Establishing a schoolwide micro-community:

Students view their micro-community as their town and themselves as its officers. Their jobs and businesses have personal value to them and are perceived as a means of learning about the real world. They feel confident that they are learning the skills and knowledge they will need to become successful adults

bers, selection processes, duties, responsibilities, powers, etc. Service providers (e.g., environmental protection, health and building code departments, post office, etc.) and businesses are authentically run as well.

situational skills appropriate to the settings. In preparation for each such entity, an experienced member of that entity has provided firsthand information (through "being there" visitations and on-campus presentations by current position-holders) about his/her role and the work of that organization. In the area of commerce, similar training is provided for each classroom business—training by community people who actually operate that kind of business.

and valued citizens. They perceive school as not only connected to real life but as a part of real life. Every classroom has either a governmental function to perform or a business to run. Students fill all roles; adults serve as advisors only.

Time for curriculum and team planning is provided for during the regular school day on a regular basis.

Such time is devoted solely to curriculum planning individually and with team colleagues. Other business is handled at other times.

A minimum of half-a-day every two weeks is provided. Resources, such as curriculum coaching and resource people, are available to make most productive use of time.

Governance

Training and Implementing	Expectations	Indicators
Consistent with the "use it or lose it" principle from brain research for students and the need for staff time for training and planning together, the school calendar has been modified.	The school year is year-round for students with no break longer than four weeks so that students' mental wiring of learning is not lost due to lack of use.	Each break in the school year is used for both staff vacation and for reflection time—analysis of what worked and didn't work, further training, and individual and team planning time.
Staff have become aware that governance within a bureaucracy with its top-down authoritarianism is not congruent with governance in a democratic society. Thus, school governance has changed, becoming a fluid flow of consensus planning and decision-making between the Committee-as-a-whole (all staff and involved parents), the School Improvement Committee, and various short-term work committees.	In big ways and small, staff members are making the transition from a culture of "they said I have to" or "they won't let me" to a workplace culture characterized by personal responsibility for aligning both personal and professional behavior with best knowledge and best practice.	There is a strong sense of individual professionalism and group collegiality and a pervasive sense of "we." People have the authority, group and individual, to change what doesn't work. Decisions within the governance processes and within individual classrooms are made based upon what's best for students according to the brain research concepts used in the ITI Decision-Making Template. Staff model continuous learning and productive citizenship for students and each other. Comments such as the following are common: "Teaching and working here has even changed my personal life." "I've grown, I'm no longer the same person."

The school curriculum leadership team, with involvement and support of the district office staff, has created a process by which all teachers can re-think the curriculum content for their grade level.

Staff use the ITI Decision-Making Template to analyze critical schoolwide and classroom curriculum and instruction policies and practices—those which need to be abandoned in light of best knowledge and best practice and those that need to be added. The template is also used to analyze allocation of resources using a zero-based budgeting perspective in order to focus discussion upon what is truly needed next to continue the journey toward a fully brain-compatible learning environment versus continuing what has been.

The process for adopting/adapting/developing such curriculum is a model for future curricular areas.

Resource acquisition and use have changed to allow for more time for collaborative planning and other resources needed to support implementation of brain-compatible learning. Talents and resources of parents, businesses, and community groups have been identified and are being integrated into the school program (on and off campus). The focus for staffing is on training and supporting regular classroom teachers and current staff to provide a fuller brain-compatible learning environment rather than on adding auxiliary certificated and classified staff, e.g., Chapter 1 specialists, classroom aides, etc.

Staff agree that the process, with the improvements already agreed to, will work for analyzing and adopting/adapting/developing schoolwide curriculum for future areas.

The process of allocating new resources involves all interested staff members and involved parents and includes the use of the ITI Decision-Making Template. All staff development opportunities, including those provided by district office resources, support implementation of brain-compatible education. Educational goals and/or methodologies inconsistent with the agreed upon schoolwide principles of best knowledge and best practice are being eliminated. Resources are aimed at solving underlying problems, not symptoms of problems.

Before beginning Stage 4, the staff, parents, and community members meet to discuss, and celebrate, their progress to date and to formally recommit to becoming a brain-compatible school using best knowledge and best practice. This analysis and recommitment process includes a thorough brain-compatibility audit as well as a review of relevant data about student growth and achievement. The school mission statement is revisited and revised as appropriate as is each individual's personal mission statement; the school's improvement plan is also revised as needed.

Stage 3

Toward a Common Vocabulary

Because education is such an old field of endeavor, most of the terms used within it have become freighted with special and often highly personalized meanings. As the saying goes, there are as many definitions for an educational term as there are people in the room. Thus, one of the earliest and most important tasks of any group is to come to terms with its vocabulary so that members can feel confident that what they said is what gets heard. To assist in the task of common vocabulary-building, important terms from Stage 3 of this rubric are defined here in alphabetical order. Many definitions are accompanied by recommended books for further reading.

Age-appropriateness — widely used with varying meanings, the term age-appropriate here is used to denote an awareness that the human brain develops through stages which have been described by Piaget and others. The ITI model uses the version of stages described by Dr. Larry Lowery, University of California, Berkeley, in *Thinking and Learning: Matching Developmental Stages with Curriculum and Instruction.*

Best knowledge and best practice — a term coined by John Champlin to describe a mindset dedicated to acquiring the best available knowledge about how learning takes place (brain research and its implications for curriculum and instructional practices) and commitment to full and rigorous use of such information in design and execution of curriculum and instructional practice (also implies a commitment to root out all current practice that does not align with best knowledge)

Brain-Compatibility Audit — an analysis, conducted annually, of the curriculum, instructional strategies, and administrative policies and procedures of the school using the ITI Decision-Making Template. The purpose of the audit is to determine what elements of the current program are inconsistent with the school's written statement of best knowledge and best practice in order to identify what resource allocations (time, effort, money) should be eliminated or altered thus creating time and money for implementing the school's improvement plan.

Brain-compatible curriculum — brain-compatible curriculum is conceptually-based curriculum that identifies important concepts to be learned, as distinguished from lists of "The student will...." or lists of factoids. It is curriculum that is consistent with learning as a two-step process (patterns and programs) and has been agreed to schoolwide through a thoughtful and thorough adoption/adaptation/development process. All teachers have been involved in the process to varying degrees. The final vote is as a Committee-as-a-whole. For an example of brain-compatible curriculum for teachers to use in developing curriculum for their classroom, see *A Continuum of Science Concepts*.

Bureaucracy — the nature of bureaucracy—its affect on people, policy-making, and faceless lack of personal responsibility—is chillingly described by Dr. Michael Katz, historian, in *Class, Bureaucracy, and the Schools*. His is a must-read historical account of the roots of our public schools, inextricably enmeshed in bureaucracy. The effects of bureaucracy on people's behavior is profound and rarely positive or even neutral. To succeed at significant school improvement efforts, staff and parents must be alert to the impact of bureaucracy, mindful of its massive inertia, and alert to its antipathy toward excellence.

Chosen content area of focus — in an ideal environment for ITI teachers, the school/district would be able to provide a single, comprehensive, integrated statement of concepts to be learned that would include all of the areas of traditional curriculum. Until then, development of conceptual curriculum will likely proceed by re-thinking and improving curriculum one traditional area at a time. As these unfold, teachers can then select from them to integrate curriculum and skills at the classroom level.

Citizenship — the ultimate goal of the ITI model, to produce adults who are ready (skill and knowledge) and willing (have a sense of commitment to the success of the community not just their own) to undertake their responsibilities to nurture and support our democratic way of government and life. Citizenship to maintain and nurture our democratic society should be the core goal of education. For an excellent discussion of citizenship as the goal of education, see Carl Glickman's *Renewing America's Schools: A Guide for School-Based Action.* (*Renewing America's Schools: A Guide to School-Based Action*, pp. 155-156).

Congeniality versus Collegiality — a distinction drawn by Carl Glickman in *Renewing America's Schools: A Guide for School-Based Action*. According to Glickman, "congenial schools are characterized by an open, social climate for adults. Communications are friendly, [people] socialize easily with one another. Faculty meetings are pleasant, holiday parties are great, refreshments at meetings are plentiful, and faculty members spend time together away from school. Members describe their school as a nice place where everyone gets along well. Collegial schools are characterized by purposeful, adult-level interactions focused on the teaching and learning of students.

People do not necessarily socialize with one another but they respect their differences of opinion about education. Mutual respect comes from the belief that everyone has the students' interest in mind. The result of such respect is seen in school meetings, where the school community members debate, disagree, and argue before educational decisions are made. Even in the hottest of debates, people's professional responses for others supersedes personal discomfort. People believe that differences will be resolved and that students will benefit. Social satisfaction is a by-product of professional engagement and resolution, of seeing how students benefit, and of the personal regard in which adults hold one another. They become colleagues in the deep sense of being able to work and play together, and each side of the relationship strengthens the other. Being collegial means being willing to move beyond the social facade of communication, to discuss conflicting ideas and issues with candor, sensitivity, and respect. For many schools, the first job is to move from being conventional to being congenial, but the big job for public education is to become collegial, so that social satisfaction is derived mainly from the benefits derived from efforts on behalf of students." (*Renewing America's Schools: A Guide to School-Based Action*, pp. 22).

Curriculum Leadership Team — the Curriculum Leadership Team is as much a process as a group of people. Its purpose is to ensure that the vote of the Committee-as-a-whole is an informed vote by each person. This is critically important because few issues affect a teacher in the classroom more intimately or more fundamentally than the selection of what students are to learn.

Factoids — a term to describe curriculum content that is loaded with facts rather than concepts, facts to be memorized and repeated back for a test which do not allow for transfer to other learning or empower students when faced with real-life situations. The fundamental deficiency of factoid-based curriculum is that it is extremely difficult to learn because facts have few attributes that the brain's pattern-seeking process can use. This is especially devastating if the area is unfamiliar to a student and he/she has no prior information to call up in order to give the factoid some context.

ITI Decision-Making Template — a process and format to assist in analyzing program operations and resource allocations to determine if they are consistent with the goals of providing a brain-compatible learning experience for students (and adults). For more information, see Appendix A.

Key points and inquiries — two key ITI structures for developing curriculum at the classroom level. Key points state what students are expected to understand. Inquiries provide opportunities for students to practice what they understand in real-life settings in order to solve real-life problems and/or create real products. For more information, see the ITI book(s) relevant to your grade levels: *ITI: The Model* or *Kid's Eye View of Science* (for elementary grades), *The Way We Were . . . The Way We CAN Be: A Vision for the Middle School* (for middle school grades) or *Synergy: Transformation of America's High Schools* (for high school).

Levels of Use — the levels of use, developed by Gene Hall and Susan Loucks at the University of Texas in the 1970s, describe the process of implementing a particular skill. The seven steps provide a predictable roadmap and thus remind us that we are on a common journey rather than an individual nightmare. The levels are: Non-use, orientation, preparation, mechanical use, routine use, refinement, and renewal. For a useful description of how these levels apply to the design and implementation of staff development, see *Mentor Teacher Role: Owners' Manual*, Chapter 4, pages.

Linear, sequential curriculum — the format for most traditional curriculum, based on the belief that the brain, like a computer, learns in a sequential, linear manner. Now understood to be more brain-antagonistic than brain-compatible. According to Leslie Hart in *Human Brain and Human Learning*, "Perhaps there is no idea about human learning harder to accept for people familiar with classroom schools than this: that the ideal of neat, orderly, closely-planned, sequentially logical teaching will, in practice with young students, guarantee severe learning failure for most." Why? Because one person's sense of sequential logic differs from another and the "pattern" of what defines the sequence is not understood until after a great deal is understood about the topic. Thus, linear, sequential curriculum is meaningful for the expert (and the teacher), but not for the beginner. See discussion about brain-compatible curriculum, page S3-8.

Looping — a student assignment structure in which the teacher moves with his/her students to the next grade level(s). The purpose of looping is to enhance the sense of family/community and to improve student achievement

Mission — a written statement of what the school community intends to have happen for students. It emerges from the written statement of best knowledge and best practice that the school has committed itself to and directly addresses the real work of the school, not platitudes. It is updated yearly to ensure it remains a working document that guides people's on-going planning and discussion.

Multi-age grouping — a student assignment structure which includes heterogeneous, multi-aged students (preferably three years or more) in a classroom taught by the same teacher throughout the years of the age span. The purpose of multi-age grouping is to enhance the sense of family/community and to improve student achievement.

New definition of learning — The new definition of learning used in the ITI model is based on brain research over the past 20 years. Leslie Hart articulated it as a two-step process. Step one: extraction from confusion of meaningful patterns by first recognizing and then understanding the pattern and its attributes. Step two: the acquisition of useful programs for using what is understood, first at an unskilled level using short-term memory and then moving to expert application wired into long-term memory. Other students of brain research such as Carl Perkins use different vocabulary but point to the same functional processes.

Patterns and programs — two of the six concepts from brain research that form the basis of the ITI model. Taken from Leslie Hart's work, *Human Brain and Human Learning*, these two are especially important for curriculum development, both when creating conceptual curriculum at the schoolwide level and when developing key points and inquiries at the classroom level. Patterns and programs are the basis of the two-part definition of learning used by the ITI model. (See *New Definition of Learning*.)

School calendar — the current school calendar is a creation of our agrarian society more than 100 years ago in which all hands, young and old, turned out to harvest and make the necessary preparations for surviving through the next winter. Child labor laws make this calendar obsolete. Brain research informs us that one of the basic principles of the biology of learning is "use it or lose it," i.e., neural networks required for mental programs just being established will disappear during long periods of non-use, a waste of time and energy of both student and teacher. Thus, the traditional long summer break "undoes" much learning in progress, especially by lower achieving students as seen when comparing fall and spring testing over the years. An all too familiar pattern is that students' test results in the fall are significantly lower than their results from the prior spring. Even worse are the statistics about victimization, which increases during long periods of minimal supervision by families in which both parents work, and the growth in gang activity by youth who grow bored and vulnerable during long periods of unstructured time. Further, conversations with teachers mid-year too often reflect exhaustion, lack of time to reflect on and learn from prior successes and failures, and a general sense of being overwhelmed combined with a "can't wait until the end of the year" attitude. Year-round schools are needed, not to make maximal use of facilities, but to make maximal growth in learning.

Schoolwide micro-community — the micro-community is a multi-faceted structure of the ITI model for pulling together a number of goals: daily experiences in citizenship, meaningful applications of basic skills on a daily basis, exploration of personal aptitudes and interests, creating and nurturing a sense of community schoolwide, and opportunities to learn about the world of commerce and develop personal finance skills.

Site visitations — more than a field trip site, site visitations or "study trips" to "being there" locations are the heart of the ITI model's curriculum development and integration processes; they are also instructional strategies to maximize sensory input from the 19 senses.

Social and situational skills — development of social skills in the ITI model occur through daily application of the Lifelong Guidelines and LIFESKILLS (the definition of personal best). Learning situational skills occurs through the rich variety of experiences posed through the micro-community and "being there" experiences.

Social/political action projects — an integral and key part of the ITI model, social/political action projects are an important means for structuring outreach into the community, for providing students a vehicle for applying what they learn to real world problems, and providing opportunities to practice citizenship related to issues students care about. As the name implies, the projects can be social, such as assisting at a food bank or a home for the elderly or creating a community garden, or they can be political, such as a lobbying effort to obtain a traffic light at the corner near the school, drawing attention to the plight of ocean mammals, etc. In all cases, such projects are a natural extension of what the students are currently studying and often are the culminating project. Typically, there is at least one project for each monthly component. Projects can be for the class as a whole, for a learning club, or individual. For more information, see the ITI book appropriate for your grade level(s).

Transitions — William Bridges, in his book *Transitions: Making the Most of Change*, makes an important distinction between change and transitions. According to Bridges, "It isn't the changes that do you in, it's the transitions." Change, he says, is situational (e.g., a new principal or school board, shifting to a different grade level, converting from textbooks to integrating curriculum based on physical locations, etc.). On the other hand, transition is "the psychological process people go through to come to terms with the new situation." "Change is external; transition is internal."

Zero-based budget perspective — zero-based budgeting is a mindset and discussion process that assumes nothing, starts every budget category with zero dollars and asks the question, "What is most needed to take the next step toward full brain-compatibility?" With this mind-set, what has been—successes as well as non-results—must be put aside. For example, if little or no growth in student achievement and growth toward citizenship has occurred over the past two years, major re-budgeting is needed. Expenditures for categories such as classroom aides or any other category that could be classified as "business as usual" must be abandoned in order to free up monies for implementation strategies that will improve achievement and citizenship. Look for expenditures that have had negligible or even negative impact on implementing a brain-compatible environment. Be honest with yourselves and each other. Don't expect this process to be comfortable. If improving education were easy, we would already have done it!

Most recommended books are available from Books For Educators, Inc.
Toll Free 1-888-777-9827   Fax 253/630-7215   www.books4educ.com

APPENDIX C—RESOURCES

One of the most comprehensive models for translating brain research into action—taking into account the full spectrum of classroom and school life—is the ITI model created by Susan Kovalik & Associates. Curriculum and instruction are changed in light of five ITI Learning Principles from brain research:

- *Intelligence* as a function of experience
- Learning is an inseparable partnership between *brain* and *body*
  - Emotions is the gatekeeper to learning and performance
  - Movement enhances learning
- There are *multiple intelligences* or ways for solving problems and producing products
- Learning is a *two-step process:*
  - Step one: Making meaning through pattern seeking
  - Step two: Developing a mental program for using what we understand and wiring itinto long-term memory
- *Personality* impacts learning and performance

Listed below are but a few of the books, videos, and other materials available. The first four books provide an overview of the above concepts from brain research and practical, step-by-step instructions for creating a bodybrain-compatible learning environment and integrating all basic skills and content areas. They provide lots of examples and tips.

BOOKS—

Exceeding Expectations: User's Guide to Implementing Brain Research in the Classroom
by Susan Kovalik with Karen D. Olsen

Transformations: Leadership For Brain-Compatible Learning
Contributing Editor Jane Rasp McGeehan

What's Worth Teaching? Selecting, Organizing, and Integrating Knowledge by Marion Brady

ITI Classroom Stages of Implementation by Susan Kovalik and Karen D. Olsen

ITI Schoolwide Stages of Implementation by Susan Kovalik and Karen D. Olsen
Science Continuum of Concepts, K-6 by Karen D. Olsen

Anchor Math: The Brain-Compatible Approach to Learning by Leslie A. Hart

VIDEOS—

Getting Started Video Set:
Stage 1 of the ITI Rubric: First Things First
LIFESKILLS: Creating a Class Family
by Susan Kovalik & Associates, Inc.

Stage 2 of the ITI Rubric: Intelligence Is a Function of Experience by Susan Kovalik & Associates, Inc. (video)

Stage 3 of the ITI Rubric: Creating Conceptual Curriculum by Susan Kovalik & Associates, Inc. (video)

I Can Divide and Conquer: A Concept-in-a-Day
by Martha Miller-Kaufeldt (video)

Classroom of the 21st Century
by Robert Ellingson (video & handbook)

Jacobsonville: A ITI Micro Society
by Susan Kovalik & Associates, Inc.

These materials are available from Books For Educators, Inc.
Call toll free 1-888-777-9827 for a free catalog
Fax 253/630-7215 www.books4educ.com

For more information about the Kovalik ITI model and trainings, contact:
Susan Kovalik & Associates, Inc.
17051 SE 272nd St., Suite 17•Covington, WA 98042
Phone: 253/631-4400 Fax: 253/631-7500
E-mail: skovalik@oz.net   www.kovalik.com

GLOSSARY

These entries are offered to assist readers in quick review of terms used. Since the language is compressed, it is suggested that the more explicit main text be used for any quotations or references. Items that strongly express a Proster Theory viewpoint are marked by asterisk.

*ABORT. A program that is interrupted or fails to achieve the intended goal is said to abort.

ACTIVITY. In a schooling situation, what a learner, or teacher, actually does.

ADDRESS. Where information stored can be reached for recall. In a file drawer,the label on the folder; in a computer, the coded location; in the brain, relevant uses. See MEMORY.

AGGRESSIVE TEACHING. Instruction that a teacher decides to give unilaterally, without learner request or evidence of desire or interest.

AMBIANCE. Atmosphere prevailing in the immediate environment.

ANALOG. An approximate representation, in contrast to DIGITAL. A clock with hands is an analog device.

BEHAVIORISM. General term for the psychology dominant in the United States through most of the 20th century, heavily using such terms as *stimulus response, reward, reinforcement, motivation, mediation,* etc.

*BIASES. The upper and lower settings for HOMEOSTASIS; also all the factors affecting choice of PROGRAM in a PROSTER.

BODYBRAIN PARTNERSHIP. Coining the term "bodybrain partnership" attempts to capture or represent several key concepts from the new brain biology. First, there is no hyphen in bodybrain, just as there is no way to separate the functions of the two as generator and receptor of the dozens of information substances. Second, both are physical entities, not conceptual models such as "mind." Both can be studied concretely, scientifically, to the cellular and molecular levels. Third, both come to school and sit before us; we must learn to deal with them as they are, not as may be convenient for the system. Fourth, connection is too passive a term. Survival—for which learning is the first line of offense and defense—requires a proactive, committed collaboration of body and brain—a true "body-brain partnership."

BRAIN. The main, central mass of the nervous system housed in the skull, comprising 95 percent or more of the entire human NERVOUS SYSTEM.

BRAIN BASED. Utilizing scientific knowledge of the brain, especially the human brain.

BRAIN BIOLOGY. A term used to denote the research into learning linked to actual physiological changes and processes in the brain.

*BRAIN-COMPATIBLE. Fitting well with the nature or shape of the human brain as currently understood; in contrast to brain-antagonistic.

BRAIN STEM. Those parts of the brain rising from the spinal cord, from and around which more complex portions developed during evolution.

*CATEGORIZING DOWN. The process of making finer and finer classifications, as: vehicle, car, sedan, Plymouth, Horizon, 1982 liftback model, etc.

CEREBELLUM. The "little brain" near the back of the neck, long-known to be concerned with coordinating muscular activity and recently believed to play an important role in learning.

CEREBRUM. The new mammalian brain, composed of two largely mirror-image hemispheres, in humans about 5/6 of the entire brain. See TRIUNE BRAIN.

CLASSROOM. An organizational device by which a group of students, often 20-35, are confined in one room with one teacher over long periods of sessions, frequently a school year. If graded, as is conventionally the case, the students are purported to be sufficiently alike to benefit by grouping in a grade, in spite of massive evidence to the contrary.

*CLUE. An attribute used by the brain in pattern recognition. See PROBABILITY.

CONCEPT. A general term for any consistent portion of an individual's progress in "making sense of the world"; a working hypothesis.

CONSCIOUS. Brain activity of which a person is aware is said to be conscious, as opposed to SUBCONSCIOUS activity going on at many levels. Awareness may be compared to a spotlight which illuminates one area after another. The brain is not sharply divided into a conscious portion and an unconscious or subconscious portion.

CORPUS CALLOSUM. Large bundle of nerve fibers forming a two-way bridge between the left and right cerebral HEMISPHERES.

CORTEX. The "bark" or outside layers of brain lobes; the gray matter of the brain in which THINKING proceeds. The CEREBRAL CORTEX, around the two hemispheres, is a multi-layered sheet in which each area has a dominant function, and represents the main power of the brain. It can be estimated to contain 25 billion NEURONS.

*DIGITAL. Expressed in units or numbers, and in that sense precise rather than approximation or analog. The brain is very strongly analog and typically handles digital material poorly and reluctantly. See ANALOG.

*DOWNSHIFTING. A shift in control of an individual's activities from a higher (newer) brain to a lower (older) brain. See TRIUNE BRAIN. Particularly, inhibition of use of the new mammalian brain under THREAT, interfering with learning or use of what has been learned and stored there. (See also EMOTIONAL OVERRIDE.)

*EMOTION. A shift in BIASES, changing the range of HOMOSTASIS, to adjust to a different perceived situation, AMBIANCE, or THREAT.

EMOTIONAL OVERRIDE. Replaces the term, "downshifting," and refers to an intensity of emotion which "preoccupies" the brain, thus reducing functioning of the cerebral cortex.

ETHOLOGY. The study of creatures in more or less their natural environments, rather than in laboratories, with emphasis on SPECIES WISDOM.

EVOLUTION. Development and/or changes in genetic programs, resulting in changes in the structure and behavior of creatures, usually over periods of many thousands or millions of years.

Evolution produces individual differences which may permit species to survive environmental changes.

*FEEDBACK. The return of information or report to the brain on how well a PROGRAM is working to achieve its GOAL. In opening a door, for example, feedback may indicate that the pushing effort is greater than needed, or not enough.

FEEDFORWARD. Information projected within a system as an estimate of what may be needed.

FORMAL OPERATIONS. Broadly, effort to use LOGIC. Within Proster Theory, not regarded as the highest form of mental activity, nor as generally useful.

FRONTAL LOBES. Portions of the CEREBRUM close to the forehead. (**PREFRONTAL**, most anterior.) Human frontal portions are exceptionally well developed and important in directing the brain as a whole and in longer-term planning. MYELINATION is completed very late.

*GOAL. The aim, objective, or purpose of a PROGRAM. In general, the program goal is clearly determined before the brain institutes the program. Achievement toward the goal is pleasurable as the program proceeds and contributes to confidence; ABORTION of a program short of goal produces alarm or other EMOTION and likely DOWNSHIFTING/EMOTIONAL OVERRIDE.

*GRAND IDEAS. CONCEPTS of importance which have value in several or many areas of application; unifying ideas. The fractionating effect of courses may inhibit formation of grand ideas.

HEMISPHERES. The left and right portions of the CEREBRUM, roughly mirror-images. The left in most people handles language, the right spatial, nonverbal matters; but the division of functions is highly individual and complex, and the CORPUS CALLOSUM provides pathways for massive exchanges. (Discussion of hemispheric functions in recent years has tended to be simplistic, overstated, inaccurate, and conjectural to a misleading degree.)

HOLISTIC. Taking a large, overall view, rather than attending to details or only certain aspects. Hence MACRO.

HOMEOSTASIS. The balancing of interacting body systems within limits set by current BIASING, to produce a relatively steady state suited to the current situation of the person.

HORMONE. A "chemical messenger" carried by the bloodstream to various organs and controls, in a slower and more diffuse way than messages via the nervous system. Some hormones may alter BIASES within a second or less, others may have effect over years, as for body growth.

HUMAN. A member of the species HOMO SAPIENS, the only surviving species. Other species of humans existed perhaps as recently as some tens of thousands of years ago. One definition of human involves: (1) standing erect, (2) living in social groups, (3) using language, (4) using tools.

INFORMATION. The content of any form of message, or PROGRAM, or stored program (without regard to right or wrong.)

INFORMATION SUBSTANCES. The basic units of a language used by cells throughout the organism to communicate across systems such as the endocrine, the neurological, the gastrointestinal, and the immune.

*INPUT. The total INFORMATION offered to the brain in a given situation; the raw material from which individual brains extract PATTERNS, without regard to quality. An individual human brain selects what input it will receive, moment to moment, and determines how far it will process it. Settings can vary enormously in the level of input they offer, and instructors can provide more or less; but each individual learner controls how much and what input will be admitted to that brain and how it will be processed. To best facilitate learning, input should be varied, in part repetitive, presented randomly, and in great volume. High input does not automatically produce learning, but low or restricted input tends to prevent learning.

*KNOWLEDGE. See INFORMATION. Knowledge almost always takes the form of stored programs or pattern recognition.

KNOWLEDGE STRUCTURE. A hierarchy of levels, from common knowledge to higher and higher specific, detailed, technical, broad and theoretical, professional levels.

*LEARNING. A two-step process:
- The extraction from confusion of meaningful PATTERNS (which can subsequently often be recognized by MATCH) **AND**
- The acquisition of useful PROGRAMS (useful from the view of the individual learner).

LIGAND. Is the term used for any natural or manmade substance that binds selectively to it's own specific receptor on the surface of a cell. Comes from the Latin ligare, "that which binds," sharing its origin with re*lig*ion. Used here it refers specifically to three kinds of molecules known as "information substances."

Included are the neurotransmitters found at the synaptic gap, steroids, and peptides.

LIMBIC SYSTEM. A complex group of brain structures more or less below the cerebrum, largely concerned with what are commonly called emotional matters. The term may be equated with OLD MAMMALIAN BRAIN for most purposes. Portions are involved in ROTE learning.

LINEAR. Arranged in a line, or simple sequence; single path as opposed to MULTIPATH.

*LOGIC. Broadly, unnatural, contrived style of reasoning. Logical is commonly used to imply orderly, neat, arranged in some scheme, in contrast with HOLISTIC, intuitive, RANDOM, recursive. Logic is often assumed to mean Greek-type, LINEAR progression from point A to point B to point C to compose a logical chain, or "sound thinking" as popularly understood and traditionally admired in spite of its general uselessness and tendency to lead to simple wrong answers. Many modern logics, complex and not linear, have highly useful special applications. See MULTI-CHANNEL, SYSTEM.

MACRO. A large, HOLISTIC approach, as opposed to MICRO concentration on parts or details.

MANIPULATION. Literally, handling physical objects or materials, in contrast to using words or representations. Manipulation can greatly aid learning in many situations, especially for younger learners.

MASTERY. The concept of allowing as much time as necessary for an individual to learn thoroughly, in contrast to giving a score or grade for learning achieved in a fixed period of time, such as a semester. An implication is that every student is capable of learning, given time.

MATCH. A sufficiently good fit between incoming input and some stored pattern permit probably correct recognition or identification. Many CLUES would be those expected, with absence of strong negative clues. For example, four legs, fur, tail, visible ears would match dog; horns or wrong size would be negative clues, preventing that match. See PROBABILITY.

*MEMORY. A convenience term; the brain has no separate part or place for memory, which appears to be stored at many points in the brain and body. Within Proster Theory, memory is seen as one tense of PROGRAM: a program used in the past is seen as memory, the same program to be used in the future is seen as plan. To recall "how much is 6 times 7" the program for answering that question is located and actuated.

MIND. A vague term, used as a convenience.

MODEL. A hypothetical concept of how the parts of some entity or pattern are interrelated; its "shape."

MOLECULES OF EMOTION. Term coined by Candace Pert to encompass the "information substances" that are the chemical basis of emotion.

MULTICHANNEL, MULTIPATH. In contrast to LINEAR, moving along many pathways rather than one, usually simultaneously. The channels or pathways may be discrete, extending in many directions, or they can be parallel, or they can form a network. FEEDBACK and FEEDFORWARD may be involved. The brain is characteristically designed for multichannel processing. This gives the brain huge advantages over digital electronic computers, which thus far tend to be linear.

MULTIMODAL. Utilizing more than one mode, such as sight, hearing, touch, motion, song or music, etc. Multimodal INPUT appears to greatly accelerate learning.

MYELINATION. The process by which nerves are insulated by acquiring a coating, wrapped around by special cells. The pathway then carries messages faster and with less loss. Myelination continues to about age 20, with timing and sequence highly variable by individual. The apparent maturity of a child's behavior may relate to the progress of myelination.

NERVE. General term for specialized fibers that carry electro-chemical messages.

NERVOUS SYSTEM. The extremely elaborate, complex system by which external or internal information is brought to the main part of the system, the BRAIN, where some input may be analyzed and interpreted in the light of experience. The brain makes decisions on action and on regulating the many body systems, such as those for breathing, pumping blood, digestion, etc. The brain sends out instructions to muscles and organs, and controls, along with INFORMATION SUBSTANCES, all emotions as commonly called. (See EMOTION.) An autonomous system, not under the brain's control, was long thought to exist, but this concept has been dropped. (See literature on "bio-feedback.")

NEURON. The specialized cell of the NERVOUS SYSTEM, which has 30 billion or more. There are a number of categories of neurons, with different shapes and functions. Essentially neurons are sophisticated switches, in a sense equivalent to diodes and transistors in electronic computers, but much more complex and subtle. A newborn child has at birth or shortly after almost a lifetime supply of neurons, few of which get replaced as they die. The long human growth period is necessary to allow time for organization of neuronal structures.

NEUROSCIENCES. Those that are concerned with physical, direct study of the brain, in contrast to psychiatry and psychologies which stay outside the skull.

NEW MAMMALIAN BRAIN. In MacLean's scheme of the TRIUNE BRAIN, the CEREBRUM, in evolutionary terms the newest, and by far the largest, brain. Language and use of symbols are functions of this brain, to which the great bulk of formal education is addressed.

NOISE. In communication theory, unintended signals that do not carry meaning, such as interference on radio or television.

OLD MAMMALIAN BRAIN. In MacLean's scheme of the TRIUNE BRAIN, the middle brain in point of age and size; roughly the LIMBIC SYSTEM.

*PATTERN. An entity, such as an object, action, procedure, situation, relationship or SYSTEM, which may be recognized by substantial consistency in the CLUES it presents to a brain, which is a pattern-detecting apparatus. The more powerful a brain, the more complex, finer, and subtle patterns it can detect. Except for certain SPECIES WISDOM patterns, each human must learn to recognize the patterns of all matters dealt with, storing the LEARNING in the brain. See process of LEARNING. Pattern recognition tells what is being dealt with, permitting selection of the most appropriate PROGRAM in brain storage to deal with it. The brain tolerates much variation in patterns (we recognize the letter a in many shapes, sizes, colors, etc.) because it operates on the basis of PROBABILITY, not on DIGITAL or LOGIC principles. Recognition of PATTERNS accounts largely for what is called insight, and facilitates transfer of learning to new situations or needs, which may be called creativity.

PEPTIDE. Any of various natural or synthetic compounds containing two or more amino acids linked by the carboxyl group of one amino acid and the amino group of another. By definition, polypeptides are the larger peptides, usually those with in excess of 100 amino acids. But they are smaller than the proteins, which may have 200 or more amino acids as well as other attached molecules, such as sugars or lipids.

*PROBABILITY. The principle by which the brain recognizes PATTERNS on the basis of receiving a number of CLUES which combine to suggest a probable conclusion. The assortment of clues may vary at any given time. This permits the brain to recognize as "chair" furniture of widely varying design, or to detect the word, "water," spoken in many different ways, or to recognize a friend despite different clothing, hair style, change in weight, etc. The human brain *naturally* uses this principle.

*PROGRAM. A sequence of steps or actions, intended to achieve some GOAL, which once built is stored in the brain and "run off" repeatedly whenever need to achieve the same goal is perceived by the person. A program may be short, for example giving a nod to indicate "yes," or long, as in playing a piece on the piano which requires thousands of steps, or raising a crop of wheat over many months. A long program usually involves a series of shorter subprograms, and many parallel variations that permit choice to meet conditions of use. Many such programs are needed, for instance to open different kinds of doors by pushing, pulling, turning, actuating, etc. Language requires many thousands of programs, to utter each word, type it, write it in longhand, print it, etc. Frequently used programs acquire an "automatic" quality: they can be used, once selected, without thinking, as when one puts on a shirt. Typically, a program is CONSCIOUSLY selected, then run off at a subconscious level. See LEARNING, PATTERN, PROSTER, ABORT. In general, humans operate by selecting and implementing programs one after another throughout waking hours.

PROSTER. A diagrammatic concept, based on the physical arrangement of cortical brain cells, which suggests how PROGRAMS may be stored in the brain as if they were grouped as alternatives for achieving some broad GOAL. For example, a locomotion proster provides alternatives such as walking, running, going up stairs or down, etc. An arithmetic proster provides programs for addition, subtraction, multiplying, etc. Successful selection of a program from a proster first requires recognition of the PATTERN to be dealt with. Only one program from a proster can be used at a time, and selection can only be from those already stored and available. BIASING of the switches in a proster leads to choice of what the brain considers the most appropriate program; unless the biases change, the same program will be selected again. The term proster derives from program structure. The concept seeks to clarify many aspects of human behavior and learning.

*RANDOM. In chance or jumbled order, as opposed to some logical approach or a conventional sequence. The sounds of letters of the alphabet can be taught in sequence A, B, C, D, or in random order such as M, O, W, R. Since life presents input in random order, the brain prefers random to alternatives.

*REAL. As found in life, in contrast to what has been prepared, ordered, analyzed, simplified, or fragmented in conventional formal education. Real objects, situations, etc., usually involve complexities and present more INPUT.

REINFORCEMENT. A key concept of BEHAVIORISM which holds that a behavior that is rewarded will more likely be repeated more often. Contrary evidence is now strong; reward is difficult to define, especially for humans. Proster Theory emphasizes that a GOAL is always evident before the program is implemented, so the idea of reward appears unnecessary and artificial in real life.

REPTILIAN BRAIN. In MacLean's scheme of TRIUNE BRAIN, the oldest and smallest brain, concerned with operating many systems of the body essential to life, some crude "fight or flee" emotions, and probably with genetically transmitted schemata. See SPECIES WISDOM.

RETINA. The inner lining of the eye, on which light falls to begin the nervous system processes of vision.

RIGHT ANSWER. An official or approved answer to a question, examination item, or problem, etc., often viewed as the only acceptable answer. The assumption is made that one, simple, right answer does in fact exist.

*RISK. The need felt by humans, because of their evolution, to take chances and compete, in activities such as travel, skiing, games, gambling, and many others. Risk, in contrast to THREAT, is taken voluntarily by the individual, by intent, to a selected degree. Risk shifts BIASES to settings for more alertness, faster consumption of energy, etc.

RITUAL. A program, or group of programs, conducted as conventional behavior, without regard to how well stated GOALS are achieved. Example: a rain dance. How well, long, or elaborately the ritual is performed has no bearing on the outcome avowedly intended.

SCHEMA, SCHEMATA (plural) A term used for PROGRAMS which are not learned after birth but are genetically transmitted. *Example:* a bird "knows" how to build a nest. In humans schemata may be vague, to be refined by the culture. Some, such as sucking at the breast and taking interest in human faces, have great importance for the neonate's survival. See SPECIES WISDOM.

*SETTING. For each individual those aspects, more than transient, of an environment that have direct, continuing effect or influence.

*SMORGASBORD. By analogy with elaborate buffet, the principle of offering learners a wide, appealing choice of INPUT or ACTIVITIES.

SPECIES WISDOM. PROGRAMS or SCHEMATA transmitted with the genes from parents to offspring. Recognition of certain PATTERNS is included. Contrasts with learning after birth. (Relates to instincts, a term rarely used scientifically today.) The importance of species wisdom in humans has been little investigated, but may be profound. Most is probably stored in the REPTILIAN or oldest brain. See TRIUNE BRAIN.

*STIMULUS. An old and perhaps obsolete behaviorist psychology term, very difficult to define. The brain chooses whether or not, and how much, it will respond to a stimulus, which makes the term questionable.

SYNAPSE. The connection between one NEURON and another; actually a tiny gap across which neurotransmitters act. Since a single neuron may connect with 10,000 or more others, synapses in a human brain run into vast numbers.

SYSTEM. An arrangement of components or subsystems in which there is interaction in various directions. Any living creature is a system; so is any social entity. Characteristically a system has no starting point and cannot be dealt with by LINEAR LOGIC. Systems are inherently complex; the human brain is by far the most intricate.

*TEACH. In practice, the term has two meanings: (1) to carry on a RITUAL called teaching which may have little, no, or negative effect on student learning; (2) to carry on BRAIN-COMPATIBLE activities which directly or indirectly (via SETTING and INPUT arranged)

*TEST. In schools, typically use of some instrument of evaluation which directs students to give RIGHT ANSWERS to selected questions. A test rarely evaluates what 8 student can do or does when undirected.

*THINKING. Switching processes in the brain to make SYSTEMS decisions. The brain does not use LOGICAL or LINEAR thinking except under duress to do so.

*THREAT. The imminent prospect of harm, in the view of the individual. The degree of harm perceived may range from minor to loss of life, and DOWNSHIFTING produced will relate to the seriousness and imminence.

*TRIUNE BRAIN. A concept of brain architecture based on evolutionary knowledge, propounded notably by Paul D. MacLean of the National Institute of Mental Health. It views the human brain (excluding the CEREBELLUM) as composed of a very old REPTILIAN BRAIN, around and above which is a larger, more recent old mammalian brain (LIMBIC SYSTEM), around and above which in turn is the massive new mammalian brain (CEREBRUM, HEMISPHERES), the newest brain. This approach is highly useful for gaining more insight into behavior and learning, and why findings derived from work with small laboratory animals which lack the giant human cerebrum can be seriously misleading. See DOWNSHIFTING.

BIBLIOGRAPHY

ABC News *Prime Time,* "Your Child's Brain" with Diane Sawyer, January 25, 1995.

Begley, Sharon. "How to Build a Baby's Brain," *Newsweek, Special Edition, Your Child,* Spring/Summer, 1997.

Begley, Sharon. "Your Child's Brain," *Newsweek,* February 19, 1996.

Bell, Nanci. *Visualizing and Verbalizing for Improved Language Comprehension and Thinking.* Paso Robles, California: Academy of Reading Publications, 1991. Revised edition.

Bergland, Richard. *The Fabric of Mind.* Australia: Penguin Books, 1988.

Caine, Renata and Geoffrey. *Making Connections: Teaching and the Human Brain.* Menlo Park, California: Innovative Learning Publications, 1994.

Calvin, William. *How Brains Think: Evolving Intelligence, Then and Now.* New York: Basic Books, 1996.

Calvin, William H. *"The Mind's Big Bang and Mirroring,"* unpublished manuscript. Seattle, WA: University of Washington, 2000.

Childre, Doc and Martin, Howard with Beech, Donna. *The HeartMath Solution.* San Francisco: Harper, 2000.

Damasio, Antonio. *Descartes' Error: Emotion, Reason, and the Human Brain.* New York: G. P. Putnam Sons, 1994.

Damasio, Antonio. "Thinking About Emotion," presentation at Emotional Intelligence, Education, and the Brain: A Symposium, Chicago, Illinois, December 5, 1997.

Dehaene, Stanislas. *The Number Sense: How the Mind Creates Mathematics.* New York: Oxford University Press, 1997.

Diamond, Marian and Hopson, Janet. *Magic Trees of the Mind: How to Nurture Your Child's Intelligence, Creativity, and Healthy Emotions from Birth Through Adolescence.* New York: A Dutton Book, 1998.

Gardner, Howard. *Frames of Mind: Theory of Multiple Intelligences.* New York: Basic Books, 1985.

Gardner, Howard. *The Unschooled Mind: How Children Think and How Schools Should Teach.* New York: BasicBooks, 1991.

Goldberg, Elkhonon. *The Executive Brain: Frontal Lobes and the Civilized Mind.* Oxford: University Press, 2001.

Goodlad, John I. and Klein, M. Frances, *Looking Behind the Classroom Door.* Belmont, California: Charles A. Jones, 1974.

Goodlad, John I. and Anderson, Robert H. *The Nongraded Elementary School.* New York: Teachers College Press, 1987. Revised edition.

Gopnik, A., A. Meltzoff, and Patricia Kuhl. *The Scientist in the Crib: Minds, Brains, and How Children Learn.* New York: William Morrow and Company, 1999.Greenspan, Stanley I. with Benderl, Beryl Lieffy. *The Growth of the Mind and the Endangered Origins of Intelligence.* New York: Addison-Wesley Publishing Company, 1997.

Gibbs, Jeanne. *Tribes: A New Way of Learning Together.* Santa Rosa, California: Center Source Publications, 1994.

Glickman, Carl D. *Renewing America's Schools: A Guide for School-Based Action.* San Francisco: Jossey-Bass Publishers, 1993.

Hart, Leslie A. "A Classroom Is a Classroom Is a Classroom—and Invisible," *Toronto Education Quarterly,* Autumn, 1971.

Hart, Leslie A. *The Classroom Disaster.* New York: Teachers College Press, 1969.

Hart, Leslie A. "Classrooms Are Killing Learning," *Principal,* May, 1981.

Hart, Leslie A. *How The Brain Works.* New York: Basic Books, 1975.

Healy, Jane. *Endangered Minds: Why Children Don't Think — and What We Can Do About It.* New York: Simon & Schuster, 1990.

Healy, Jane. *Failure to Connect: How Computers Affect Our Children's Minds — And What We Can Do About It.* New York: Simon & Schuster, 1998.Jensen, Eric. *Teaching with the Brain in Mind.* Alexandria, Virginia: ASCD, 1998.

Katz, Michael. *Class, Bureaucracy, and the Schools: The Illusion of Educational Change in America.* New York: Praeger Publishers, 1971.

Keirsey, David. *Please Understand Me II: Temperament Character Intelligence.* Del Mar, CA: Prometheus Nemesis Book Company, 1998.

Kohn, Alfie. *Beyond Discipline: From Compliance to Community.* Alexandria, Virginia: ASCD, 1996.

Kohn, Alfie. *Punished by Rewards: The Trouble with Gold Stars, Incentive Plans, A's, Praise, and Other Bribes.* New York: Houghton Mifflin, 1993.

Kotulak, Ronald. *Inside the Brain: Revolutionary Discoveries of How the Mind Works .* Kansas City, Missouri: Andrews McMeel, 1996.

Kovalik, Susan and Olsen, Karen D. *ITI Classroom Rubric.* Kent, Washington: Susan Kovalik & Associates, 1998.

Kovalik, Susan and Olsen, Karen D. *ITI Schoolwide Rubric.* Kent, Washington: Susan Kovalik & Associates, 1998.

Kunzig, Robert. "A Head for Numbers," *Discover,* July, 1997 and *Newsweek, Special Edition, Your Child: From Birth to Three,* Spring/Summer, 1997.

LeDoux, Joseph. "The Emotional Brain," presentation at *Emotional Intelligence, Education, and the Brain: A Symposium,* Chicago, Illinois, December 5, 1997.

LeDoux, Joseph. *The Emotional Brain: The Mysterious Underpinnings of Emotional Life.* New York: Simon and Schuster, 1996.

Lindamood, Charles and Patricia. *The Auditory Discrimination in Depth.* Allen, Texas: DLM Teaching Resources, 1969.

Luria, A. R. *The Working Brain.* New York: Basic Books, 1975.

Lustad, Hugh S. and Knapp R. Benjamin. "Controlling Computers with Neural Signals," *Scientific American*, October, 1996.

Olsen, Karen D. *A Science Continuum of Concepts, Grades K-6*. Kent, Washington: Center for the Future of Public Education, 1995.

Pearsal, Paul. *The Heart's Code: Tapping the Wisdom and Power of Our Heart Energy*. New York: Broadway Books, 1998.

Pribram, Karl and Rozman, Deborah. "Early Childhood Development and Learning: What New Research on the Heart and Brain Tells Us About Our Youngest Children," an unpublished paper, 1998.

Perkins, David. *Outsmarting IQ: The Emerging Science of Learnable Intelligence*. New York: Free Press, 1995

Pert, Candace. *Molecules of Emotion: Why You Feel the Way You Feel*. New York: Scribner, 1997.

Pinker, Steven. *How the Mind Works*. New York: W. W. Norton & Co., 1997.

Private Universe, Santa Monica, California: Pyramid Media.

Ramachandran, V. S. *Mirror Neurons and Imitation Learning As the Driving Force Behind "The Great Leap Forward" in Human Evolution*. www.edge.org/documents/archive/edge69.html

Ratey, John J. *A User's Guide to the Brain: Perception, Attention, and the Four Theaters of the Brain*. New York: Pantheon Books, 2001.Samples, Bob. *Open Mind, Whole Mind*. San Diego, California: Jalmar Press, 1987.

Shaywitz, Sally E. "Dyslexia," *Scientific American*, November, 1996.

Sylwester, Robert. *A Celebration of Neurons: An Educator's Guide to the Human Brain*. Alexandria, Virginia: ASCD, 1995.

Sylwester, Robert. "The Neurobiology of Self-Esteem and Aggression," *Educational Leadership*, February, 1997, Volume 54, No. 5.

Sylwester, Robert. "The Role of the Arts in Brain Development and Maintenance." An unpublished paper, 1998.

INDEX